Chronic Disease Management

T0259129

Guest Editors

BROOKE SALZMAN, MD
LAUREN COLLINS, MD
EMILY R. HAJJAR, PharmD, BCPS, BCACP, CGP

PRIMARY CARE: CLINICS IN OFFICE PRACTICE

www.primarycare.theclinics.com

Consulting Editor
JOEL J. HEIDELBAUGH, MD

June 2012 • Volume 39 • Number 2

SAUNDERS an imprint of ELSEVIER, Inc.

W.B. SAUNDERS COMPANY
A Division of Elsevier Inc.

1600 John F. Kennedy Boulevard, Suite 1800 • Philadelphia, PA 19103-2899

http://www.theclinics.com

PRIMARY CARE: CLINICS IN OFFICE PRACTICE Volume 39, Number 2
June 2012 ISSN 0095-4543, ISBN-13: 978-1-4557-3924-0

Editor: Yonah Korngold

Primary Care: Clinics in Office Practice (ISSN: 0095–4543) is published quarterly by Elsevier Inc., 360 Park Avenue South, New York, NY 10010-1710. Months of issue are March, June, September, and December. Periodicals postage paid at New York, NY and additional mailing offices. Subscription prices are $216.00 per year (US individuals), $353.00 (US institutions), $108.00 (US students), $264.00 (Canadian individuals), $415.00 (Canadian institutions), $169.00 (Canadian students), $329.00 (international individuals), $415.00 (international institutions), and $169.00 (international students). Foreign air speed delivery is included in all *Clinics* subscription prices. All prices are subject to change without notice. POSTMASTER: Send address changes to *Primary Care: Clinics in Office Practice*, Elsevier Periodicals Customer Service, 11830 Westline Industrial Drive, St. Louis, MO 63146. Customer Service Health Sciences Division, Subscription Customer Service, 3251 Riverport Lane, Maryland Heights, MO 63043. **Customer Service: 1-800-654-2452 (U.S. and Canada); 314-447-8871 (outside U.S. and Canada). Fax: 314-447-8029. E-mail: journalscustomerservice-usa@elsevier.com (for print support); journalsonlinesupport-usa@elsevier.com (for online support).**

Reprints. For copies of 100 or more, of articles in this publication, please contact the Commercial Reprints Department, Elsevier Inc., 360 Park Avenue South, New York, NY 10010-1710. Tel. (212) 633-3812; Fax: (212) 482-1935; E-mail: reprints@elsevier.com.

Primary Care: Clinics in Office Practice is covered in *MEDLINE/PubMed (Index Medicus)* and *EMBASE/Excerpta Medica, Current Contents/Clinical Medicine,* and *ISI/BIOMED.*

Printed and bound by CPI Group (UK) Ltd, Croydon, CR0 4YY

Transferred to digital print 2012

Contributors

CONSULTING EDITOR

JOEL J. HEIDELBAUGH, MD
Clinical Assistant Professor and Clerkship Director, Department of Family Medicine;
Clinical Assistant Professor, Department of Urology, University of Michigan Medical
School, Ann Arbor, Michigan

GUEST EDITORS

BROOKE SALZMAN, MD
Assistant Professor, Department of Family and Community Medicine, Division of Geriatric
Medicine, Thomas Jefferson University, Jefferson Medical College, Philadelphia,
Pennsylvania

LAUREN COLLINS, MD
Assistant Professor, Department of Family and Community Medicine, Division of Geriatric
Medicine, Thomas Jefferson University, Jefferson Medical College, Philadelphia,
Pennsylvania

EMILY R. HAJJAR, PHARMD, BCPS, BCACP, CGP
Associate Professor, Thomas Jefferson University, Jefferson School of Pharmacy,
Philadelphia, Pennsylvania

AUTHORS

MELINDA K. ABRAMS, MS
Vice President, Patient-Centered Coordinated Care Program, The Commonwealth Fund,
New York, New York

TYSON M. BAIN, MS
Health Services Researcher, Diabetes Health and Wellness Institute; Department of
Quantitative Sciences, Baylor Health Care System, Institute for Health Care Research and
Improvement, Dallas, Texas

FREDERICK J. BLOOM Jr, MD, MMM
Associate Chief Quality Officer, Geisinger Health System, Wyoming, Pennsylvania

KAREN BOYER, MSN, RN
Director, Diabetes Health and Wellness Institute, Dallas, Texas

CRAIG BRAMMER, BA
Office of the National Coordinator, US Department of Health and Human Services,
Washington, DC

RICKIE BRAWER, PhD, MPH
Associate Director, Center for Urban Health, Thomas Jefferson University and Hospitals; Assistant Professor, Department of Family and Community Medicine, Jefferson Medical College, Thomas Jefferson University, Philadelphia, Pennsylvania

MELINDA B. BUNTIN, PhD
Division of Health and Human Resources, Congressional Budget Office, Washington, DC

CHRISTOPHER V. CHAMBERS, MD
Professor, Department of Family and Community Medicine, Philadelphia, Pennsylvania

KATIE COLEMAN, MSPH
Research Associate, MacColl Center for Health Care Innovation, Group Health Research Institute, Seattle, Washington

MARY THOESEN COLEMAN, MD, PhD
Professor of Family Medicine, Department of Family Medicine, Louisiana State University School of Medicine; Director, Community Health, Louisiana State University Health Science Center Office of the Dean, New Orleans, Louisiana

ASHLEY COLLINSWORTH, MPH, ELS
Director, Center for Health Care Research, Baylor Health Care System, Institute for Health Care Research and Improvement, Dallas, Texas

DUANE E. DAVIS, MD
VP, Chief Medical Officer, Geisinger Health Plan, Danville, Pennsylvania

GINA DESEVO, PharmD
Assistant Professor, Department of Pharmacy Practice, Jefferson School of Pharmacy, Thomas Jefferson University, Philadelphia, Pennsylvania

NEIL S. FLEMING, PhD, CQE
Vice President & COO, The STEEP Global Institute, Baylor Health Care System, Dallas, Texas

THOMAS R. GRAF, MD
Associate Chief Medical Officer, Population Health Initiatives; Chairman, Community, Practice Service Line, Geisinger Health System, Danville, Pennsylvania

JACQUELINE KLOOTWYK, PharmD, BCPS
Assistant Professor, Department of Pharmacy Practice, Jefferson School of Pharmacy, Thomas Jefferson University, Philadelphia, Pennsylvania

PATRICK T. MCGOWAN, PhD
Centre on Aging, Professor, University of Victoria, Victoria; Ladner Office, Director of Self-Management Programs, University of Victoria, Delta, British Columbia, Canada

AARON MCKETHAN, PhD
Office of the National Coordinator, US Department of Health and Human Services, Washington, DC

ESTERIA MILLER, MBA
Director, Diabetes Health and Wellness Institute, Dallas, Texas

GEOFFREY D. MILLS, MD, PhD
Assistant Professor, Departments of Family and Community Medicine and Physiology, Jefferson Medical College, Philadelphia, Pennsylvania

MIJUNG PARK, PhD, RN
Postdoctoral Fellows in Geriatric Mental Health Services Research, Department of Psychiatry and Behavioral Sciences, University of Washington, Seattle, Washington

RYAN H. PASTERNAK, MD, MPH
Assistant Professor of Clinical Pediatrics, Section Chief, Adolescent Medicine, Department of Pediatrics, Louisiana State University Health Science Center, New Orleans, Louisiana

KATHRYN PHILLIPS, MPH
Safety Net Medical Home Initiative Director, Qualis Health, Seattle, Washington

JAMES PLUMB, MD, MPH
Professor, Department of Family and Community Medicine, Jefferson Medical College, Thomas Jefferson University; Director, Center for Urban Health, Thomas Jefferson University and Hospitals, Philadelphia, Pennsylvania

SHALINE RAO, MD
Office of the National Coordinator, US Department of Health and Human Services, Washington, DC

ROBERT J. REID, MD, PhD
Associate Investigator, Group Health Research Institute; Associate Medical Director of Health Services Research & Knowledge Translation, Group Health Permanente, Seattle, Washington

DONNA RICE, MBA, RN, CDE, FAADE
President, Diabetes Health and Wellness Institute, Dallas, Texas

MICHAEL P. ROSENTHAL, MD
Professor of Family and Community Medicine, Thomas Jefferson University, Chair, Department of Family and Community Medicine, Christiana Care Health System, Wilmington, Delaware

KEVIN SCOTT, MD
Instructor, Department of Family and Community Medicine, Jefferson Medical College, Thomas Jefferson University, Philadelphia, Pennsylvania

JONATHAN R. SUGARMAN, MD, MPH
President and CEO, Qualis Health, Seattle, Washington

JANET TOMCAVAGE, RN, MSN
Chief Clinical Transformation Officer, Geisinger Insurance Operations, Geisinger Health Plan, Danville, Pennsylvania

JÜRGEN UNÜTZER, MD, MPH, MA
Professor and Vice Chair of Psychiatry, Department of Psychiatry and Behavioral Sciences, University of Washington, Seattle, Washington

GEORGE VALKO, MD
Gustave and Valla Amsterdam Professor of Family and Community Medicine, Vice-Chair for Clinical Programs, Department of Family and Community Medicine, Jefferson Medical College, Thomas Jefferson University, Philadelphia, Pennsylvania

EDWARD H. WAGNER, MD, MPH
Director Emeritus, MacColl Center for Health Care Innovation, Group Health Research Institute, Seattle, Washington

LARA CARSON WEINSTEIN, MD, MPH
Assistant Professor, Department of Family and Community Medicine, Jefferson Medical College, Thomas Jefferson University, Philadelphia, Pennsylvania

RICHARD C. WENDER, MD
Alumni Professor, Chair, Department of Family and Community Medicine, Jefferson Medical College, Thomas Jefferson University, Philadelphia, Pennsylvania

MICHELE Q. ZAWORA, MD
Instructor, Medical Director, Department of Family and Community Medicine, Jefferson Family Medicine Associates, Jefferson Medical College, Thomas Jefferson University, Philadelphia, Pennsylvania

Contents

The need for improved models of chronic care is great and will become critical over the next years as the Medicare-aged population doubles. Many promising models have been developed by outstanding groups across the country. This article reviews key strategies used by successful models in chronic disease management and discusses in detail how Geisinger has evolved and organized its cohesive delivery model.

In 2007, the major primary care professional societies collaboratively introduced a new model of primary care: the patient-centered medical home (PCMH). The published document outlines the basic attributes and expectations of a PCMH but not with the specificity needed to help interested clinicians and administrators make the necessary changes to their practice. To identify the specific changes required to become a medical home, the authors reviewed literature and sought the opinions of two multi-stakeholder groups. This article describes the eight consensus change concepts and 32 key changes that emerged from this process, and the evidence supporting their inclusion.

The concept of the patient-centered medical home (PCMH) has been widely embraced as a foundation for the transformation of health care delivery. Recent evaluations of PCMH pilots validate the initial hypothesis that care provided in the PCMH has the potential to result in better health outcomes at lower cost. However, earning recognition or certification as a PCMH can be a daunting task. This article discusses the process of developing the potential to function as a PCMH, earning formal recognition, and implementing a system of continuous quality improvement to enable the establishment of a mature, sustainable PCMH.

Strategies that are most effective in both prevention and management of chronic disease consider factors such as age, ethnicity, community, and technology. Most behavioral change strategies derive their components from application of the health belief model, the theory of reasoned action/ theory of planned behavior, transtheoretical model, and social cognitive theory. Many tools such as the readiness ruler and personalized action plan form are available to assist health care teams to facilitate healthy behavior change. Primary care providers can support behavior changes by providing venues for peer interventions and family meetings and by making new partnerships with community organizations.

With the changing health care environment, prevalence of chronic health conditions, and burgeoning challenges of health literacy, obesity, and homelessness, self-management support provides an opportunity for clinicians to enhance effectiveness and, at the same time, to engage patients to participate in managing their own personal care. This article reviews the differences between patient education and self-management and describes easy-to-use strategies that foster patient self-management and can be used by health care providers in the medical setting. It also highlights the importance of linking patients to nonmedical programs and services in the community.

Adoption of health information technology (HIT) is a key effort in improving care delivery, reducing costs of health care, and improving the quality of health care. Evidence from electronic health record (EHR) use suggests that HIT will play a significant role in transforming primary care practices and chronic disease management. This article shows that EHRs and HIT can be used effectively to manage chronic diseases, that HIT can facilitate communication and reduce efforts related to transitions in care, and that HIT can improve patient safety by increasing the information available to providers and patients, improving disease management and safety.

A significant portion of the adult population uses one or more medications on a regular basis to manage chronic conditions. As the number of medications that patients are prescribed increases, an increase in pharmacologic-related issues and complications may occur, such as polypharmacy, inappropriate prescribing, medication nonadherence and nonpersistence, and adverse drug reactions and events. Risk factors and consequences of these issues have been identified and are discussed in this article. In addition, a review is presented of the numerous methods that have been evaluated to help prevent and minimize these pharmacologic issues in the management of chronic disease.

Many patients with diabetes do not have access to clinical care or medications, resulting in cases of undiagnosed diabetes or uncontrolled diabetes, especially in patients of low socioeconomic status. Given these considerations, new strategies are needed to control the rampant growth of diabetes and prevent new cases. This article discusses effective strategies for improving the management of diabetes in underserved populations, with special reference to the Juanita J. Craft Diabetes Health and Wellness Institute, a unique partnership between a large, urban integrated health care system, the City of Dallas, and a South Dallas community.

Childhood asthma is at historically high levels, with significant morbidity and mortality. Despite more than two decades of improved understanding of childhood asthma care and the evolution of beneficial medications, widespread control remains poor, leading to suboptimal patient outcomes and quality of life. This lack of control results in excessive emergency department use, hospitalizations, and inappropriate and/or unnecessary costs to the health care system. Advanced practice models that incorporate community-based approaches and services for childhood asthma are needed. Innovative, community-included methods of care to address the burden of childhood asthma may provide examples for care of other chronic diseases.

The purpose of this article is to provide resources for primary care physicians to manage heart failure as a chronic disease. We review evidence-based interventions that can be adopted in primary care practices to improve adherence to available guidelines for medication use, promotion of self-care behaviors, transitions of care in acute decompensated heart failure, and end of life care. This information will be valuable to primary care providers who care for patients with heart failure in all care settings but is focused on the management of heart failure in the outpatient setting.

Effective management of depression in the primary care setting requires a systematic, population-based approach, which entails systematic case finding and diagnosis, patient engagement and education, use of evidence-based treatments, including medications and/or psychotherapy, close follow-up to ensure patients are improving, and a commitment to adjust treatments or consult with mental health specialists until depression is

PRIMARY CARE:
CLINICS IN OFFICE PRACTICE

DOWNLOAD
Free App!

Review Articles
THE CLINICS

NOW AVAILABLE FOR YOUR iPhone and iPad

Foreword

Teaching Strategies Behind the Principles

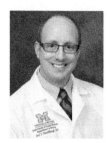

Joel J. Heidelbaugh, MD
Consulting Editor

In my role as a family medicine clerkship director, every four weeks I facilitate a case conference discussion for the respective cohort of third-year medical students. The goal of this exercise is for each student to present a patient whom they have encountered in one of our ambulatory clinic practices, focusing on a particular chronic disease, discussing both treatment goals and their inherent challenges in appropriate management. Last month, I dazzled the students with the terms "patient-centered medical home (PCMH)," "pay-for-performance," "population management," and "motivational interviewing." The blank stares and deafening silence were suddenly broken when one MD/MBA candidate (and future subspecialty surgeon) asked, "Why does any of this matter? If patients don't want to follow our advice, then why are we responsible for their outcomes? Aren't these 'goals' just a bunch of numbers anyway?"

My first internal response to those comments was that we aren't teaching medical students (read: the next generation of physicians) these salient concepts of patient care. The next thought I had was that, despite being a family physician for over 15 years, I'm still trying to make sense of how to master these concepts in my own everyday practice! Since the clinician can't be the sole coordinator of chronic disease management, who is helping us? Are the insurance companies working with us or against us and the patients? Of course, I'm not alone in admitting these thoughts and challenges....

What is so exciting about the gravitation toward the PCMH model for chronic disease management is that collectively patients and clinicians stand to benefit substantially, with regard to clinical outcomes and financial implications. If we possess the right knowledge and ancillary support, coupled with the most current recommended guidelines for clinical care, then patient care teams consisting of clinicians, nurses, and complex care managers will engage in better relationships and overall health care.

This volume of *Primary Care: Clinics in Office Practice* provides readers with a detailed and comprehensive overview of the concepts behind the PCMH model,

Prim Care Clin Office Pract 39 (2012) xiii–xiv
doi:10.1016/j.pop.2012.03.012   **primarycare.theclinics.com**

predicated on chronic disease management. Specific models with proven success for chronic disease management are highlighted, with a focus on effective strategies to motivate our patients toward positive behavioral changes. Articles on health information technology, how to assist practices in qualifying as a PCMH, and self-management education and support will serve as detailed primers for our practices in moving forward through the complex framework of managed care demands. Impressively, articles dedicated to addressing effective strategies to improve asthma, diabetes, depression, heart failure, and inherent pharmacologic issues in chronic disease management in our patients provide evidence-based guidelines for utilization in everyday practice and in the instruction of our learners.

I would like to bestow significant kudos to Dr Brooke Salzman for her initiative and outstanding achievement in creating this unique, timely, and invaluable volume of articles on chronic disease management. The concepts presented within this edition of *Primary Care: Clinics in Office Practice* compile a true curriculum for students, residents, and practitioners alike in their quest for delivering the best cost-effective and patient-centered care for our patients with chronic diseases—an absolute "must have" on the smartphones, tablets, laptops, and shelves for today's health care provider.

Joel J. Heidelbaugh, MD
Ypsilanti Health Center
200 Arnet Street, Suite 200
Ypsilanti, MI 48198, USA

E-mail address:
jheidel@umich.edu

Preface

Chronic Disease Management: The Changing Landscape of Primary Care

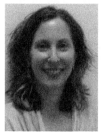 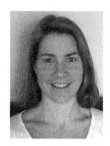 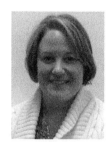

| Brooke Salzman, MD | Lauren Collins, MD | Emily R. Hajjar, PharmD, BCPS, BCACP, CGP |

Guest Editors

INTRODUCTION

Over the past several decades, the health care needs of the US population have been shifting from predominantly acute, episodic care to care for chronic conditions.[1] Accounting for 7 of 10 leading causes of death in the United States, chronic diseases have emerged as the principal cause of morbidity and mortality in the 21st century.[2] More than 145 million people in the United States, nearly half of the population, have one or more chronic conditions, and chronic diseases account for the vast majority of health care spending.[3]

The predominance of chronic disease is a distinct change from the major causes of death and illness in the early 20th century that mostly involved infectious diseases such as tuberculosis, pneumonia, and influenza.[4] In addition, new medications and medical procedures developed over the century have converted once-fatal diseases to chronic, life-long conditions. This dramatic shift from acute to chronic disease has altered the landscape of health and illness in this country, and yet, the present health care system is largely based on models of care designed to cope with managing acute illness. As a result, the management of chronic disease has been woefully inadequate and has largely contributed to the nation's health care problems, namely, suboptimal quality and excessive costs.

While the Unites States spends more per capita than any other nation on health care, approximately 16% of the gross domestic product or $2.2 trillion, the US health care system ranks 37th overall among 191 countries examined by the World Health Organization.[5–7] Chronic disease accounts for 84% of total health care spending,

---

Prim Care Clin Office Pract 39 (2012) xv–xxi
doi:10.1016/j.pop.2012.04.002
0095-4543/12/$ – see front matter © 2012 Elsevier Inc. All rights reserved.

and yet, chronically ill patients receive only about half of clinically recommended services.[8,9] Suboptimal health care quality disproportionately affects minority populations and low-income groups.[10]

Over the next 20 years, approximately 11,000 people per day will turn 65. With higher rates of chronic disease in those over age 65 and increasing overall life expectancy, the current health care system is not prepared to handle the growing number of older people, the multitude of chronic illness, and the increasing complexity of care. Improving chronic disease management must be at the forefront of health care reform. Multiple leading organizations including the Agency for Healthcare Research and Quality have consistently documented major deficiencies and disparities in this country in regards to health care for chronic conditions.[10] Over 10 years ago, the Institute of Medicine's landmark report, *Crossing the Quality Chasm*, recognized that the current health care system cannot provide Americans with the quality of care they need, want, and deserve. Instead, only a fundamentally redesigned system that focuses on effective delivery of care for people with chronic conditions could significantly improve quality.[1]

Increasingly, evidence suggests that an effective health care delivery system not only centers on addressing chronic disease, but also requires a solid basis in primary care.[11,12] Extensive data have shown that health care systems with robust primary care provide better quality care at lower costs.[13] As primary care clinicians provide a majority of the care for patients with chronic diseases, a health care system that emphasizes a strong foundation in primary care is integral to providing optimal chronic disease prevention and management.[12-14]

This article and others in this volume of *Primary Care Clinics in Office Practice* will elaborate fully on the need to transform systems of care to improve chronic disease management and the overall health of our population. This series will highlight successful strategies in practice redesign that can lead to better, sustainable results, as well as underscore the critical role of primary care in leading and achieving health care delivery transformation.

CHRONIC DISEASE—DEFINITION AND EPIDEMIOLOGY
Definition

Chronic disease has been defined as a long-lasting condition that can be controlled but not cured.[15] Others have described chronic disease as including conditions that are expected to last a year or longer, limit what one can do, and/or may require ongoing medical care.[3] Examples include heart disease, stroke, diabetes, cancer, obesity, arthritis, chronic respiratory diseases (asthma and COPD), mental disorders, vision and hearing impairment, and oral diseases. Chronic conditions are common for people at all ages, but leading causes of chronic illness vary among different age groups. For people ages 65 and older, major chronic conditions include hypertension (60%), dyslipidemia (41%), arthritis (28%), heart disease (25%), and opthalmologic disorders (23%). For people ages 18 to 64, leading chronic conditions are hypertension (30%), dyslipidemia (20%), respiratory diseases (19%), and diabetes (12%). For children, principal causes of chronic illness are asthma (30%) and other upper respiratory disease (36%).[3]

Epidemiology

As of 2009, over half of the US population lives with at least one chronic condition, and this number is rising at an alarmingly fast pace.[3] In 2006, 28% of all Americans had two or more chronic conditions, and this percentage is also increasing exponentially.[3] As the prevalence of chronic conditions increases with age, the majority of older adults have multimorbidity (the simultaneous presence of more than one type of illness); in fact, three of every four persons aged 65 and older have multiple chronic conditions.[3]

There are several contributing factors to the rising prevalence of chronic disease in the United States. Advances in medical science and technology have enabled the treatment of acute illnesses that have resulted in people living longer. The average life expectancy has increased over the past century from 47.3 years in 1900 to 78.7 years in 2010.[2,16] As Americans are living longer, more people are growing older and developing chronic conditions that are often associated with advanced age. In addition, as those of the baby-boomer generation are reaching the age of 65, the number and proportion of older Americans are rising dramatically. The nation's 65-year-and-older population will expand from 35 million in 2000 to 71 million in 2040.[17] By 2040, at least 20% of the population will comprise people age 65 and older. Even more astounding is the rising rate of the population ages 85 and older. The number of US residents over the age of 85 years is projected to grow by more than 300% over the next 40 years.[3,17] In addition, the current epidemic and rising rate of obesity in this country plays a significant role in the increasing prevalence of chronic disease.[18]

Impact of Chronic Disease

Chronic conditions are associated with significant morbidity and frequently cause people to develop significant functional limitations, particularly if their illness is not well managed.[19] More than 25% of people with chronic conditions have one or more daily activity limitations, such difficulty walking or requiring assistance with dressing or bathing.[20] Independent activities of daily living, such as grocery shopping, paying bills, and taking medications correctly, are also commonly affected in those with chronic disease. Depression, a common chronic condition, is also frequently seen as a comorbid condition in people with chronic diseases.[21,22] Nearly 30% of stroke patients develop depression and up to 65% of patients suffering from a myocardial infarction experience depressive symptoms.[23–25] Evidence suggests not only that having a chronic illness may be a risk factor for depression, but that depression significantly affects chronic disease management and related health outcomes.[26–28]

Chronic disease not only accounts for the leading causes of death and disability in the United States but is also associated with 84% of total health care spending, nearly 99% of Medicare spending, and about 80% of Medicaid spending.[3] Nearly 50% of all health care dollars are spent on treating the sickest 5% of the population.[9] Health care spending is approximately three times greater for someone with one chronic condition as compared to a person without a chronic illness, and about seventeen times greater for someone with five or more chronic conditions.[3,9]

Risk Factors and Root Causes of Chronic Disease

A small number of common, modifiable risk factors are responsible for most of the main chronic diseases.[19] Such modifiable risk factors account for a significant portion of disability and premature death related to chronic conditions. Modifiable risk factors include unhealthy diet, lack of exercise, obesity, tobacco use, and excessive alcohol intake.[20] In fact, it is estimated that at least 80% of all heart disease, stroke, and diabetes could be prevented and over 40% of cancer are potentially avoidable with risk factor modification.[19] Primary care providers may help modify risk factors for chronic disease by effecting behavior change and providing self-management support. However, health-related behaviors are difficult for many individuals to change without adequate resources, education, guidance, and support.[19]

In 2007, only one-quarter of adults reported eating five or more servings of fruits and vegetables per day and 60% of children and adolescents exceeded the dietary guidelines for saturated fat.[20] Less than 50% of adults met current guidelines for physical activity. In addition, despite the availability of effective interventions for smoking cessation, more than 20% of adults, approximately 43 million people, continue to smoke, a number which has remained consistent for the past 5 years.[20] Further, one-third of adults report consuming four or more drinks in one setting approximately four times per month.[20] Almost one-half of high-school students have reported drinking in the past month with 60% reporting binge drinking.[20] More than one-third (36%) of adults in this country are considered obese; in addition, about 17% of children are obese.[28] There are significant racial and ethnic disparities in obesity prevalence among US adults, children, and adolescents, including higher rates of obesity in African Americans and Hispanic populations.[28]

Older age, hereditary, race, and ethnicity are some examples of nonmodifiable factors associated with chronic disease. Several other broader societal issues determine health in general and contribute to the prevalence of chronic disease, such as underlying socioeconomic, cultural, political, and environmental factors.[19]

CHRONIC DISEASE MANAGEMENT—DEFINITION, CHALLENGES, AND OPPORTUNITIES
Definition

The failure of traditional methods of health care delivery to address the growing burden of chronic disease has necessitated the development of new strategies for the care of chronic conditions. The new model of chronic disease management (CDM) consists of an organized, proactive, multicomponent, patient-centered approach to health care delivery that involves all members of a defined population who have a specific disease entity or a population with specific risk factors.[29]

Challenges and Opportunities in Chronic Disease Management

Challenges in the redesign of health care delivery to address the care needs of patients with chronic disease are numerous, resulting from a growing number of patients with chronic conditions as well as increased complexity of care needs. Four deficiencies in the infrastructure of primary care have been identified as contributing to the failure of our current health care system to adequately address the burden of chronic disease: (1) primary care providers and many other health professionals are not trained to work in teams to provide complex chronic care; (2) advanced health information technologies, such as interoperative electronic health records, telemonitoring devices, and patient portals that could facilitate the necessary processes of chronic care, are not widely available or utilized; (3) most current public and private health insurers' payment policies are based on fee-for-service payments that do not support the supplemental services needed to provide complex chronic care; and (4) the payment and provision of medical and social services are not integrated.[30]

Other critical issues that require attention in the reorganization of health care delivery to improve CDM include the current lack of care coordination between various providers and sites of care particularly during transitions in care, the growing shortage of primary care providers and declining recruitment into primary care, and the need for performance and outcome measurements for quality and accountability.

This volume of *Primary Care Clinics in Office Practice* is dedicated to tackling these challenges and exploring new opportunities in CDM in the primary care practice setting. In *Value Based Reengineering: 21st Century Chronic Care Models*, the authors identify key strategies and novel approaches to practice redesign and illustrate the process of health care delivery transformation at the Geisinger health care system. In *The Changes Involved in Patient-Centered Medical Home Transformation*, Dr Edward Wagner and his team delve into the patient-centered medical home (PCMH), defining its rationale, composition, organization, and capabilities to improve health care quality for populations with chronic illness. The authors of *A "How To" Guide to Creating a Patient-Centered Medical Home* take an evidence-based practical approach to developing a PCMH and provide a blueprint for primary care practices that want to transform their practice. Articles in this series also focus on how to integrate key aspects of transformed health care delivery systems into practice, detailing evidence-based strategies for influencing behavior change, providing self-management education and support, and utilizing innovations in health information technology. In *Pharmacologic Issues of Chronic Disease Management*, Dr DeSevo explores pharmacologic issues that are critical in CDM. Disease-based articles discuss practice redesign in relation to specific key conditions including diabetes, congestive heart failure, childhood asthma, and depression. Finally, in the article, *Community-Based Partnerships for Improving Chronic Disease Management*, the authors focus on the need to prioritize and develop community-based partnerships and coalitions for improving CDM.

CONCLUSION

Recognition that US health care is fragmented, inefficient, and unaffordable has sparked the growing national debate over how best to reorganize this system. To better address the needs of the population, the provision of quality care for persons with chronic disease must be at the forefront of health care reform. Effective CDM requires fundamental, comprehensive system changes that entail more than simply adding new features to an unchanged system focused on acute care.[31] Supporting a strong foundation in primary care is integral to providing optimal management of chronic disease, reshaping health care delivery, and creating sustainable improvements in health care quality.

Brooke Salzman, MD
Department of Family and Community Medicine
Division of Geriatric Medicine
Thomas Jefferson University
Jefferson Medical College
1015 Walnut Street, Suite 401
Philadelphia, PA 10107, USA

Lauren Collins, MD
Department of Family and Community Medicine
Division of Geriatric Medicine
Thomas Jefferson University
Jefferson Medical College
1015 Walnut Street, Suite 401
Philadelphia, PA 10107, USA

Emily R. Hajjar, PharmD, BCPS, BCACP, CGP
Thomas Jefferson University
Jefferson School of Pharmacy
130 South 9th Street, Suite 1540
Philadelphia, PA 19107, USA

E-mail addresses:
Brooke.Salzman@jefferson.edu (B. Salzman)
lauren.collins@jefferson.edu (L. Collins)
Emily.hajjar@jefferson.edu (E.R. Hajjar)

REFERENCES

1. Committee on Quality Health Care in America. Institute of Medicine. Crossing the quality chasm: a new health system for the 21st century. Washington, DC: National Academies Press; 2001.
2. Murphy SL, Xu J, Kochanek KD. Deaths: Preliminary Data for 2010. National Vital Statistics Reports 2012;60(4):1–68. Available at: http://www.cdc.gov/nchs/data/nvsr/nvsr60/nvsr60_04.pdf. Accessed April 22, 2012.
3. Robert Wood Johnson Foundation. Chronic Care: Making the Case for Ongoing Care. 2010. Available at: http://www.rwjf.org/files/research/50968chronic.care.chartbook. pdf. Accessed April 20, 2012.
4. Leading Causes of Death, 1900-1998. National Office of Vital Statistics, available at: http://www.cdc.gov/nchs/data/dvs/lead1900_98.pdf. Accessed April 20, 2012.
5. World Health Organization. Countries: United States of America, Statistics. Available at: http://www.who.int/countries/usa/en/. Accessed April 22, 2012.
6. The World Health Report 2000—Health systems: Improving performance. Geneva: World Health Organization; 2000. Available at: http://www.who.int/whr/2000/en/index.html. Accessed April 22, 2012.
7. Murray CL, Phil D, Frenk J. Ranking 37th—Measuring the performance of the U.S. health care system. N Engl J Med 2010;362:98–9.
8. McGlynn EA, Asch SM, Adams J, et al. The quality of health care delivered to adults in the United States. N Engl J Med 2003;348(26):2635–45.
9. Health Care Costs: A Primer, Key Information on Health Care Costs and Their Impact. The Henry J. Kaiser Family Foundation, March 2009. Available at: http://www.kff.org/insurance/upload/7670_02.pdf. Accessed April 20, 2012.
10. National Healthcare Report 2011, Agency for Healthcare Research and Quality, U.S. Department of Health and Human Services, AHRQ Publication No. 12-0005, March 2012. Available at: www.ahrq.gov/qual/qrdr11.htm. Accessed April 21, 2012.
11. Landon BE, Gill GM, Antonelli RC, et al. Prospects for rebuilding primary care using the patient-centered medical home. Health Affairs 2010;29(5): 827–34.
12. Starfield B. Family Medicine Should Shape Reform, Not Vice Versa. Family Practice Management 2009. Available at: www.aafp.org/fpm. Accessed March 12, 2012.
13. Starfield B, Shi L, Macinko J. Contribution of primary care to health systems and health. Milbank Q 2005;83(3):457–502.
14. Pearson WS, Bhat-Schelbert K, Probst JC. Multiple chronic conditions and the aging of America: Challenge for primary care physicians. J Primary Care Comm Health 2012;3:51–6.

15. The Center for Managing Chronic Disease. What is Chronic Disease? Available at: http://cmcd.sph.umich.edu/what-is-chronic-disease.html. Accessed April 20, 2012.
16. Arias E. United States Life Tables, 2007. Natl Vital Statist Rep 2011;59(9):1–61. Available at: http://www.cdc.gov/nchs/data/nvsr/nvsr59/nvsr59_09.pdf. Accessed April 22, 2012.
17. Vincent GK, Velkoff VA. The Next Four Decades—The Older Population in the United States: 2010 to 2050, Population Estimates and Projections. United States Census Bureau 2010. Available at: http://www.census.gov/prod/2010pubs/p25-1138.pdf. Accessed April 22, 2012.
18. World Health Organization. Chronic diseases—Obesity and overweight fact sheet. CDM intro 4-22-12 with LC edits.doc. Available at: http://www.who.int/mediacentre/factsheets/fs311/en/index.html. Accessed April 22, 2012.
19. World Health Organization. Preventing chronic diseases: a vital investment. Geneva: WHO; 2005. Available at: http://www.who.int/chp/chronic_disease_report/full_report.pdf. Accessed April 17, 2012.
20. The Power of Prevention. Chronic disease…the public health challenge of the 21st century. National Center for Chronic Disease Prevention and Health Promotion. Centers for Disease Control and Prevention 2009. Available at: http://www.cdc.gov/chronicdisease/pdf/2009-Power-of-Prevention.pdf. Accessed April 22, 2012.
21. Wells K, Golding JM, Burnam MA. Psychiatric disorder in a sample of the general population with and without chronic medical conditions. Am J Psychiatry 1988; 145:976–81.
22. Anderson R, Freedland K, Clouse R, et al. The prevalence of comorbid depression in adults with diabetes: a meta-analysis. Diabetes Care 2001;24:1069–78.
23. Paolucci S. Epidemiology and treatment of post-stroke depression. Neuropsychiatr Dis Treat 2008;4(1):145–54.
24. Guck TP, Kavan MG, Elsasser GN, et al. Assessment and treatment of depression following myocardial infarction. Am Fam Physician 2001;64:641–8.
25. Nabi H, Shipley MJ, Vahtera J, et al. Effects of depressive symptoms and coronary heart disease and their interactive associations on mortality in middle-aged adults: the Whitehall II cohort study. Heart 2010;96:1645–50.
26. Katon WJ, Lin EHB, Con Kroff M, et al. Collaborative care for patients with depression and chronic illnesses. New Engl J Med 2010;36:2611–20.
27. Van der Feltz-Cornelis CM, Nuyen J, Stoop C, et al. Effect of interventions for major depressive disorder and significant depressive symptoms in patients with diabetes mellitus: a systematic review and meta-analysis. Gen Hosp Psychiatry 2010;32:380–95.
28. Overweight and Obesity, Centers for Disease Control and Prevention. Data and Statistics. Available at: http://www.cdc.gov/obesity/data/index.html. Accessed April 22, 2012.
29. Norris SL, Glasgow RE, Engelgau MM, et al. Chronic Disease Management: A Definition and Systematic Approach to Component Interventions, IDEAS. Available at: http://ideas.repec.org/a/wkh/dmhout/v11y2003i8p477-488.html. Accessed April 22, 2012.
30. Boult C, Wieland GD. Comprehensive primary care for older patients with multiple chronic conditions: Nobody rushes you through. JAMA 2010;304(17):1936–43.
31. Wagner EH, Austin BT, Davis C, et al. Improving chronic illness care: translating evidence into action. Health Aff (Millwood) 2001;20(6):64–78.

Value-Based Reengineering
Twenty-first Century Chronic Care Models

Thomas R. Graf, MD[a],*, Frederick J. Bloom Jr, MD, MMM[b],
Janet Tomcavage, RN, MSN[c], Duane E. Davis, MD[d]

KEYWORDS

- Chronic care models • Primary care • Medical home • Practice redesign

KEY POINTS

- There are several promising models based in primary care practice for improving the chronic care delivered in the United States. Widespread adoption of these models will be critical to changing the cost and quality trends that are driving an unsustainable trajectory.
- Geisinger has created a sustainable model to divide the population into meaningful subgroups, understand and predict the needs of each subgroup, and proactively support and engage patients in their care.
- The success of Intermountain, Johns Hopkins, Geisinger, and others will need to be rapidly expanded across the nation and reliably delivered to all patients for the full value of these innovations in chronic-disease care to be realized and for financial and quality catastrophes to be averted.

The United States' health care system is poorly placed to respond to the burgeoning need for chronic-disease care. The 2009 Organization for Economic Co-operation and Development (OECD) Health Care Quality Indicators Data report shows that, despite having the highest adjusted per capita cost, the United States has nearly three times the rate of hospitalization for acute diabetes complications than the OECD average.[1] Some 10,000 new patients are entering the Medicare system daily as the baby boomers are turning 65 years of age. This trend will continue for the next several years, driving the number of Medicare beneficiaries to 70 million. A substantially different workforce will be needed to optimally manage the health care needs of an older

Drs Graf and Bloom are part of the Speaker's Bureau for Merck on Medical Home.
[a] Population Health Initiatives, Community Practice Service Line, Geisinger Health System, 100 North Academy Avenue, Danville, PA 17821-3220, USA; [b] Geisinger Health System, 389 Wyoming Avenue, Wyoming, PA, USA; [c] Geisinger Insurance Operations, Geisinger Health Plan, 100 North Academy Avenue, Danville, PA 17821-3220, USA; [d] Geisinger Health Plan, 100 North Academy Avenue, Danville, PA 17821-3220, USA
* Corresponding author.
E-mail address: trgraf@geisinger.edu

population because most of these new Medicare beneficiaries will have multiple chronic diseases.[2–4] To assist primary care practices in retooling to provide better chronic disease care, this article reviews several promising strategies for successful chronic disease management, highlighting the practical experiences at Geisinger Health System. Value-based reengineering is the focused effort of redesigning care to reliably deliver high quality care and improve measurable health outcomes. Geisinger has been at the forefront of value-based reengineering and has managed to improve health care quality while reducing total costs of care.

A CALL FOR ACTION: WHY TRANSFORM CARE?

In 2003, several landmark studies provided support that the United States health care system was not providing optimal value for medical care provided.[5–7] According to the landmark observational RAND Corporation study, adults in the United States received 54.9% of recommended care.[8] The Dartmouth Atlas Project has examined regional variations in the practice of medicine and in spending for health care. The project clearly demonstrated that fee-for-service payment models without regard for outcomes have contributed to significant problems of overutilization and waste and, in fact, illustrated a negative correlation between cost of care and quality.[2] Health care systems that spent the most money did not provide the best care.

At the same time, studies examining the provision of primary care have shown that to perform all necessary acute, chronic, and preventive activities in a typical primary care practice would require 4.6 hours a day for acute care, 10.6 hours a day for chronic care, and 7.4 hours a day for preventive care for a total of 22.6 hours of work per day.[3,9] Clearly, no primary care physician, regardless of training or dedication, can sustain this level. The competing needs of the practice serve to overwhelm practices built for 1940s acute care needs and have not fundamentally changed to meet new demands. These needs include phone calls, medication refills, prior authorization, emergency department or specialty physician calls, test results review and communication with patients, and practice management issues and concerns.

Despite being part of an integrated delivery system and having a greater than 10-year history of electronic health record (EHR) use, health outcomes in the populations served by Geisinger primary care practices were far from ideal. The dysfunction of the prior model was evident in that over one-third of recommended preventive care was not provided to continuity patients. Quality care indicators were nearly 20% better than national averages, but there was still room for significant improvement. At Geisinger and across the nation, primary care is under severe economic pressure, in large part because of the current payment model. In addition, despite the increasing shortage of primary care physicians, fewer new graduates are choosing a career in primary care, exacerbating access issues.[10,11]

These facts, coupled with a growing recognition nationally that the United States health care system is severely fragmented and lacks a coordinated approach, underscore the fundamental need for both practice redesign and payment redesign to optimize health care delivery.[3,9] Optimization is defined by the Institute for Healthcare Improvement's Triple Aim to create value in new designs by improving the health of the population, enhance the patient experience of care, and reduce, or at least control, the total cost of care.[12]

Effective primary care redesign serves as the foundation for a patient-centered medical home (PCMH).[13] With an appropriately focused and redesigned medical home, population management can be integrated into clinical practice. At Geisinger, the redesigned model is known as ProvenHealth Navigator (PHN). A successful foundation in primary care becomes the centerpiece of a successful health care organization and provides a framework for accountable care organizations (ACOs). As ACOs strive to provide higher quality at lower cost to populations, a high-performance primary care team is required. Indeed, primary care practices compose the defining core for ACOs supported by the Centers for Medicare and Medicaid Services Innovation Center, such as Pioneer or the Medicare Shared Savings Program.

The approach Geisinger embarked on was accelerated by a true partnership between providers of care and payers of care. Providers and payers, dedicated to a common mission, combined their cultures, skill sets, tools, and measurable health outcomes data to create a collaborative, innovative partnership, referred to as the "sweet spot." The partnership was strengthened by an underlying commitment to achieve transformation of the health care delivery system and target the following deficiencies in care:

- Unjustified variation
- Fragmented care delivery
- Perverse payment incentives
  - Payment by units of work
  - Outcome irrelevant
- Passive patients as recipients of care
- Inefficient mechanisms to deliver care.

This partnership of providers and payers has created an alignment that is critical to achieving the Triple Aim Plus, which includes improving quality, improving patient experience, reducing cost, and increasing professional satisfaction.[14] Professional satisfaction is a necessary ingredient for sustained success.

GEISINGER

"Make my hospital right, make it the best," was the charge Abigail Geisinger gave Harold Foss, the first superintendent of the George F. Geisinger Memorial Hospital nearly 100 years ago. Those words continue to drive the performance of every team member at Geisinger. Over the years, it has grown and changed, but that primary mission remains the focus and foundation. As a result, a truly patient-centered, value-driven culture was created and a dramatically altered landscape of care was set in motion.

Geisinger comprises a 1000 physician medical group, three acute-care hospital campuses, an inpatient drug rehabilitation center, and a health plan. The goal was to leverage this vertical integration to innovate solutions, improve health care quality, reduce cost, and improve patient and family experience while enhancing professional pride. Providing care to nearly 3 million residents throughout 43 rural counties in Pennsylvania, Geisinger is one of the largest rural systems in the country. Some 30% of patients cared for by the Geisinger clinical enterprise are insured by Geisinger Health Plan (GHP). The remaining patients are insured by Medicare, Medicaid, regional Blue Cross, and other commercial payers.

Geisinger health insurance companies offer diversified health maintenance organization (HMO) and commercial health plans, serving 300,000 members, including 52,000 Medicare Advantage members. Geisinger medical entities provide care to 45% of these members. The remaining 55% of the Geisinger Health Plan members receive their care at 19,000 contracted physician offices and 102 hospitals across Pennsylvania.

The Community Practice Service Line (CPSL), comprising nearly a third of the medical group, has become the most innovative in the system. Its family physicians, internists, internal medicine pediatric physicians, and pediatric physicians are organized into nearly 40 offices in nine regions, which have unified physician leadership with shared goals and vision. At least 10 years have been invested in creating efficient operations at these sites by developing effective methods of communication and shared management, as well as a structured innovation and implementation process. During this time, CPSL moved from an HMO-like "doc on every corner" approach of one to two physician practices to the current hub-and-spoke model to cover the primary and secondary service areas. This model, with hub regional practices, has allowed for the concentration of a critical mass of patients and physicians that enables the deployment of advanced resources (eg, imaging, specialty outreach) close to patients' homes. The franchise-like departmental substructure uses paired physician and administrative leadership at all levels (ie, site, region, and service line) and is supported by unified goals, frequent shared decision-making meetings, and a high-performance culture to achieve optimal outcomes. Sites are regionally integrated with community or Geisinger resources and unified by shared themes and tactical approaches. These unifying themes are designed to create a meaningful difference for patients. Initial themes included "Advanced Access," "Care Systems," "Professional Reputation," and "Transparency." These themes migrated over time to the current strategies that maintain a focus on "Systems of Care" and "Professional Reputation" as well as "Systemness" (ensuring reliable delivery of optimal care through the Geisinger continuum) and "Automation." These themes, coupled with physician and administrative leadership, have allowed CPSL to rapidly advance, deploy across the network, and improve. The ability to innovate is accelerated because the physicians are fully embedded in the local communities where they live, practice medicine, and raise their families.

The compensation model is a unique blend of high performance in the traditional fee-for-service environment, quality-focused pay-for-performance compensation, and population-based payments focused on improving the health of all segments of the panels.[15] Additionally, each team member—from front desk to nurses to advanced practitioners—are measured, monitored, and rewarded on the same quality and population metrics as a team. The compensation model for CPSL physicians includes 80% of total cash compensation from a relative value unit productivity-based formula and 20% of total cash compensation tied to prevention and chronic disease management performance, as measured by the comprehensive bundle measures following.[15] With the advent of the PHN medical home model, the compensation plan added an additional 10% for population health management for a net gain to primary care physician's income. All other team members receive quality-based bonuses just as the physicians do, every 6 months, and annual quality-gated population payments. Highly competent and caring heath care workers who work alone cannot consistently produce the same superior performance as an organized and focused team with shared strategies and high performance leadership.

QUALITY PROGRAM

Value in health care is the relationship of quality to cost. Improving the quality of care provided, in addition to providing more efficient, less wasteful care, increases the value of care provided. There are now many examples of high-quality care in low-cost areas in the country.[2] Redesigned models of care often eliminate waste and, therefore, generate a higher quality, lower cost outcome. Measuring the quality of care provided is essential for demonstrating high-value health care and for demonstrating that the new model of care is not cutting cost to the detriment of patient outcomes.

Measures of quality should include an evaluation of the ability of the program to provide recommended care, of patient and provider satisfaction with the program, and of patient clinical and functional outcomes. The measures should address the Institute of Medicine's six aims for improving health care by making it more safe, effective, patient-centered, timely, efficient, and equitable.[5] In addition, recent literature on quality has emphasized the need for high reliability in health care, highlighting the importance of leadership, safety, culture, and robust process improvement.[16]

Metrics can also reflect process measures (eg, diabetic foot examination rate), intermediate outcomes (eg, blood pressure control), or patient outcomes (eg, myocardial infarction rate). Obtaining accurate data is easier for process measures but may not be correlated with the goal of improved patient outcomes. Ultimately, determining metrics for a quality program involves an analysis of available data sources, accuracy of the data, timeliness of the data, and reporting capabilities.

During the last seven years, Geisinger's CPSL has developed comprehensive systems to measure, monitor, and improve care. Patient surveys are conducted regularly to evaluate patient satisfaction with the care experience. Disease-specific bundles have been developed and are reported in an "all or none" methodology along with distinct outcome measures (**Box 1**). Regular dashboards documenting both practice-wide and individual physician results with peer comparisons are shared electronically to each team member monthly. Patient-centered measures are used with patient-specific goals and an "all-or-none" methodology to comprehensively deliver all evidence-supported care to each patient. For instance, the diabetes glucose-control goal is determined individually by the physician-patient dyad based on specific health risk factors. All-or-none care

---

Box 1
Bundles for diabetes and coronary artery disease

1. Diabetes
   a. Hemoglobin A1c (HgbA1c) every 6 months
   b. HgbA1c at patient-specific goal
   c. Low density lipoprotein (LDL) every 12 months
   d. LDL at "patient specific" goal
   e. Microalbumin screening
   f. Blood pressure (BP) less than 140/80
   g. Documentation as nonsmoker
   h. Pneumococcal vaccine
   g. Influenza vaccine

2. Coronary artery disease
   a. LDL at "patient specific" goal
   b. BP less than 140/90
   c. Body mass index documented
   d. On angiotensin-converting enzyme inhibitor or angiotensin receptor blocker for left ventricular systolic dysfunction, diabetes mellitus, hypertension
   e. On antiplatelet therapy
   f. On beta blocker if history of myocardial infarction or acute coronary syndrome
   g. Documentation as nonsmoker
   h. Pneumococcal vaccine
   i. Influenza vaccine

measures that bundle a host of related care processes and outcomes offer a new approach to clinical process improvement. The all-or-none bundle (see **Box 1**) measures the percentage of patients who achieve all of the recommended measures, rather than an average or composite of the individual measures. According to Nolan and Berwick,[17] the all-or-none measurement improves performance by:

- More closely reflecting the interests and desires of patients, insuring they receive all the care they personally need.
- Fostering a systems perspective—addressing all aspects of care through use of a health care team.
- Offering a more sensitive scale for assessing improvement.

Performance on each measure and disease bundles are collected from the EHR and continuously assessed. The information is available to the care team and patient. It is also used at a population level to drive improvements in system programs.

The all-or-none bundle is only one element of a redesigned care process.[18] This redesigned process led to more reliable and accountable team-based service. The all-or-none bundle score and all 9 process and intermediate outcomes for diabetes improved within the first year of implementation and consistently thereafter.[19] Systems of care for other chronic diseases (eg, coronary artery disease, chronic kidney disease, and hypertension) and for prevention have followed the same process of workflow redesign and all-or-none measurement.

In addition to the patient satisfaction and bundle measures, other quality metrics related to the operation of this new model were developed. CPSL and GHP leadership agree annually on 10 quality metrics to monitor and use as part of the results-share payment model. These include the preceding as well as site-based innovation projects (eg, office-based heart failure management systems including intravenous diuretic use), process of care measures (eg, percentage of patients seen after hospital discharge in fewer than 7 days), and program evolution metrics. The goal is to make the targets simultaneously important, credible, and attainable (**Tables 1–3**).[20]

PRIMARY CARE REDESIGN CORE ELEMENTS
Leadership Commitment

Designing a successful model of care begins with the leadership commitment to reengineer care to improve value. The initial lesson learned from the first National Demonstration Project testing a PCMH model included the need for leadership dedication to meaningful, whole practice transformation. This dedication involved a willingness to face anticipated and unanticipated challenges, an appreciation of the magnitude

Table 1 Improving diabetes care for 24,712 patients				
	March 2006	March 2007	March 2010	March 2011
Diabetes bundle	2.4%	7.2%	11.2%	11.5%
Influenza vaccination	57%	73%	76%	78%
Pneumococcal vaccination	59%	83%	84%	83%
Microalbumin result	58%	87%	79%	77%
HgbA1c at goal	33%	37%	48%	50%
LDL at goal	50%	52%	53%	54%
BP<130/80	39%	44%	52%	53%
Documented nonsmokers	74%	84%	85%	85%

Table 2
Improving coronary artery disease (CAD) care for 15,337 patients

	September 2006	March 2007	March 2010	March 2011
CAD bundle percentage	8%	11%	21%	23%
LDL<100 or <70 if high-risk	38%	37%	48%	52%
ACE/ARB in LVSD, DM, HTN	65%	66%	76%	78%
BP<measured	79%	86%	99%	99%
BP<140/90	74%	74%	78%	79%
Antiplatelet therapy	89%	91%	92%	92%
Beta-blocker use S/P MI	97%	97%	97%	97%
Documented nonsmokers	86%	86%	87%	87%
Pneumococcal vaccination	80%	80%	87%	86%
Influenza vaccination	60%	74%	79%	80%

Abbreviations: ACE, angiotensin-converting enzyme; ARB, angiotensin receptor blocker; DM, diabetes mellitus; HTN, hypertension; LVSD, left ventricular systolic dysfunction; MI, myocardial infarction; S/P, status post.

Table 3
Improving preventive care for 217,693 patients

	November 2007	March 2011
Adult preventive bundle	9.2%	30%
Breast cancer screening (q 2 y, age 40–49; q 1 y, age 50–74)	46%	61%
Cervical cancer screening (q 3 y, age 21–64)	64%	72%
Colon cancer screening (age 50–84)	44%	65%
Prostate cancer discussion (age 50–74)	72%	76%
Lipid screening (q 5 y: males age>35; females age>45)	75%	86%
Diabetes screening (q 3 y, age>45)	85%	90%
Obesity screening (body mass index in EPIC)	77%	96%
Documented nonsmokers	75%	78%
Tetanus diphtheria immunization (q 10 y)	35%	70%
Pneumococcal immunization (once age>65)	84%	87%
Influenza immunization (yearly age>50)	47%	61%
Chlamydia screening (yearly age 18–25)	22%	34%
Osteoporosis screening (q 3 y, age>65)	52%	73%
Alcohol-intake assessment	84%	90%

and pace of change required, and the need to develop a credible strategic approach.[21] Practice transformation begins with communicating a clear, compelling vision of the future state and the benefits to patients, providers, and payers that will be achieved. Building partnerships with the community, providers, health care facilities, and payers to align incentives and provide funding for the needed infrastructure changes in a primary care practice is necessary for the sustained success of the redesign.[22,23]

A key cultural change for primary care leaders is the move from a physician-centered practice to an evidence-based, physician-directed, team-delivered practice. It involves changing the focus of the practice from a series of individual patient encounters to the continuous management of a population of patients. Engaging a team of health care professionals, including new members such as a case manager, requires continuous learning and rapid-cycle redesign.[24]

Using Health Information Technology

An EHR is a valuable tool that can help improve the quality of care provided.[25,26] Instituting an EHR without redesigning the underlying workflows will not result in improved practice efficiencies. Improving quality and eliminating unnecessary costs from a current practice requires changing the operational workflows. Then, an EHR can help to "hardwire" the changes. It can also provide reminders and alerts that increase the reliability. The accurate clinical information that is available from an EHR can populate registries, identify patients in need of care, and allow the management of populations of patients. It can also provide timely feedback of data and performance reporting for teams making changes to their practice workflows.

Obtaining actionable data from an EHR requires attention to many variables, such as provider attribution, active patient selection, and disease identification. Validation of the information is necessary, but the process rapidly improves the accuracy of the reports and confidence in the data. The accuracy of clinical information from the EHR is often better than claims-based quality reporting and can be more timely.

Patient-Centered Care

One of the joint principles of a PCMH is that it is patient-centered.[27] This commitment to what a patient wants and needs, when a patient wants and needs it, is what helps differentiate the PCMH from prior gate-keeper models. Instead of denying care, necessary care is provided earlier and the patient is included in the decision-making process. For instance, proactive Bluetooth scale weight monitoring for patients with congestive heart failure can allow intervention at home when a patient's weight is minimally above target, rather than waiting until the patient is symptomatic and may require inpatient treatment.

Evidence supports that informed patients have better health outcomes.[28] The new model of physician-led, team-delivered care allows greater patient interaction. Patients can be better educated and involved in managing their health and illness. Case managers, office nurses, dieticians, diabetes educators, pharmacists, and other members of the care team work together to provide patients with better self-management skills to affect their health.

Population Accountability

A fundamental difference between a great primary care practice and a PCMH is the accountability for a population of patients. Providing great care to the scheduled patients each day is a hallmark of traditional practice. This is still essential in a PCMH, but the medical home makes a commitment to all patients in the practice, even those that are not on today's schedule. Population management strategies range from identifying the patient with diabetes who has missed an interval appointment and needs to be contacted for laboratory testing and follow-up, to the patient with congestive heart failure who has gained 3 lb overnight and needs to activate the diuretic titration protocol. It requires a team of health professionals who interact with the patient outside of the office encounter to provide timely, efficient, and coordinated care.

Aligning Efforts and Incentives

Health care delivery transformation must involve many participants in the "medical neighborhood" to achieve the desired outcomes of the Triple Aim.[12] Patients, physicians, hospitals, payers, and purchasers of health care have had conflicting incentives in the past, but need to align incentives and efforts. There are many examples of early success in this effort.[4,29] A recent review of seven of the largest medical home pilots revealed that, in addition to primary care redesign, four factors were essential: dedicated case managers, expanded access, performance management tools, and effective incentive payments.[30] Incorporating these into an accountable, reliable, transparent process is the new "ART" of medicine.

SYSTEMS OF CARE
Workflow Redesign

Since the chronic care model was proposed, it has been clear that developing the prepared proactive practice team would start with redesign of the primary care office.[31,32] Various frameworks for redesign have promoted the chronic care model and other innovations in primary care.[33,34] Each of these frameworks involves process redesign of the primary care workflows. At Geisinger, this workflow redesign involves five steps: eliminate, automate, delegate, incorporate, and activate.

Elimination of non–value-added work starts with understanding the current workflow and comparing it to the ideal workflow. Multidisciplinary teams that include patients can work together to create the new workflows and eliminate redundant or wasteful steps. Rapid-cycle redesign principles can test these new workflows and quickly accept or modify them for the next Plan-Do-Study-Act cycle.[35] Many aspects of before visit planning can be automated in an EHR with the needed information displayed at the appropriate time in the new workflow.

Incorporation of the new processes into reliable workflows is a critical step. Designing workflow reminders, EHR tools and alerts and other environmental prompts can "hardwire" the needed steps into place. To get to high levels of reliability, the workflow cannot be dependent on individual diligence or memory. It is accomplished by designing processes that consistently deliver all needed care—every patient, every office, every time. Providing prompt feedback to the team on performance helps to identify areas of inconsistency that need additional redesign.

Activation of the patient to be an informed partner in their health care is the ultimate goal. Patients can participate in new ways at all steps of the process: before visit preparation, kiosk registration, visit agenda-setting, shared decision-making, and after visit use of the patient EHR portal for educational resources, patient-entered data, e-mail, and e-visits.

Team-Delivered Care

The provision of all necessary services to a patient population is beyond the abilities of any one physician. It requires a multidisciplinary team, with new members and new roles, such as the case manager. It is a new model in which the physician works in new ways with other members of the health care team. The physician is still the leader but shares responsibility for patient care with many others. This new model is challenging for many established physicians and can be confusing to patients. For this new team-delivered care to work, it must be tightly integrated into the office-based workflow, with clear communication, often facilitated by the EHR, between all members. As an example, if the physician activates a chronic obstructive pulmonary disease emerging exacerbation protocol at home, the case manager should be aware and alerted to follow up by telephone in 24 to 48 hours and the scheduling staff should be aware that the patient might need an urgent appointment if the home therapy is failing. Every member of the team must consistently carry out his or her new duties. The patients should see each team member as an extension of the relationship that they have with their personal physician.

Population Management

The management of a population of patients requires accurate clinical information that can produce actionable reports. Although this is available from insurance databases, it is more timely and accurate from an EHR. Patient disease registries allow tracking of every patient in the practice and identification of needed care. Registries that self-populate based on discrete data collected from an EHR can provide very timely reporting and actionable alerts in the EHR. For example, physician alerts can draw attention to the patients last LDL date, value, and out-of-range status, prompting the physician to address the issue with the patient. Similarly, nurses should receive alerts, while the patient is in the office, that the patient needs to have blood drawn or a flu shot administered.

Generating lists of patient information or care gaps for distribution to busy physicians is rarely successful because it is not immediately actionable. Better use of the registry information is to use it to drive outreach and action by other members of the team, including nurses, case managers, patient service representatives, and call center staff. Rather than sending a list of patients who need a flu shot to their physician, the list should be sent to the call center from which patients can be scheduled. Indexing all disease registries by patient allows easy identification of all care needs for a patient and enables these to be addressed with one contact.

SUCCESSFUL MODELS OF CARE
Group Health Cooperative

Group Health is a nonprofit integrated health system based in Seattle, Washington.[36] Beginning in 2006, a PCMH model was instituted at one prototype site. The group invested in the primary care site by increasing primary care staffing and lowering panel size from 2300 to 1800. The nonprovider staffing model was enhanced at the site and visit times increased. The site had registered nurses (RNs) and clinical pharmacists participate in care management. They also instituted team huddles, increased appointment times from 20 to 30 minutes, instituted prevention outreach, expanded e-visit and telephone visits, and developed patient-specific quality deficiency reporting. The results at 2 years showed improvements in patients' experiences, quality of care, and reduction in clinician burnout. Compared with other Group Health clinics the patients in the medical home model had 29% fewer emergency room (ER) visits and 6% fewer hospitalizations. Savings were estimated at $10.30 per patient per month.

Community Care of North Carolina

Since 1998, Community Care of North Carolina has been building primary-care–based community health networks for Medicaid and low-income children.[37] The program provided care coordinators focusing on the high-cost beneficiaries. It has worked with more than 1360 practices. The physicians are paid a management fee between $2.50 and $5.00 per member per month and, in return, they agree to focus on access, preventive and chronic disease metrics, and data reporting. They also receive regular feedback on cost and quality and see their performance against national and local benchmarks. Case managers, including nurses and social workers, coordinate services, collect and report data, and access a statewide database of high-risk individuals. The program has shown 40% reductions in hospitalizations and 16% reductions in ER use. There is an estimated $516 annual total savings per patient.[22]

Vermont Blueprint for Health

Vermont Blueprint for Health is a public-private initiative that was launched in 2006 and was rolled out in three pilot sites by March 2011, covering 10% of the state population.[38] The model uses community health teams that work with primary care providers to coordinate care and provide patient registry support. The community health teams engage primary care practices, health centers, hospitals and others to meet medical and social needs of patients and their families. Payment reforms as well as statewide enhanced data access are critical components. Patients with chronic disease have greater access to care and mental health services. Hospitalizations dropped 21% and ER use declined 31% in the medical home sites.

Johns Hopkins Guided Care PCMH Model

The Guided Care PCMH model uses teams of RNs working with community-based primary care physicians.[21] The Guided Care nurse focuses on Medicare beneficiaries at greatest risk and educates the patients and families about early identification of worsening symptoms. A Guided Care nurse, working with two to five physicians, manages a panel of 50 to 60 chronically ill patients. The nurses conduct in-home assessments, promote self-management, monitor conditions monthly, and coordinate the efforts of other health care professionals. After 8 months, the 904 Guided Care patients experienced, on average, 24% fewer hospital days, 37% fewer skilled-nursing facility days, and 15% fewer ER visits. The differences in use were estimated to show an annual net savings of $75,000 per nurse, or $1364 per patient.[39]

Intermountain Health Care

Intermountain has focused on patients with multiple chronic diseases since 2003 in the Care Management Plus program.[22] This program uses a primary care redesign focused on EHRs, reminders, and care pathways. Physicians identify patients with complex care needs and engage a care manager who develops a plan of care, coordinates the care delivery, and supports self-care and patient education. Electronic messaging systems enhance the connectivity of the various health professionals, allowing less duplication of services and faster responses. The program has shown a reduction in hospitalizations, ER visits, and an estimated $640 savings per patient per year.

PHN

PHN is the Geisinger PCMH (**Box 2**). It has these five pillars or core program components: patient-centered primary care, integrated case management, medical

---

Box 2
Geisinger's PHN core components

1. Patient-centered primary care
   a. Physician-led, team-delivered care
   b. Patient and family engagement
   c. Enhanced access and scope of services
   d. Optimized preventive care and chronic disease management through care redesign and health information technology
2. Integrated population management
   a. Population segmentation and risk stratification
   b. Embedded, in-office case management
   c. Disease management
   d. Medication management
3. Medical neighborhood
   a. Microdelivery referral systems using efficient specialists
   b. 360°-care delivery systems: nursing home, emergency departments, hospitals, home health, and so forth.
4. Quality improvement
   a. Patient satisfaction
   b. Access
   c. Preventive services metrics
   d. Bundled chronic disease metrics
5. Value-based reimbursement
   a. Fee-for-service with pay-for-performance payments for quality outcomes
   b. Physician and practice transformation stipends
   c. Value-based incentive payments
   d. Payments distributed on quality performance

---

neighborhood, quality improvement, and value-based reimbursement.[8,20] These components have been described in detail previously.[24]

Patient-Centered Primary Care

Patient-centered primary care serves as the foundation of Geisinger's PHN model. The value of physician-led, team-based care is derived from the primary care physician, advanced-nurse practitioners, the practice's clinical and front desk support staff, and the case managers. As experience in the PHN model grew, practices expanded the scope of available in-office treatments. Examples include treatment of acute exacerbations of diabetes, asthma, heart failure, and chronic obstructive pulmonary disease. All team members are aware of high-risk patients and all are empowered to provide access to patients with acute problems or exacerbations of chronic illnesses. Monthly meetings with all team members are held to review avoidable hospitalizations, discuss workflow barriers, and review program operations. The team also reviews overall quality and efficiency outcome metrics provided by the clinic and the health plan.

The practices have extended evening and Saturday hours. For after-hours care, patients have round-the-clock access to telephone support from physicians and nurses. On-call physicians have direct access from their home to the EHR, ensuring that patient's medical history and treatment status are always available and considered in providing any after-hours care. Case managers are available to support physician needs for specialized service requests such as home or ER-directed skilled nursing facility (SNF) placement or emergent home care.

INTEGRATED CASE MANAGEMENT

Population management aligns resources for all patients along the health care continuum. Predictive modeling and other stratification tools identify high-risk or vulnerable patients. Integrating case management with a deliberate focus on those patients within the practice that are most at risk is a core element. Staffing ratios are established at one RN case manager for every 800 Medicare members or 5000 commercial members. Each case manager has a case load of 125 to 150 high-risk patients. The case manager works with the physician and other primary care team members to understand the population with the use of using profiling reports and team members' personal knowledge.

The case manager, working with the patient, family, and physician, develops an individualized care plan for each high-risk patient. He or she interacts daily with the rest of the team to incorporate the "whole" patient view to better design the patient care plan. Case managers also take direct patient calls, coordinate specialty physician consultations, and respond to physician requests to coordinate community services such as home care.

All patients admitted to acute care are referred to the case manager for transitions of care management. Care managers contact the inpatient team to share subtleties of the patient, to understand the hospital course, and to prepare for post-acute care. They contact all patients within 24 to 48 hours of discharge and focus on medication reconciliation, follow-up with the primary care provider within 7 days, and the design of an "action plan" for the patient and family to use for problem management.

MEDICAL NEIGHBORHOOD

To improve quality and efficiency outcomes, it is essential to address care beyond the primary care office. The goal of PHN is to keep patients in the "line of sight" of the primary care team, regardless of where services are provided. To this end, practices develop partnerships with other care systems, including home health, acute hospitals, SNFs, community pharmacists, and emergency departments. Either primary care physicians personally provide care in these alternative sites or they have identified others who share their practice approach. This connection allows for prompt identification of patient needs and improves handoffs through the care transitions. Preferred partnerships with nursing facilities and home health providers have been established to improve continuity of care management after discharge and during acute exacerbations.

Many primary care providers provide services in SNFs, none of which are Geisinger owned. A further evolution of PHN has been a new physician-nurse practitioner model dedicated to providing full-time care in these facilities The focus is on delivering care "in place" to minimize transitions, each of which is an opportunity for safety failures and quality degradation. Advanced practitioners, dedicated solely to SNFs, developed systems to connect with both inpatient facilities and outpatient care teams. The redesign of SNF care is underway despite the challenges of a burdensome regulatory environment, significant fiscal and staffing limitations, and the need to transplant a culture of innovation. Improved care begins immediately with a comprehensive admission assessment within 48 hours of admission, careful medication review, early identification of acute exacerbations, and accelerated initiation of discharge planning. Emerging results from the skilled nursing home model look promising with substantial reductions in 30-day acute care readmissions (**Table 4**).

Value Reimbursement Model

Geisinger's approach was to create a gain-sharing model layered on top of traditional payments at the primary care level. Standard fee-for-service payments as well as existing pay-for-performance programs were continued. This was designed to both reduce fear and resistance as well as encourage primary care to be as clinically active as possible. A transformation payment was created that is paid upfront to allow financial support for the sites to adopt, implement, and maintain the infrastructure and process changes necessary for the advanced medical home. This transformation payment was netted from gain-sharing payment (see later discussion) but without downside risk.

The final component of the financial model is a quality-gated gain-sharing program. It relies on a comparison between each site's per-member-per-month (PMPM) allowed amounts at the end of the year versus a target PMPM. This target PMPM is best thought of as an estimate of what the allowed amount would have been had PHN not been implemented. This includes site-specific costs over the previous 2 years as well as regression to the mean adjustments for both high and low performers. The difference between target and actual expenditures are shared with the practice based on the percentage of quality metrics achieved.

NETWORK DEPLOYMENT

Geisinger began piloting this program in late 2006, and rapidly expanded with essentially a dozen sites added each year until all sites were fully operational in the autumn of 2010. This model was expanded from three sites (two Geisinger, one private practice) to 47 (38 Geisinger, nine private practices). This created the need to develop an appropriate infrastructure and support network, appropriate strategic and tactical reporting for site and region, and overall program management and improvement. Site-based leadership is optimized by the teaming up of physician site leaders, office managers, and case-management staff. Those leadership teams focus on site-specific reporting and on identifying opportunities for improvement, as determined by weekly review of admissions, readmissions, ER use, and nursing home use. Focused improvement projects, including office-based care system development

Table 4
Early results for nursing homes look promising

Nursing Home	Baseline Readmissions 2008	Readmissions 2009	Reduction
Nursing home A	34%	18.5%	−45.5%
Nursing home B	18.5%	14.5%	−21.6%
Nursing home C	27%	9%	−66.6%
Nursing home D	44%	33%	−25%
Nursing home E	42.5%	31%	−27%
Nursing home F	27.5%	24%	−12.7%

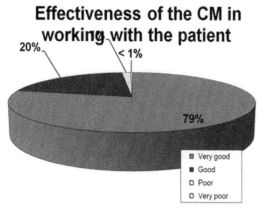

Fig. 1. Patients were asked to rate the effectiveness of working with the office-based case manager (CM); 99% rated this as "very good" or "good."

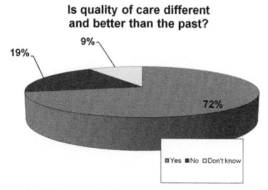

Fig. 2. Patients were asked if they noticed a change in their care 6 months after the unheralded start of PHN. Almost three-quarters noted a definite improvement.

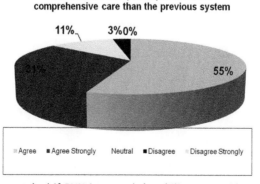

Fig. 3. Physicians were asked if PHN increased the ability to provide comprehensive care; 86% "agreed" or "strongly agreed."

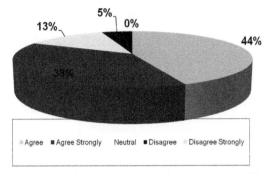

Fig. 4. Physicians were asked if they had more timely access to transitions of care information such as discharge summaries; 82% "agreed" or "strongly agreed."

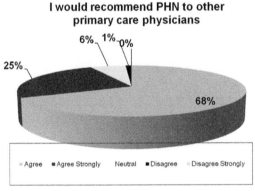

Fig. 5. Physicians were asked if they would recommend PHN to their primary care colleagues; 93% "agreed" or "strongly agreed."

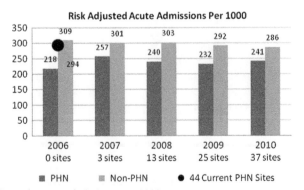

Fig. 6. Risk-adjusted acute admissions per 1000.

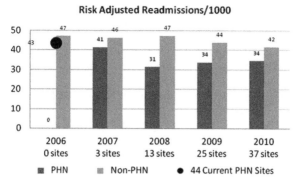

Fig. 7. Risk-adjusted readmissions per 1000.

for high-frequency problems (eg, cellulitis protocols, including outpatient intravenous antibiotics) are developed and generalized. Overall program leadership is charged with review of site, region, and program reports. System-wide and regional themes are determined; improvement goals and processes are added; reporting, tool development, or other key resource needs are assessed; and solutions developed. This ensures appropriate focus on emerging issues as well as creates the appropriate focus and convergence of improvement efforts from across the various regions.

Outcomes

PHN has improved all elements of the Triple Aim Plus. Quality measures have improved for prevention and chronic disease. In addition to improvements in process and intermediate outcome measures, there has been a significant reduction in the odds of a patient experiencing a diabetic amputation or end-stage renal disease.[40]

Patients and physicians are very satisfied with the level of communication and support that the new model delivers. Both patients and physicians recognize the change in overall orientation and effectiveness of the office by understanding their situation and proactively providing support (**Figs. 1** and **2**). The authors electronically surveyed 153 primary care physicians and, with a 78% return rate, they showed overwhelming appreciation for the new model. They value it because it allows them to improve health in ways that they were previously unable to do, as portrayed in **Figs. 3–7**. By moving to a more proactive design, better deploying resources, and coupling new systems to understand patient current status, needs, and desires, they are much more successful in improving health.

SUMMARY

There are several promising models based in primary care practice for improving the chronic care delivered in the United States. Widespread adoption of these models is critical to changing the cost and quality trends that are driving an unsustainable trajectory. The burgeoning population of patients with multiple chronic diseases will require these and other innovative approaches to the best care delivery. Geisinger has created a sustainable model to divide the population into meaningful subgroups, understand and predict the needs of each subgroup, and proactively support and engage patients in their care. This has resulted in measureable improvements in the quality of care delivered, the cost of that care, and the satisfaction of the patients and the care team. That said, there is clearly much more work to be done.

One significant challenge will be finding ways to spread these changes beyond the innovators to primary care practices at large. The success of Intermountain, Johns Hopkins, Geisinger, and others will need to be rapidly expanded across the nation and reliably delivered to all patients for the full value of these innovations in chronic disease care to be realized and the financial and quality catastrophe we are facing to be averted.

A second major challenge will be further improving the PCMH model. Patient and family activation, incorporation of patient preferences into decision-making, leveraging the experience of the entire organization relative to the care of patients in areas where other evidence is lacking, supporting patient care and the patient-care team through more personal and interactive technology, and increasing our ability to serve patients wherever they are and whenever needed will be critical areas as we continue the journey of value reengineering.

REFERENCES

1. OECD Library: Health at a Glance 2009: OECD Indicators. Available at: http://www.oecd-ilibrary.org/sites/health_glance-2009-en/00/02/index.html?contentType=&itemId=/content/chapter/health_glance-2009-2-en&containerItemId=/content/serial/19991312&accessItemIds=/content/book/health_glance-2009-en&mimeType=text/html. Accessed January 13, 2012.
2. Fisher E, Goodman D, Skinner J, et al. Health care spending, quality and outcomes. Dartmouth Institute for Health Policy and Clinical Practice: 2009. Available at: http://www.dartmouthatlas.org/downloads/reports/Spending_Brief_022709.pdf. Accessed June 30, 2011.
3. Østbye T, Yarnall KS, Krause K, et al. Is there time for management of patients with chronic diseases in primary care? Ann Fam Med 2005;3:209–14.
4. Boult C, Green AF, Boult LB, et al. Successful models of comprehensive care for older adults with chronic conditions: evidence for the Institute of Medicine's "Retooling for an Aging America" report. J Am Geriatr Soc 2009;57:2328–37.
5. Committee on the Quality of Healthcare in America, Institute of Medicine. Crossing the Quality Chasm: a new health system for the 21st Century. Washington, DC: National Academies Press; 2001.
6. Schoen C, Osborn R, Huynh P, et al. Commonwealth Fund. Primary care and health system performance: adults' experiences in five countries. Commonwealth Fund: Health Affairs Web Exclusive, October 28, 2004 W4-487-W4-504. And: Top 10 Health Policy Stories of 2004. Commonwealth Fund; 2004.
7. Anderson LM, May DS. Has the use of cervical, breast and colorectal cancer screening increased in the United States? Am J Public Health 1995;85:840–2.
8. McGlynn EA, Asch SM, Adams J, et al. The quality of health care delivered to adults in the United States. N Engl J Med 2003;348:2635–45.
9. Yarnall KS, Pollak KI, Østbye T, et al. Primary care: is there time for prevention? Am J Public Health 2003;93(4):635–41.
10. Bodenheimer T, Grumback K, Becicenson RA. A lifeline for primary care. N Engl J Med 2009;360:2693–6.
11. Goodman DC, Grumback K. Does having more physicians lead to better health system performance? JAMA 2008;299(3):335–7.
12. Fisher ES. Building a medical neighborhood for the medical home. N Engl J Med 2008;359(12):1202–5.
13. A toolkit for redesign in health care. Available at: http://www.ahrq.gov/qual/toolkit/tkappa.htm. Accessed January 13, 2012.

14. Improving health worker performance: In Search of Promising Practices. Available at: http://www.who.int/hrh/resources/improving_hw_performance.pdf. Accessed January 13, 2012.
15. Pierdon S, Eckrote B. Changing compensation plans. Moving beyond last year's, this year's and next year's. Physician Exec 2004;30(1):26.
16. Chassin MR, Loeb JM. The ongoing quality improvement journey: next stop, high reliability. Health Aff (Millwood) 2011;30(4):559–68.
17. Nolan T, Berwick D. All-or-none measurement raises the bar on performance. JAMA 2006;295:1168–9.
18. Bloom FJ, Graf T, Anderer T, et al. Redesign of a diabetes system of care using an all-or-none diabetes bundle to build teamwork and improve intermediate outcomes. Diabetes Spectr 2010;23(3):165–9.
19. Weber V, Bloom F, Pierdon S, et al. Employing the electronic health record to improve diabetes care: a multifaceted intervention in an integrated delivery system. J Gen Intern Med 2008;23(4):379–82.
20. Gilfillan RJ, Tomcavage JF, Rosenthal MB, et al. Value and the medical home: effects of transformed primary care. Am J Manag Care 2010;16(8):607–14.
21. Nutting PA, Miller WL, Crabtree BF, et al. Initial lessons from the first National Demonstration Project of practice transformation to a patient-centered medical home. Ann Fam Med 2009;7(3):254–60.
22. Shih A, Davis K, Schoenbaum S, et al. Organizing the U.S. health care delivery system for high performance. New York (NY): The Commonwealth Fund; 2008.
23. Merrell K, Berenson RA. Structuring payment for medical home. Health Aff (Millwood) 2010;29(5):852–8.
24. Steele GD, Haynes JA, Davis DE, et al. How Geisinger's advanced medical home model argues the case for rapid-cycle innovation. Health Aff (Millwood) 2010; 29(11):2047–53.
25. Cebul RD, Love TE, Jain AK, et al. Electronic health records and quality of diabetes care. N Engl J Med 2011;365(9):825–32.
26. Buntin MB, Burke MF, Hoaglin MC, et al. The benefits of health information technology: a review of the recent literature shows predominately positive results. Health Aff (Millwood) 2011;30(3):464–71.
27. Patient Centered Primary Care Collaborative. Joint principles of the patient centered medical home. February 2007. Available at: http://www.pcpcc.net/content/joint-principles-patient-centered-medical-home. Accessed January 13, 2012.
28. Hibbard JH. Engaging health care consumers to improve the quality of care. Med Care 2003;41(Suppl 1):I61–70.
29. Grumbach K, Grundy P. Outcomes of implementing patient centered medical home interventions: a review of the evidence from prospective evaluation studies in the United States. Patient Centered Primary Care Collaborative. Available at: http://www.pcpcc.net/files/evidence_outcomes_in_pcmh.pdf. Accessed January 13, 2012.
30. Fields D, Leshen E, Patel K. Driving quality gains and cost savings through adoption of medical homes. Health Aff (Millwood) 2010;28(5):819–26.
31. Wagner EH, Austin BT, Van Korf M. Organizing care for patients with chronic illness. Milbank Q 1996;74(4):511–44.
32. Bodenheimer T, Wagner EH, Grumbach K. Improving primary care for patients with chronic illness: the Chronic Care Model, part 2. JAMA 2002;288:1909–14.
33. Improving Chronic Illness Care. Steps for improvement manual. Available at: http://www.improvingchroniccare.org/downloads/improving_your_practice_manual_icic.doc. Accessed January 14, 2012.

34. Kabcenell AI, Langley J, Hupke C. Innovations in Planned Care. Innovation Series. Cambridge (MA): Institute for Healthcare Improvement; 2006. Available at: www.IHI.org. Accessed January 14, 2012.

35. Plan-Do-Study-Act (PDSA) Cycle. AHRQ. Available at: http://innovations.ahrq.gov/content.aspx?id=2398. Accessed January 14, 2012.

36. Reid RJ, Coleman K, Johnson EA, et al. The Group Health medical home at year two: cost savings, higher patient satisfaction, and less burnout for providers. Health Aff (Millwood) 2010;29(5):835–43.

37. Community Care of North Carolina. Community Care of North Carolina disease and care management initiatives. Raleigh (NC): CCNC; 2007.

38. Bielaszka-Duvernay C. Vermont's blueprint for medical homes, community health teams, and better health at lower cost. Health Aff (Millwood) 2011;30(3):383–6.

39. Leff B, Reider L, Frick K, et al. Guided care and the cost of complex healthcare: a preliminary report. Am J Manag Care 2009;15(8):555–9.

40. Maeng D, Graf T, Davis D, et al. Can a patient-centered medical home lead to better patient outcomes? The quality implications of Geisinger's ProvenHealth Navigator. Am J Med Qual 2011. Published online August 19, 2011. Available at: http://ajm.sagepub.com/content/early/2011/08/17/1062860611417421.full.pdf+html. Accessed January 15, 2012.

The Changes Involved in Patient-Centered Medical Home Transformation

Edward H. Wagner, MD, MPH[a],*, Katie Coleman, MSPH[a],
Robert J. Reid, MD, PhD[b,c], Kathryn Phillips, MPH[d],
Melinda K. Abrams, MS[e], Jonathan R. Sugarman, MD, MPH[d]

KEYWORDS

- Chronic illness • Primary care • Patient-centered medical home

KEY POINTS

- In 2007, the major primary care professional societies collaboratively introduced a new model of primary care: the patient-centered medical home (PCMH).
- The basic attributes and expectations of a PCMH are outlined, but not with the specificity needed to help interested clinicians and administrators make the necessary changes to their practice.
- To identify the specific changes required to become a medical home, literature was reviewed and consensus with two multistakeholder groups was sought. This article describes the eight consensus change concepts and 32 key changes that emerged from this process, and the evidence supporting their inclusion.

The Patient Protection and Affordable Care Act makes it clear that building a strong primary care sector is now a major goal of American health care policy.[1] Underlying this focus on primary care is the premise that more effective care will reduce costs for individuals with chronic illness by improving the quality, experience, and efficiency of their care. The focus on chronically ill patients stems from the fact that beneficiaries with multiple chronic conditions account for "virtually all" of the recent growth in

The work was supported by a grant from The Commonwealth Fund. The views presented here are those of the authors and not necessarily those of The Commonwealth Fund, its directors, officers, or staff.

The authors have nothing to disclose.

[a] MacColl Center for Health Care Innovation, Group Health Research Institute, 1730 Minor Avenue, Suite 1600, Seattle, WA 98101, USA; [b] Group Health Research Institute, 1730 Minor Avenue, Suite 1600, Seattle, WA 98101, USA; [c] Group Health Permanente, 1730 Minor Avenue, Suite 1600, Seattle, WA 98101, USA; [d] Qualis Health, 10700 Meridian Avenue North, #100, Seattle, WA 98133, USA; [e] Patient-Centered Coordinated Care Program, The Commonwealth Fund, One East 75th Street, New York, NY 10021, USA
* Corresponding author.
E-mail address: wagner.e@ghc.org

Medicare spending.[2] Agreement is now widespread that traditionally organized primary care practices must redesign their infrastructure and the way they organize and deliver care if they hope to achieve more effective, less costly care.[1,3] In an effort to foster practice transformation and reform payment, the major primary care professional societies proposed a new model of primary care,[4] which couples practice transformation with payment reform. They labeled this new model the patient-centered medical home (PCMH).

The PCMH has many roots: earlier work defining primary care[3] and patient-centered care,[5] the observation that children with major health problems benefit from a general pediatric medical home,[6] and the Chronic Care Model.[7] The *Joint Principles of the Patient-Centered Medical Home* (February 2007) wove these threads into the PCMH and added payment reform.[4] The PCMH represents an amalgamation of two well-established models: the Pediatric Medical Home model[8] and the Chronic Care Model.[9] The Pediatric Medical Home model clearly places the accountability on the generalist physician team for assuring that care is comprehensive, continuous, accessible, coordinated, and patient- and family-centered. The elements of the Chronic Care Model comprise structural and functional modifications to practice that support patient activation and planned proactive care, and produce better patient outcomes.[9]

The two models are complementary: one describes what patients should expect and how the practice can meet those expectations; the other describes how care should be structured and delivered. Both, however, emphasize the centrality of the relationship between the primary care team and the patient/family. Furthermore, both advocate for the empowerment of patients and their families so that they play a greater role in their health and health care. Although the Joint Principles describe basic attributes and expectations of a PCMH, they do not provide a definition or description of a PCMH that is sufficiently operational to help interested practices and clinicians understand and implement the requisite changes in practice structure and function. To meet this need, the authors sought to define the characteristics of fully transformed medical homes and the changes to practice infrastructure, organization, and care delivery needed to get there. This article describes the consensus change concepts and key changes that emerged from this process, and the evidence supporting their inclusion.

METHODS

Defining the practice changes to become a PCMH from an operational perspective was an important early step in the Commonwealth Fund's Safety Net Medical Home Initiative (SNMHI). The initiative is helping 65 community health centers or other safety net practices in five different regions (Colorado, Idaho, Massachusetts, Oregon, and Pittsburgh) implement the PCMH and evaluate its impacts. The methods used to develop the changes have been described in more detail elsewhere.[10]

To define the characteristics of a PCMH for the SNMHI, project staff reviewed literature related to the definitions and characteristics of a PCMH,[11–20] including definitions of patient-centered care,[7,21–23] descriptions of the Pediatric Medical Home[8,24] and Chronic Care models,[21–23,25,26] and related topics. They also studied related practice transformation initiatives.[16,18,20,27–29] Because the efforts to become a PCMH should be guided by the goals of the transformation, the authors first considered the objectives of becoming a medical home. They then tried to identify high level change concepts, which are general notions or approaches to change found to be useful in developing specific ideas for changes that lead to improvement,[30] and then identified more specific key changes under each change concept. Both change concepts and key changes describe general directions for practice transformation to encourage creativity and adaptation to local resources and circumstances.

The authors then convened a panel of experts and stakeholders in the delivery of primary care, including provider, health plan, patient, and research representatives, to review and edit the preliminary change concepts. A second panel, convened for another PCMH transformation project, reviewed the changes approved by the first panel.

Preliminary Characterization of a PCMH

Based on the literature review and study of transformation efforts already underway or completed, the authors developed a preliminary list of features of a PCMH and related change concepts. They suggested that, to become fully developed medical homes, practices would have to implement changes in eight areas. These areas would begin with ensuring (1) engaged leadership and (2) an effective quality improvement strategy, and (3) linking patients with specific providers and care teams (empanelment). Then, through (4) continuous, team-based relationships, patients would receive (5) organized, evidence-based care and (6) patient-centered interactions. PCMHs would assure that patients would get the care they need when they need it in the practice through (7) enhancing access and, from outside the practice, by more effectively (8) coordinating care. Within each of these eight areas or change concepts, the authors suggested three to five more specific features or key changes.

RESULTS
The Goals of PCMH Transformation

Broad agreement was reached that effective PCMHs should improve patient experience, the quality of clinical care especially for patients with chronic illness, and the work satisfaction of physicians and other primary care staff. Both panels believed that the sustainability of the PCMH model and rationale for increased primary care payments hinged on its ability to reduce health care costs. They emphasized the importance of improved care for patients with multiple chronic conditions because of their high health care costs. Cost data and emerging evidence from pilot evaluations suggested that PCMH-like interventions have the potential to decrease total health care costs principally through reducing emergency room use and hospitalizations for ambulatory care–sensitive conditions.[29,31,32]

The Change Concepts

Engaged leadership
Leadership support of any initiative is obviously helpful, but it is pivotal when the initiative involves major changes in a practice's culture and usual ways of working.[33] Implementing the PCMH often requires disruptive changes to the culture, roles, and routines of a practice.[28] Active involvement of senior leaders in the change process seems to be crucial. In one study, experts in clinical system redesign reported that "direct involvement of top- and middle-level leaders" was most critical to success.[34] Leaders must also recognize that creating and sustaining PCMHs takes considerable time and will engender frustration and unrest.

A useful model for leading transformational change in primary care suggests that effective leaders have knowledge and skills in three important domains: (1) systems thinking, or the capacity to understand the practice as a series of interrelated processes that determine performance; (2) envisioning change, or recognizing the gap between current and optimal practice and promising changes to close the gap; and (3) change management, or implementing proven strategies for quality improvement and engaging staff in the process.[35] The authors' suggested key changes reflect these domains.

Specific activities and changes recommended under engaged leadership are as follows:

- Provide visible and sustained leadership to lead overall cultural change and specific strategies to improve quality and spread and sustain change.
- Ensure that the PCMH transformation effort has the time and resources needed to be successful.
- Ensure that providers and other care team members have protected time to conduct activities beyond direct patient care that are consistent with the medical home model.
- Incorporate the practice's values regarding creating a medical home for patients in staff hiring and training processes.

The first and second key changes recognize leadership's essential role in transformation, including the establishment and support of a quality improvement strategy and infrastructure. Effective leaders can support culture change through increasing the involvement of patients and staff in the process, assuring support from the Board of Directors, and using data and success stories to sustain enthusiasm.[36] Because primary care practices are complex adaptive systems, changes have impacts that ripple throughout the organization.[37] Therefore, effective leaders ensure that boundaries and communication barriers among staff are eliminated; all components of the practice are involved in improvement and transformation; and staff development inculcates the values of providing a medical home for patients.

Quality improvement strategy

Implementing something as complex as the eight change concepts of the PCMH is very different from changing a process; it fundamentally changes a practice's culture and operations, and affects most staff and clients. Change of this magnitude has been called "practice transformation." Based on their evaluation of a national PCMH implementation pilot, Nutting and colleagues[28] suggested that this transformation requires "epic whole-practice reimagination and redesign." Successful practices seemed to have "adaptive reserve," or the leadership and capacity to fundamentally redesign their organization, and an explicit quality improvement (QI) strategy or approach. Studies have confirmed the link between high performance and an explicit QI strategy.[38] To establish an effective strategy, a practice should

- Choose and use a formal model for quality improvement
- Establish and monitor metrics to evaluate routinely improvement efforts and outcomes; ensure all staff members understand the metrics for success
- Ensure that patients, families, providers, and care team members are involved in quality improvement activities
- Optimize use of health information technology to meet meaningful use criteria.

The key changes mentioned collectively create a sustainable continuous QI program that relies on involvement of staff and patients, proven methods for testing ideas for change, and performance measurement. Most successful practice organizations use QI methods that rely on rapid cycles of change and continuous measurement.[30,39,40] Little rigorous evaluative or comparative research is available to help practices choose among these approaches.[41] Considerable experience now suggests that selecting a QI strategy and integrating it into the organization's culture and operations are more important than worrying about which one to choose.

Trying to improve quality without a trusted measurement system has generally proven futile. Audit and feedback of relevant quality indicators has been shown to improve practice performance.[42] The work of the National Quality Forum is providing care delivery organizations with a carefully vetted, consensus menu of potential measures.[43] But many challenges exist to obtaining and interpreting clinical performance measures, especially in smaller practices.[44] Given the importance of patients with multiple chronic illnesses in adult primary care, measuring performance among this group raises additional considerations, such as the appropriateness of recommended clinical targets or the need for generic measures, such as functional status.[45] The involvement of staff in improvement activities provides a grounded perspective on current processes and ideas for change, and may make changes more acceptable.

The final key change, optimizing use of information technology, has now been defined by the Meaningful Use criteria established by the Office of the National Coordinator of Information Technology.[46] These criteria define the data and functions that should be included in an effective electronic medical record (EMR). Although the implementation of EMRs has accelerated, many practices still do not use them to their full capacity.[47]

Empanelment

The foundation of the PCMH is the longitudinal relationship between patients and providers and the practice team. When patients visit the same practitioner, greater compliance with prescribed medications, improved identification of medical problems, increased patient and provider satisfaction, fewer hospital admissions, and lower overall costs are seen.[48] In many fee-for-service practices, no explicit process links a patient with a specific provider. Because key features of a medical home, such as continuous team-based healing relationships, enhanced access, population-based care, and care coordination, depend on the existence of strong patient-provider relationships, establishment of these linkages (empanelment) must be an early step in the transformation to a PCMH.

To create patient-provider relationships consistent with the preferences of both parties, a practice should

- Assign all patients to a provider panel and confirm assignments with providers and patients; review and update panel assignments on a regular basis
- Assess practice supply and demand, and balance patient load accordingly
- Use panel data and registries to proactively contact and track patients according to disease status, risk status, self-management status, and community and family needs.

The decision to link a patient with a provider begins with an examination of the past use of the practice by each patient.[49] In general, patients who tend to see a particular provider are initially assigned to that provider, and others with less consistent use patterns are assigned after discussion among relevant providers.[50] These tentative links should then be reviewed by the provider and the patient and adjusted accordingly. This empanelment process may be especially challenging in safety net practices, though it has been effectively accomplished in these organizations.[49]

The process of empanelment provides practices with important information concerning workloads that can help to balance demand among providers. Review of panel data at Group Health Cooperative showed that many primary care panels were too large to provide high-quality care, and they were reduced.[51] Although many patients had to be reassigned to different providers, with well-designed patient information and thoughtful management, satisfaction did not decline among the reassigned patients.[52]

Patient panels and information systems with registry functionality enable staff to identify and reach out to patients with unmet needs. For example, a practice can review its patients with diabetes to identify who may be out of control or missing preventive or chronic care services, and schedule them for a planned visit. Defined panels also enable the measurement and feedback of performance at the individual provider level.

Continuous and team-based healing relationships

A primary goal of empanelment is to establish patient-provider continuity, which has been linked to better health outcomes, especially among patients with chronic illness.[53,54] An effective medical home reinforces this relational continuity and organizes its systems and processes to support it. However, growing evidence shows that the best care is provided by well-organized teams, not isolated clinicians. To provide continuous team-based healing relationships, effective PCMHs should

- Establish and provide organizational support for care delivery teams that are accountable for the patient population/panel
- Link patients to a provider and care team so both patients and provider/care teams recognize each other as partners in care
- Assure that patients are able to see their provider or care team whenever possible
- Define roles and distribute tasks among care team members to reflect the skills, abilities, and credentials of team members.

Although the relationship between clinician and patient is crucial, growing evidence suggests that clinical care improves when other practice team members help meet the clinical needs of patients. For example, team involvement in care has been shown to be among the most efficacious interventions for improving disease control in patients with diabetes,[55] hypertension,[56] and depression.[57] Researchers have estimated that providing care to a patient panel consistent with consensus chronic disease and preventive care guidelines would take a primary care provider 18 hours each practice day.[58] But work volume is not the only factor that necessitates team care; many of the services chronically ill and other patients need do not require physician involvement, and some, such as self-management counseling or care coordination, are often better performed by team members other than the physician.[59] A recent European review suggests that enhancing the collective clinical expertise of the team improves processes of care, but also confirms how little is known about the determinants and characteristics of effective teamwork.[60]

The PCMH should reinforce the ongoing patient-provider link at every opportunity. Abundant evidence confirms that seeing the same clinician over time leads to higher patient satisfaction, more complete preventive care, and better outcomes among people with chronic illnesses.[54,61–64] Three aspects of continuity have been described in the literature: continuity of clinical information, continuity of management, and continuity of relationship.[63] Continuity of clinical information and management continuity (consistency of clinical approach) have been improved through the use of shared electronic records that incorporate decision support. However, the real power of continuity resides in continuity of the relationship between patient and provider.[65] The question is, though, are the benefits of seeing the same provider jeopardized when a patient has an interaction with someone else on the team? One study suggests that no decrease in patient satisfaction occurs when a patient sees someone else on the practice team as long as the patient perceives the provider to be part of a well-functioning team with good communications.[66]

Care teams seem to function best when each member has clearly defined roles that are made transparent to patients. Involving staff in clinical care does not come naturally to many clinicians. It can be facilitated by a deliberate process of delineating and matching the tasks involved in meeting a panel's needs with the skills, credentials, and interests of staff members. The goal is to have every member of a practice team working "at the top of their license," providing all the care their license or certification allows. Innovative practices have shown that talented medical assistants can do more than take vital signs and room patients, including providing self-management support,[67] reviewing registries, and reaching out to high risk patients needing service. When assigning tasks or roles, practices should ensure that the staff is appropriately trained for their designated functions. Given the high turnover in staff positions, cross-training is also prudent.

Organized evidence-based care
Considerable evidence now suggests that implementation of the elements of the Chronic Care Model improves the quality of care for patients with chronic conditions.[9,68] Important elements of the CCM, such as team care, patient activation and self-management support, and linkage to community resources, are included in other PCMH change concepts. **Table 1** shows how the key elements of the Chronic Care Model have been included in the eight change concepts. The changes included in organized evidence-based care largely address the underuse of proven preventive interventions, clinical assessments, and treatments, which continues to be a major problem in chronic illness care. The Institute of Medicine report, *Crossing the Quality Chasm*,[69] primarily attributes the failure to provide scientifically proven services to deficiencies in systems of care, not in the providers working in those systems. Providers are frequently unaware when their patients are in need of a given test or treatment, and, if aware, may not get around to addressing it in a rushed problem-related visit. To routinely deliver organized evidence-based care, PCMHs should

- Use planned care according to patient need
- Identify high-risk patients and ensure they are receiving appropriate care and case management services
- Use point-of-care reminders based on clinical guidelines
- Enable planned interactions with patients by making up-to-date information available to providers and the care team before the visit.

Many of the services proven beneficial to chronically ill patients are periodic and predictable, such as foot examinations in patients with diabetes and forced expiratory volume in the first second of expiration (FEV_1) or peak flow monitoring in patients with asthma, and their administration can be planned. Planned visits are organized to ensure that all needed services are identified before the visit and delivered at the visit. Although limited formal study has been performed of planned care, except for group visits, considerable quality improvement experience suggests its value.[70–72] These visits can be initiated through identifying patients in need of services from registries or other data sources, inviting them in for a visit, and obtaining needed test results before the visit. Alternatively, planned care can be delivered during patient-initiated encounters if information systems can efficiently identify needed services and practice teams review the data before the visit and organize their work so that identified service needs are met.

Table 1
Inclusion of chronic care model elements into PCMH change concepts

Change Concept	Key Changes	Chronic Care Model Elements
Engaged leadership	Visible leadership for culture change and QI	Health care organization
Quality improvement strategy	Use formal QI model Establish metrics to evaluate improvement Optimize use of health information technology	Health care organization Information systems
Empanelment	Use panel data to manage population	Information systems Proactive care
Continuous, team-based relationships	Establish and support care delivery teams Distribute roles and tasks among team	Practice redesign (team care)
Organized evidence-based care	Use planned care according to patient need Use patient data to enable planned interactions Use point-of-care reminders	Practice redesign (planned care) Decision support Information systems
Patient-centered interaction	Encourage patient involvement in health and care Provide self-management support at every encounter	Activate patients Self-management support
Enhanced access		
Care coordination	Link patients with community resources Provide care management services	Community resources Practice redesign (care management)

High-risk patients with multiple problems often need more intensive clinical support in addition to assistance with navigating the health care system. The provision of more intensive follow-up and clinical management, in addition to help with care coordination, has generally been called *care* or *case management*. Nurse care managers can improve outcomes and reduce costs for elderly and complex chronically ill populations when closely integrated with or embedded in primary care.[32,55,56,73,74] Because nurse care managers focus on a very small segment of the practice panel at highest risk of major morbidity, they cannot be expected to meet all of the care coordination needs of a practice. To systematically ensure that patients receive the services they need in a timely way, the practice must know what evidence-based guidelines apply to a specific patient at that time. Provider reminder systems reflecting evidence-based guidelines and embedded in an EMR have been shown to increase the likelihood that recommended services are delivered.[75]

Patient-centered interactions

Crossing the Quality Chasm includes patient-centeredness as one of the six goals of high-quality health care.[69] Patient-centered care involves patients in decisions about their care and in the process of care to ensure that it is consistent with the patient's preferences, values, and culture. Other definitions of patient-centered care emphasize: the patient "as a whole person" rather than a set of diseases or risk factors,[76] the patient's own role in managing health and illness,[77] the social and emotional aspects of illness and care, and the provision of clear and comprehensible information.[5] Taking a broader view of patient-centeredness, the authors recommend five key changes that a practice can implement to facilitate patient-centered interactions:

1. Respect patient and family values and expressed needs.
2. Encourage patients to expand their role in decision-making, health-related behaviors, and self-management.
3. Communicate with patients in a culturally appropriate manner, in a language and at a level that the patient understands.
4. Provide self-management support at every visit through goal setting and action planning.
5. Obtain feedback from patients/families about their health care experience and use this information for quality improvement.

The quality of care from the perspective of patients and their families generally depends on the extent to which their care is consistent with their needs, preferences, values, and expectations.[78] Despite this seemingly obvious relationship, medical care has generally not placed much emphasis in eliciting this information from patients. Although people vary in the extent to which they want to make decisions about their care, most want the opportunity to discuss treatment options and share their preferences and concerns about treatment.[79] Interventions to increase patient involvement in decision-making, primarily decision aids, are now widely available. They seem to have positive effects on patient satisfaction and adherence to treatment, and can influence treatment choices, especially related to discretionary surgery.[80]

Roughly one-half of patients leaving medical encounters do not comprehend what was recommended[81,82] by the provider; these patients are, therefore, less likely to adhere to treatment recommendations and generally have worse outcomes than those who can recount the provider's advice.[83,84] Making certain that patients and their providers understand each other is an essential goal of a patient-centered practice. Practices with significant non–English-speaking clientele should have reliable translation services or language-concordant staff. Routine assessment of health literacy and use of teach-back or "closing the loop" (asking patients to recount what they have been asked to do) can substantially increase comprehension of medical advice and recommendations.[85]

The ability of patients to effectively manage (self-management) their chronic illnesses is an important determinant of good outcomes. Evidence now indicates that most patients can acquire the skills to become competent self-managers with appropriate support. Most of the published evidence on the effectiveness of self-management support interventions pertains to time-limited group or individual interventions.[86–88] Because the challenges of self-managing most chronic illnesses fluctuate in content and intensity over time, most experts now recommend that self-management support be an ongoing process best performed in the context of clinical interactions.[89,90] This function necessitates the availability of practice team members trained to help patients set self-management goals, identify and solve problems in reaching goals, and develop realistic action plans. A new role, the health coach, is emerging to meet the need for self-management support in primary care.[91] Medical assistants and even lay people have, with appropriate training, proven to be effective health coaches.[91]

Measurement of the effectiveness of a PCMH is incomplete without assessing patient experience. Many health care organizations routinely measure patient satisfaction, but often the measures and methods used do not allow the practice to use the data to identify improvement opportunities and evaluate successes. Patient experience measures differ from traditional satisfaction instruments in that they assess key behaviors or activities that occurred during patients' interactions with the health care provider or system, thus providing a clearer path for intervention and quality improvement. The use of valid instruments and scientifically based sampling methods increase the usefulness of patient experience data.[92,93] Several studies show that positive patient experience is significantly associated with better clinical quality outcomes, greater adherence to clinicians' advice, reduced malpractice risk, and increased patient loyalty to the practice or provider.[93–96]

Enhanced access
Accessibility, which is the ability to receive acceptable medical care whenever one needs it, is a defining element of high-quality primary care. In reality, however, many Americans have difficulty seeing their doctor when they feel ill, during or outside of traditional office hours. Recent Commonwealth Fund surveys suggest that access to primary care is worse in the United States than in the other 10 developed countries studied. Only one in four American adults with chronic illness could get an appointment the same day if they were sick.[97] A survey of primary care physicians found that less than one-third of American primary care doctors reported that they provide after-hours care, the lowest of the 11 countries surveyed.[98] Barriers to accessing primary care, such as limited urgent care appointments, or after-hours care, contribute to costly avoidable hospitalizations and emergency room use.[99] Therefore, a PCMH should

- Promote and expand access through ensuring that established patients have 24/7 continuous access to their care teams via phone, e-mail, or in-person visits
- Provide scheduling options that are patient and family-centered and accessible to all patients
- Help patients attain and understand health insurance coverage.

Patients should be able to communicate 24 hours a day, 7 days a week with a provider who knows them and has access to their clinical information. Developing enhanced telephone access to the practice during and after clinic hours is an important element. Telephone access to providers during office hours can be improved through more efficient management of incoming calls.[31] Telephone access after hours through triage or consultation services has increased clinician satisfaction and reduced clinical workload, but patients express dissatisfaction if they view the service as a barrier to being seen.[100–102] A variety of community-based approaches have been used to provide after-hours primary care services.[103] Community-based primary care cooperatives in the Netherlands and other countries provide telephone triage and in-person care after hours to the patients of the participating primary care physicians. One evaluation indicated that the cooperative reduced emergency department use by more than 50%.[104] Whatever the coverage arrangement, it should be carefully explained to clients of a medical home so that after-hours coverage meets expectations.

Practices must implement flexible appointment systems to accommodate varying patient needs, including: same-day appointments for patients who wish to be seen that day; longer appointments for patients with more complex issues; and appointments made in advance to address preventive services and follow-up. Open- or advanced-access appointment scheduling has been proposed as a way to better meet patients' needs.[105] A recent review suggests that implementing advanced access improves appointment waiting time and reduces no-show rates, but effects on patient satisfaction are inconclusive.[106] An early step in the implementation of advanced access is to ensure that the practice has the capacity to meet the demand for its services. Balancing supply and demand, a key step in the empanelment process, is crucial to improving access.

Medical homes, especially those serving lower-income populations, should develop the capacity to help their patients understand or obtain health insurance. Estimates show that as many as 20% of Medicaid-eligible children and 12% of Medicaid-eligible children with major chronic conditions are uninsured because their parents lacked the necessary information or were intimidated by the enrollment process.[107,108]

Care coordination

High-quality medical care now requires that many patients, especially those with chronic illness, receive medical and nonmedical services from multiple providers and organizations. However, breakdowns in communication between providers and organizations limit the effectiveness of these services and contribute to medical errors, unnecessary hospitalizations, duplicate procedures, inappropriate drug regimens, and gaps in follow-up care.[109–111] Problems after discharge of patients from the hospital highlight this issue. One in five Medicare recipients discharged from the hospital are readmitted within 30 days after discharge[112]; approximately one-half will return to the hospital without having seen a physician in the community. The lack of follow-up is not surprising given that many primary care physicians are not made aware that their patients have been hospitalized.[113]

Although coordinating care is everyone's responsibility, the PCMH should protect its patients from the damage associated with fragmentation of care. They should help patients access important community services, make key referrals, clarify expectations for prereferral and postreferral care, and facilitate timely transfer of information. To better coordinate care, the PCMH should

- Link patients with community resources to facilitate referrals and respond to social service needs
- Integrate behavioral health and specialty care into care delivery through co-location or referral agreements
- Track and support patients when they obtain services outside the practice
- Follow up with patients within a few days of an emergency room visit or hospital discharge
- Communicate test results and care plans to patients.

Medical homes have an obligation to identify high-quality patient-friendly organizations and programs in their community. For critical services such as cardiology, behavioral health, or weight loss, it helps to have general working agreements in place with the providers and their organizations. The goals of these agreements are shared expectations that could reduce the chances of ineffective or failed referrals, duplicate testing, breakdowns in communication, or other misunderstandings.

Many patients will need more than a referral slip to have a safe and satisfying referral or transition; they may need help securing an appointment, figuring out how to pay for the service, or making certain that all of their providers are well informed. To identify and remedy problems in the referral or transition process, the PCMH should have the capacity to identify and track patients as they move across settings and disciplines. Electronic referral systems that are part of shared EMRs or separate

Web-based programs can facilitate appointment making and referral tracking, and improve the quality and timeliness of the communication.[114]

Care management of patients recently discharged from the hospital reduces morbidity and prevents readmissions.[115–118] Although these transition management activities begin in the hospital, they must be followed by effective follow-up care in the PCMH. Recent research found that one-half of discharged medical patients, most of whom had a primary care physician, failed to have timely follow-up appointments with their PCP.[119] Those without timely primary care experienced higher rates of hospital readmission.[119] Therefore, PCMHs should contact their patients shortly after discharge from the emergency department or hospital. Because many hospitals seem to make little effort to identify a patient's primary care physician, PCMHs will have to initiate conversations with the hospitals and emergency departments that commonly serve their patients.

Finally, an important element of care coordination is timely communication of test results and care plans with patient. Patients clearly want to know the results of tests performed. Preference studies indicate that most patients find timely mail or electronic communication of normal results to be acceptable, but strongly prefer a telephone call for abnormal results.[120]

Implementing the Changes

Epic whole-practice reimagination and redesign will not become a reality unless practices start with a stable "core structure,"[28] which includes reliable business and clinical operations, limited staff turnover, and established information systems. QI experience strongly suggests that practices have great difficulty making changes while in the throes of implementing an EMR or dealing with key staff turnover.

The change concepts and key changes build on one another, suggesting that sequential implementation will be most practical and effective. Meaningful practice change is unlikely unless an organization has the internal capacity to learn and change, or "adaptive reserve."[121] Adaptive reserve largely seems to be a function of unified leadership that can envision a future, facilitate staff involvement in a strategy for getting there, and devote time to plan, make, and evaluate changes. Engaged leadership and putting in place an effective QI strategy should therefore be initial priorities. Most of the remaining change concepts assume a primary patient-provider relationship, so empanelment should be tackled next. Once patients are in panels, practice teams should begin work on changing the way they deliver care. This step usually involves selected changes from three change concepts: continuous and team-based healing relationships, patient-centered interactions, and organized evidence-based care. Early changes include establishing practice teams and defining roles, using data systems to begin planning care, and developing the capacity to routinely provide self-management support. Care coordination is a critical practice function that should be addressed when team role assignments are considered. Access has two major components: after-hours coverage and a more patient-friendly appointment system. The former should be undertaken early, because it may be critical to assuring continuity and reducing emergency room use. The latter can be arduous, and might best be addressed after care teams and delivery have been reorganized. The SNMHI Web site includes guides for implementing each of the change concepts (http://www.qhmedicalhome.org/safety-net/about.cfm).

The change concepts are intended to guide the formulation and testing of specific practice changes reflective of the unique needs, capabilities, and culture of each practice organization. They serve as the goals of practice change, not the specific methods through which to reach the goals. The key changes, although more actionable, generally are also not specific or concrete enough to implement as such. They should be viewed as opportunities for innovation and adaptation rather than prescriptions for implementation. As practices use and test the key changes and evidence accumulates, they will become more specific and useful.

SUMMARY

The components of the PCMH identified collectively capture the major features of the Medical Home and Chronic Care Models.

The change concepts described also correlate closely with other definitions of the PCMH[4,20] and with the National Committee on Quality Assurance's PCMH recognition program criteria.[122] These criteria focus more on the availability of electronic data than do the change concepts, which place more emphasis on the functions of information systems (whether electronic or paper) in patient care, such as using patient data for outreach and care planning, performance measurement, and clinician reminders.

The authors believe that implementation of the PCMH as defined earlier best meets the needs of patients with chronic illness. In addition to receiving care from a provider and practice team that knows them as a person and is organized in accord with the Chronic Care Model, chronically ill patients will be more likely to have the continuity of care, enhanced access, and care coordination that will help them avoid unnecessary emergency room visits and hospitalizations. As the number of a patient's chronic conditions increases, the number of physicians seen, health care costs, reported medical errors, and coordination problems also increase. A well-organized PCMH should help to avoid this expensive and potentially dangerous spiral.

The authors wrestled with the question as to whether the change concepts and their more specific changes should only include items supported by robust evidence showing that they contribute to reaching the PCMH goals. Although the recommended changes should adhere to evidence as much as possible, the reality is that the evidence supporting some of the essential and defining features of primary care, such as after-hours coverage or care coordination, is limited. Therefore, the more specific recommendations embedded in many of the key changes should be viewed as provisional, subject to change as new evidence emerges. The change concepts and key changes described are providing the guiding framework for statewide PCMH transformation efforts in Washington, Massachusetts, and Montana in addition to the SNMHI. As experience grows, more insight should be gained into how this model can better serve as a template for transformed primary care.

REFERENCES

1. Goodson JD. Patient Protection and Affordable Care Act: promise and peril for primary care. Ann Intern Med 2010;152(11):742–4.
2. Berenson RA, Hammons T, Gans DN, et al. A house is not a home: keeping patients at the center of practice redesign. Health Aff (Millwood) 2008;27(5): 1219–30.
3. Committee on the Future of Primary Care, Division of Health Care Services, Institute of Medicine. Defining primary care: an interim report. Washington, DC: Institute of Medicine; 1994.
4. American Academy of Family Physicians. Joint principles of the patient-centered medical home. Del Med J 2008;80(1):21–2.
5. Stewart M. Towards a global definition of patient centred care. BMJ 2001; 322(7284):444–5.

6. General principles in the care of children and adolescents with genetic disorders and other chronic health conditions. American Academy of Pediatrics Committee on Children with Disabilities. Pediatrics 1997;99(4):643–4.

7. Wagner EH, Austin BT, Davis C, et al. Improving chronic illness care: translating evidence into action. Health Aff (Millwood) 2001;20(6):64–78.

8. Cooley WC, McAllister JW. Building medical homes: improvement strategies in primary care for children with special health care needs. Pediatrics 2004; 113(Suppl 5):1499–506.

9. Coleman K, Austin BT, Brach C, et al. Evidence on the Chronic Care Model in the new millennium. Health Aff (Millwood) 2009;28(1):75–85.

10. Wagner EH, Coleman K, Reid RJ, et al. Guiding transformation: how medical practices can become patient-centered medical homes. The Commonwealth Fund 2012.

11. Carrier E, Gourevitch MN, Shah NR. Medical homes: challenges in translating theory into practice. Med Care 2009;47(7):714–22.

12. Bailit M, Hughes C, National Business Coalition on Health. The patient-centered medical home: a purchaser guide. Understanding the model and taking action. Patient-Centered Primary Care Collaborative Web site. Available at: http://www.pcpcc.net/files/PurchasersGuide/PCPCC_Purchaser_Guide.pdf. Accessed March 27, 2012.

13. Ferrante JM, Balasubramanian BA, Hudson SV, et al. Principles of the patient-centered medical home and preventive services delivery. Ann Fam Med 2010; 8(2):108–16.

14. Friedberg MW, Lai DJ, Hussey PS, et al. A guide to the medical home as a practice-level intervention. Am J Manag Care 2009;15(Suppl 10):S291–9.

15. Kellerman R, Kirk L. Principles of the patient-centered medical home. Am Fam Physician 2007;76(6):774–5.

16. O'Malley AS, Peikes D, Ginsburg PB. Making medical homes work: moving from concept to practice: qualifying a physician practice as a medical home. Policy Perspective: Insights into Health Policy Issues. Center for Studying Health System Change 2008;(1):1–19.

17. Rittenhouse DR, Shortell SM. The patient-centered medical home: will it stand the test of health reform? JAMA 2009;301(19):2038–40.

18. Rosenthal TC. The medical home: growing evidence to support a new approach to primary care. J Am Board Fam Med 2008;21(5):427–40.

19. Sidorov JE. The patient-centered medical home for chronic illness: is it ready for prime time? Health Aff (Millwood) 2008;27(5):1231–4.

20. Stange KC, Nutting PA, Miller WL, et al. Defining and measuring the patient-centered medical home. J Gen Intern Med 2010;25(6):601–12.

21. Wagner EH. Chronic disease management: what will it take to improve care for chronic illness? [editorial]. Eff Clin Pract 1998;1(1):2–4.

22. Bodenheimer T, Wagner EH, Grumbach K. Improving primary care for patients with chronic illness. JAMA 2002;288(14):1775–9.

23. Bodenheimer T, Wagner EH, Grumbach K. Improving primary care for patients with chronic illness: the chronic care model, Part 2. JAMA 2002;288(15):1909–14.

24. American Academy of Pediatrics Medical Home Initiatives for Children With Special Needs Project Advisory C. Policy statement: organizational principles to guide and define the child health care system and/or improve the health of all children. Pediatrics 2004;113(Suppl 5):1545–7.

25. Wagner EH, Austin BT, Von Korff M. Organizing care for patients with chronic illness. Milbank Q 1996;74(4):511–44.

26. Glasgow RE, Orleans CT, Wagner EH. Does the chronic care model serve also as a template for improving prevention? Milbank Q 2001;79(4):579–612, iv–v.

27. Barr MS. The need to test the patient-centered medical home. JAMA 2008; 300(7):834–5.

28. Nutting PA, Miller WL, Crabtree BF, et al. Initial lessons from the first national demonstration project on practice transformation to a patient-centered medical home. Ann Fam Med 2009;7(3):254–60.

29. Grumbach K, Bodenheimer T, Grundy P. The Outcomes of Implementing Patient-Centered Medical Home Interventions: a Review of the Evidence on Quality, Access and Costs from Recent Prospective Evaluation Studies, August 2009. Washington, DC: Patient-Centered Primary Care Collaborative; 2009.

30. Langley GJ, Nolan KM, Nolan TW, et al, editors. The improvement guide: a practical approach to enhancing organizational performance. San Francisco (CA): Jossey-Bass; 1996.

31. Reid RJ, Coleman K, Johnson EA, et al. The Group Health Medical Home at year two: cost savings, higher patient satisfaction, and less burnout for providers. Health Aff (Millwood) 2010;29(5):835–43.

32. Gilfillan RJ, Tomcavage J, Rosenthal MB, et al. Value and the medical home: effects of transformed primary care. Am J Manag Care 2010;16(8):607–14.

33. Reinertsen JL. Physicians as leaders in the improvement of health care systems. Ann Intern Med 1998;128(10):833–8.

34. Wang MC, Hyun JK, Harrison M, et al. Redesigning health systems for quality: lessons from emerging practices. Jt Comm J Qual Patient Saf 2006;32(11): 599–611.

35. Taylor HA, Greene BR, Filerman GL. A conceptual model for transformational clinical leadership within primary care group practice. J Ambul Care Manage 2010;33(2):97–107.

36. Reinertsen JL, Bisognano M, Pugh MD. Seven leadership leverage points for organization-level improvement in health care. 2nd edition. IHI Innovation Series white paper. Cambridge (MA): Institute for Healthcare Improvement; 2008.

37. Plsek PE, Greenhalgh T. Complexity science: the challenge of complexity in health care. BMJ 2001;323(7313):625–8.

38. Shortell SM, Gillies R, Siddique J, et al. Improving chronic illness care: a longitudinal cohort analysis of large physician organizations. Med Care 2009;47(9):932–9.

39. Going Lean in Health Care. IHI Innovation Series white paper. Cambridge (MA): Institute for Healthcare Improvement; 2005.

40. Deckard GJ, Borkowski N, Diaz D, et al. Improving timeliness and efficiency in the referral process for safety net providers: application of the Lean Six Sigma methodology. J Ambul Care Manage 2010;33(2):124–30.

41. Vest JR, Gamm LD. A critical review of the research literature on Six Sigma, Lean and StuderGroup's Hardwiring Excellence in the United States: the need to demonstrate and communicate the effectiveness of transformation strategies in healthcare. Implement Sci 2009;4:35.

42. Jamtvedt G, Young JM, Kristoffersen DT, et al. Audit and feedback: effects on professional practice and health care outcomes (2003). Cochrane Database Syst Rev 2003;3:CD000259.

43. National Voluntary Consensus Standards for Ambulatory Care - Reports: National Quality Forum. Available at: http://www.qualityforum.org/publications/reports/ambulatory_care.asp. Accessed January 2007.

44. Landon BE, Normand SL. Performance measurement in the small office practice: challenges and potential solutions. Ann Intern Med 2008;148(5):353–7.

45. Werner RM, Greenfield S, Fung C, et al. Measuring quality of care in patients with multiple clinical conditions: summary of a conference conducted by the Society of General Internal Medicine. J Gen Intern Med 2007;22(8):1206–11.
46. Office of the National Coordinator for Health Information Technology, Department of Health Human Services. Health information technology: initial set of standards, implementation specifications, and certification criteria for electronic health record technology. Final rule. Fed Regist 2010;75(144):44589–654.
47. Miller RH, Sim I. Physicians' use of electronic medical records: barriers and solutions. Health Aff (Millwood) 2004;23(2):116–26.
48. Starfield B, editor. Primary care: concept, evaluation, and policy. New York: Oxford University; 1992.
49. Marx R, Drennan MJ, Johnson EC, et al. Creating a medical home in the San Francisco department of public health: establishing patient panels. J Public Health Manag Pract 2009;15(4):337–44.
50. Murray M, Davies M, Boushon B. Panel size: how many patients can one doctor manage? Fam Pract Manag 2007;14(4):44–51.
51. Reid RJ, Fishman PA, Yu O, et al. Patient-centered medical home demonstration: a prospective, quasi-experimental, before and after evaluation. Am J Manag Care 2009;15(9):e71–87.
52. Coleman K, Reid RJ, Johnson E, et al. Implications of reassigning patients for the medical home: a case study. Ann Fam Med 2010;8(6):493–8.
53. Cabana MD, Jee SH. Does continuity of care improve patient outcomes? J Fam Pract 2004;53(12):974–80.
54. Saultz JW, Lochner J. Interpersonal continuity of care and care outcomes: a critical review. Ann Fam Med 2005;3(2):159–66.
55. Shojania KG, Ranji SR, McDonald KM, et al. Effects of quality improvement strategies for type 2 diabetes on glycemic control: a meta-regression analysis. JAMA 2006;296(4):427–40.
56. Walsh JM, McDonald KM, Shojania KG, et al. Quality improvement strategies for hypertension management: a systematic review. Med Care 2006;44(7):646–57.
57. Gilbody S, Bower P, Fletcher J, et al. Collaborative care for depression: a cumulative meta-analysis and review of longer-term outcomes. Arch Intern Med 2006; 166(21):2314–21.
58. Ostbye T, Yarnall KS, Krause KM, et al. Is there time for management of patients with chronic diseases in primary care? Ann Fam Med 2005;3(3):209–14.
59. Wagner EH. The role of patient care teams in chronic disease management. BMJ 2000;320(7234):569–72.
60. Bosch M, Faber MJ, Cruijsberg J, et al. Review article: Effectiveness of patient care teams and the role of clinical expertise and coordination: a literature review. Med Care Res Rev 2009;66(Suppl 6):5S–35S.
61. Turner D, Tarrant C, Windridge K, et al. Do patients value continuity of care in general practice? An investigation using stated preference discrete choice experiments. J Health Serv Res Policy 2007;12(3):132–7.
62. Fan VS, Burman M, McDonell MB, et al. Continuity of care and other determinants of patient satisfaction with primary care. J Gen Intern Med 2005;20(3):226–33.
63. Haggerty JL, Reid RJ, Freeman GK, et al. Continuity of care: a multidisciplinary review. BMJ 2003;327(7425):1219–21.
64. Guthrie B, Saultz JW, Freeman GK, et al. Continuity of care matters. BMJ 2008; 337:a867.
65. Starfield B, Horder J. Interpersonal continuity: old and new perspectives. Br J Gen Pract 2007;57(540):527–9.

66. Rodriguez HP, Rogers WH, Marshall RE, et al. Multidisciplinary primary care teams: effects on the quality of clinician-patient interactions and organizational features of care. Med Care 2007;45(1):19–27.

67. Bodenheimer T, Laing BY. The teamlet model of primary care. Ann Fam Med 2007;5(5):457–61.

68. Coleman K, Mattke S, Perrault PJ, et al. Untangling practice redesign from disease management: how do we best care for the chronically ill? Annu Rev Public Health 2009;30:385–408.

69. Institute of Medicine. Crossing the quality chasm: a new health system for the 21st century. Washington, DC: National Academy Press; 2001.

70. Bodenheimer T. Planned visits to help patients self-manage chronic conditions. Am Fam Physician 2005;72(8):1454–6.

71. Sadur CN, Moline N, Costa M, et al. Diabetes management in a health maintenance organization. Efficacy of care management using cluster visits. Diabetes Care 1999;22(12):2011–7.

72. Davis AM, Sawyer DR, Vinci LM. The potential of group visits in diabetes care. Clin Diabetes 2008;26:58–62.

73. Boyd CM, Reider L, Frey K, et al. The effects of guided care on the perceived quality of health care for multi-morbid older persons: 18-month outcomes from a cluster-randomized controlled trial. J Gen Intern Med 2010;25(3): 235–42.

74. Katon WJ, Lin EH, Von Korff M, et al. Collaborative care for patients with depression and chronic illnesses. N Engl J Med 2010;363(27):2611–20.

75. Shojania KG, Jennings A, Mayhew A, et al. The effects of on-screen, point of care computer reminders on processes and outcomes of care. Cochrane Database Syst Rev 2009;3:CD001096.

76. Starfield B, Lemke KW, Bernhardt T, et al. Comorbidity: implications for the importance of primary care in 'case' management. Ann Fam Med 2003;1(1):8–14.

77. Von Korff M, Gruman J, Schaefer J, et al. Collaborative management of chronic illness. Ann Intern Med 1997;127(12):1097–102.

78. Epstein RM, Fiscella K, Lesser CS, et al. Why the nation needs a policy push on patient-centered health care. Health Aff (Millwood) 2010;29(8):1489–95.

79. Levinson W, Lesser CS, Epstein RM. Developing physician communication skills for patient-centered care. Health Aff (Millwood) 2010;29(7):1310–8.

80. O'Connor AM, Bennett CL, Stacey D, et al. Decision aids for people facing health treatment or screening decisions. Cochrane Database Syst Rev 2009; 3:CD001431.

81. Bodenheimer T, MacGregor K, Sharifi C, et al. Helping patients manage their chronic conditions. California Health Care Foundation; 2005.

82. Paasche-Orlow MK, Parker RM, Gazmararian JA, et al. The prevalence of limited health literacy. J Gen Intern Med 2005;20(2):175–84.

83. National Research Council. Front matter. Health literacy: A prescription to end confusion. Washington, DC: The National Academies Press; 2004.

84. Marcus EN. The silent epidemic–the health effects of illiteracy. N Engl J Med 2006;355(4):339–41.

85. Schillinger D, Piette J, Grumbach K, et al. Closing the loop: physician communication with diabetic patients who have low health literacy. Arch Intern Med 2003;163(1):83–90.

86. Norris SL, Lau J, Smith SJ, et al. Self-management education for adults with type 2 diabetes: a meta-analysis of the effect on glycemic control. Diabetes Care 2002;25(7):1159–71.

87. Chodosh J, Morton SC, Mojica W, et al. Meta-analysis: chronic disease self-management programs for older adults. Ann Intern Med 2005;143(6):427–38.

88. Lorig KR, Holman H. Self-management education: history, definition, outcomes, and mechanisms. Ann Behav Med 2003;26(1):1–7.

89. Gibson PG, Powell H, Coughlan J, et al. Self-management education and regular practitioner review for adults with asthma. Cochrane Database Syst Rev 2007;1:CD001117.

90. Bodenheimer T, Lorig K, Holman H, et al. Patient self-management of chronic disease in primary care. JAMA 2002;288(19):2469–75.

91. Bennett HD, Coleman EA, Parry C, et al. Health coaching for patients with chronic illness. Fam Pract Manag 2010;17(5):24–9.

92. Browne K, Roseman D, Shaller D, et al. Analysis & commentary. Measuring patient experience as a strategy for improving primary care. Health Aff (Millwood) 2010;29(5):921–5.

93. Fremont AM, Cleary PD, Hargraves JL, et al. Patient-centered processes of care and long-term outcomes of myocardial infarction. J Gen Intern Med 2001; 16(12):800–8.

94. Keating NL, Green DC, Kao AC, et al. How are patients' specific ambulatory care experiences related to trust, satisfaction, and considering changing physicians? J Gen Intern Med 2002;17(1):29–39.

95. Hickson GB, Clayton EW, Githens PB, et al. Factors that prompted families to file medical malpractice claims following perinatal injuries. JAMA 1992;267(10): 1359–63.

96. Wilson IB, Rogers WH, Chang H, et al. Cost-related skipping of medications and other treatments among Medicare beneficiaries between 1998 and 2000. Results of a national study. J Gen Intern Med 2005;20(8):715–20.

97. Schoen C, Osborn R, How SK, et al. In chronic condition: experiences of patients with complex health care needs, in eight countries, 2008. Health Aff (Millwood) 2009;28(1):w1–16.

98. Schoen C, Osborn R, Doty MM, et al. A survey of primary care physicians in eleven countries, 2009: perspectives on care, costs, and experiences. Health Aff (Millwood) 2009;28(6):w1171–83.

99. Bindman AB, Grumbach K, Osmond D, et al. Preventable hospitalizations and access to health care. JAMA 1995;274(4):305–11.

100. O'Connell JM, Stanley JL, Malakar CL. Satisfaction and patient outcomes of a telephone-based nurse triage service. Manag Care 2001;10(7):55–6, 59–60, 65.

101. Leibowitz R, Day S, Dunt D. A systematic review of the effect of different models of after-hours primary medical care services on clinical outcome, medical workload, and patient and GP satisfaction. Fam Pract 2003;20(3):311–7.

102. Belman S, Chandramouli V, Schmitt BD, et al. An assessment of pediatric after-hours telephone care: a 1-year experience. Arch Pediatr Adolesc Med 2005; 159(2):145–9.

103. Huibers L, Giesen P, Wensing M, et al. Out-of-hours care in western countries: assessment of different organizational models. BMC Health Serv Res 2009;9:105.

104. van Uden CJ, Winkens RA, Wesseling G, et al. The impact of a primary care physician cooperative on the caseload of an emergency department: the Maastricht integrated out-of-hours service. J Gen Intern Med 2005;20(7):612–7.

105. Murray M, Berwick DM. Advanced access: reducing waiting and delays in primary care. JAMA 2003;289(8):1035–40.

106. Rose KD, Ross JS, Horwitz LI. Advanced access scheduling outcomes: a systematic review. Arch Intern Med 2011;171(13):1150–9.

107. Stuber J, Bradley E. Barriers to Medicaid enrollment: who is at risk? Am J Public Health 2005;95(2):292–8.
108. Haley J, Kenney G. Low-income uninsured children with special health care needs: why aren't they enrolled in public health insurance programs? Pediatrics 2007;119(1):60–8.
109. Bodenheimer T. Coordinating care: a major (unreimbursed) task of primary care. Ann Intern Med 2007;147(10):730–1.
110. Mehrotra A, Forrest CB, Lin CY. Dropping the baton: specialty referrals in the United States. Milbank Q 2011;89(1):39–68.
111. O'Malley AS, Cunningham PJ. Patient experiences with coordination of care: the benefit of continuity and primary care physician as referral source. J Gen Intern Med 2009;24(2):170–7.
112. Jencks SF, Williams MV, Coleman EA. Rehospitalizations among patients in the Medicare fee-for-service program. N Engl J Med 2009;360(14):1418–28.
113. Roy CL, Kachalia A, Woolf S, et al. Hospital readmissions: physician awareness and communication practices. J Gen Intern Med 2009;24(3):374–80.
114. O'Malley AS, Tynan A, Cohen GR, et al. Coordination of care by primary care practices: strategies, lessons and implications. Res Briefs 2009;(12):1–16.
115. Coleman EA, Berenson RA. Lost in transition: challenges and opportunities for improving the quality of transitional care. Ann Intern Med 2004;141(7):533–6.
116. Parrish MM, O'Malley K, Adams RI, et al. Implementation of the care transitions intervention: sustainability and lessons learned. Prof Case Manag 2009;14(6):282–93 [quiz: 294–5].
117. Naylor MD. Transitional care for older adults: a cost-effective model. LDI Issue Brief 2004;9(6):1–4.
118. Phillips CO, Wright SM, Kern DE, et al. Comprehensive discharge planning with postdischarge support for older patients with congestive heart failure: a meta-analysis. JAMA 2004;291(11):1358–67.
119. Misky GJ, Wald HL, Coleman EA. Post-hospitalization transitions: examining the effects of timing of primary care provider follow-up. J Hosp Med 2010;5(7):392–7.
120. Grimes GC, Reis MD, Budati G, et al. Patient preferences and physician practices for laboratory test results notification. J Am Board Fam Med 2009;35:670–6.
121. Nutting PA, Crabtree BF, Miller WL, et al. Transforming physician practices to patient-centered medical homes: lessons from the national demonstration project. Health Aff (Millwood) 2011;30(3):439–45.
122. Patient-centered Medical Home. Available at: http://www.ncqa.org/tabid/631/Default.aspx. Accessed April 8, 2012.

A "How To" Guide to Creating a Patient-Centered Medical Home

George Valko, MD[a],*, Richard C. Wender, MD[b],
Michele Q. Zawora, MD[c]

KEYWORDS

- Patient-centered medical home • PCMH • NCQA-certified PCMH
- Practice transformation • Primary care medical home • PCMH recognition

KEY POINTS

- Care provided in the patient-centered medical home (PCMH) has the potential to result in better health outcomes at lower cost.
- Primary care clinicians are feeling growing pressure to transform their practices and to be formally recognized as a PCMH by the National Committee for Quality Assurance or a comparable certifying organization.
- An ongoing process is developing the potential to function as a PCMH, earning formal recognition, and implementing a system of continuous quality improvement to enable the establishment of a mature, sustainable PCMH.

The concept of the patient-centered medical home (PCMH) has been widely embraced as a foundation for the transformation of health care delivery.[1] The central role for the PCMH emerges from the growing body of data demonstrating that systems of care based on a strong foundation of primary care outperform systems of care based on specialty practices.[2,3] Recent evaluations of PCMH pilots validate the initial hypothesis that care provided in the PCMH has the potential to result in better health outcomes at lower cost.[4] As the PCMH model gains momentum, primary care clinicians are feeling growing pressure to transform their practices, and to be formally recognized as a PCMH by the National Committee for Quality Assurance (NCQA) or a comparable certifying organization. However, earning recognition or certification as a PCMH can be a daunting task.

The authors have nothing to disclose.
[a] Department of Family and Community Medicine, Jefferson Medical College, Thomas Jefferson University, 833 Chestnut Street, Suite 301, Philadelphia, PA 19107, USA; [b] Department of Family and Community Medicine, Jefferson Medical College, Thomas Jefferson University, 1015 Walnut Street, Suite 401, Philadelphia, PA 19107, USA; [c] Department of Family and Community Medicine, Jefferson Family Medicine Associates, Jefferson Medical College, Thomas Jefferson University, 833 Chestnut Street, Suite 301, Philadelphia, PA 19107, USA
* Corresponding author.
E-mail address: George.valko@jefferson.edu

Prim Care Clin Office Pract 39 (2012) 261–280
doi:10.1016/j.pop.2012.03.003
0095-4543/12/$ – see front matter © 2012 Elsevier Inc. All rights reserved.

This article discusses how a practice can lay the groundwork to become a PCMH from earning broad support within the practice, to creating teams and instituting new systems of care, to the application and recognition process, and finally to complete care transformation. The process of developing the potential to function as a PCMH, earning formal recognition, and finally ingraining a system of continuous quality improvement to enable the establishment of a mature, sustainable PCMH is discussed. References are provided to demonstrate successful implementation of each aspect of the PCMH model.

WHAT IS A PATIENT-CENTERED MEDICAL HOME?

The PCMH is a team-based approach to providing comprehensive primary care, involving multiple levels of medical providers, which may include medical assistants, nurses, physicians, physician extenders, social workers, pharmacists, and behavioral health providers. The PCMH facilitates and relies on partnerships between individual patients, their personal physicians, the health care team and, when appropriate, the patient's family.

According to the Agency for Healthcare Research and Quality (AHRQ), the medical home model holds promise as a way to improve health care in America by transforming how primary care is organized and delivered.[5] The medical home is not simply a place, but a model of health care that is designed to reliably and reproducibly implement the core functions of primary health care.

The medical home concept was first introduced in 1967 by the American Academy of Pediatrics (AAP) as the way to keep medical records in a central location for all medical specialists' visits.[6] The concept was expanded in 2002 by the AAP to include principles that all care be accessible, continuous, comprehensive, family centered, coordinated, compassionate, and culturally effective.[7]

In 2004, following a comprehensive strategic planning process called the Future of Family Medicine, the American Academy of Family Physicians (AAFP) released its own medical home model to improve patient care.[8] In 2006, the American College of Physicians (ACP) published and promoted the concept of the "advanced medical home."[9] The American Academy of Pediatrics (AAP), AAFP, and ACP joined with the American Osteopathic Association (AOA) to develop the Joint Principles of the Patient-Centered Medical Home. In 2007 these 4 organizations, representing approximately 333,000 physicians, released these joint principles to describe the characteristics of the PCMH[10]: These principles are listed in **Table 1**.

Several alternative names have been proposed as potential substitutes for the term PCMH, including terms such as "advanced primary care" and "comprehensive primary care." Although these alternative names do provide useful descriptors of the PCMH concept and may be used interchangeably, the term PCMH has been widely embraced by government, insurers, employers, and health care agencies.[11] The complementary concepts, such as the "medical neighborhood," have also been introduced to encompass a broader reconception of health care delivery, but PCMH remains the preferred term to describe the redesign of primary care practices to improve population health at a more affordable price.[12]

WHY SHOULD A PRACTICE BECOME A PCMH?

This question is often posited to both stimulate dialogue within a practice contemplating change and as a legitimate query: is the effort to become a PCMH worth the reward? Within practices, some individuals are likely to cite well-motivated reasons to not pursue PCMH transformation: change of any kind is very demanding; the

Table 1
Joint principles of a patient-centered medical home (PCMH)

Principle	Description	Example, Benefits
Personal physician	Each patient has an ongoing relationship with a personal physician trained to provide first contact, continuous and comprehensive care	Benefit of trusting, collaborative relationship with own physician
Physician-directed medical practice	Personal physician leads an interdisciplinary team of individuals responsible for the ongoing care of the patient	Comprehensive care is a team effort; involving all levels of medical professionals as physician extenders
Whole person orientation	Personal physician is responsible for providing all of the patient's health care needs or taking responsibility for appropriately arranging care with other qualified professionals	All stages of life included, acute care, chronic care, preventive services, end of life care
Care is coordinated and/or integrated	Personal physician ensures care is coordinated across all elements of the health care system and patient's community. Care is facilitated by registries, information technology, health information exchange	Subspecialty care, hospitals, home health agencies, nursing homes
Quality and safety are hallmarks	Practice advocate for their patients to support the attainment of optimal, patient-centered outcomes.	Evidence-based medicine and clinical decision support tools Physicians accept accountability for CQI Patients actively participate in decision making Feedback sought to ensure patient needs are being met IT used to support optimal patient care, performance measurement, education, communication Practices undergo a voluntary recognition process to ensure they have the elements to provide patient centered care Patients and families participate in QI activities at the practice level

(continued on next page)

Table 1
(continued)

Principle	Description	Example, Benefits
Enhanced access to care	Practice seeks to create/implement options to improve access	Open access scheduling Expanded office hours New options for communication
Payment	Payment should appropriately recognize the added value of caring for patients in a PCMH	Values physician and team-based care management work that happens outside of face-to-face interactions Pays for services associated with coordination of care Supports adoption and use of HIT for quality improvement Supports provision of enhanced communication access through email and telephone Recognizes the value of physician work in remote monitoring of clinical data using technology Allows for separate fee-for-service payments for face-to-face visits Recognizes case-mix differences in patient population Allows physicians to share in savings from reduced hospitalizations Allows for additional payments for achieving measurable and continuous quality improvements

Abbreviations: CQI, continuous quality improvement; HIT, health information technology; IT, information technology; QI, quality improvement.
Adapted from American Academy of Family Physicians (AAFP), American Academy of Pediatrics (AAP), American College of Physicians (ACP), American Osteopathic Association (AOA). Joint principles of the patient-centered medical home. 2007. Available at: http://www.acponline.org/pressroom/pcmh.htm.

practice is already thriving so there is no need to improve it; patients are already well cared for; there is no time to undertake a major overhaul of the practice; human and financial resources are far too scant to support such a sweeping change.

In light of these commonly held spoken, and often unspoken, beliefs, practice leaders will often confront the need to "sell" the PCMH concept to their coworkers and external stakeholders. The fundamental argument derives from the unquestioned fact that our current health care delivery and payment system is unsustainable. New reimbursement models based on delivery and measurement of high-quality care are rapidly emerging. Virtually every practice needs to be ascertaining how to improve the care it is delivering to all of its enrolled patients, not only for the benefit of the population it serves, but to maximize reimbursement for its very survival. As noted previously, the benefits of transforming a practice into a PCMH have been well documented.[4] Many practices can claim that they are a PCMH; however, formal recognition by the NCQA, or similar a organization, is required to certify that the practice has the structure in place to function as a true PCMH.

WHY DOES SEEKING CERTIFICATION FOR YOUR PCMH MATTER?

Many practices have made the transformation and function as a PCMH; however, receiving certification from a national agency has additional benefits and implications.

PCMHs Improve Care and Efficiency and Reduce Costs

Numerous studies have demonstrated that medical homes improve care and access, and reduce unnecessary medical costs. A few studies also cited by the Patient-Centered Primary Care Collaborative (PCPCC) can be found in **Table 2**.[13–17]

PCMHs Receive Enhanced Payments

Because of improved care and lower cost, insurance companies are starting to increase payments for PCMH. Independence Blue Cross (IBC) in Philadelphia

Table 2	
PCMHs improve care, efficiency, and access, and reduce cost	
Health System	**Specific Findings**
Geisinger, Pennsylvania	1. 14% reduction in hospital admissions and "trend toward a 9% reduction in medical costs" 2. Statistically significant improvement in quality of preventive, coronary artery disease and diabetes care
Group Health Cooperative, Puget Sound	1. 29% reduction in ER visits and 11% reduction in ambulatory sensitive care admissions 2. 4% increase in patients achieving target levels on HEDIS quality measures
Genessee Health Plan, Michigan	1. 50% reduction in ER visits and 15% reduction in hospitalizations 2. 137% increase in mammogram screening rates 3. 36% reduction in smoking
Health Partners Medical Group, Minnesota	1. 39% reduction in ER visits and 24% reduction in hospitalizations 2. 129% increase in patients receiving optimal diabetes care 3. 48% increase in patients receiving optimal heart disease care

Abbreviations: ER, emergency room; HEDIS, Healthcare Effectiveness Data Information Set.

increased its per-member per-month payments to any of its primary care practices for receiving NCQA PCMH certification. As of spring of 2011, IBC boasts more than 100 primary care practices with more than 1000 physicians now qualifying for such a bonus.[18]

Other insurance companies are following this lead by providing monetary recognition as more and more states take the lead in helping primary care practices become PCMHs.

Many regions have embarked on PCMH pilot programs that link enhanced payment to implementation of some elements of the medical home.[4,13,19]

PCMHs are Good for Business

Work derived from Barbara Starfield and from the Dartmouth Atlas Project has proved that regions with a high concentration of primary care provide higher quality and more affordable health care, observations that have been validated by the PCMH experiments described.[2,3,20] The PCPCC has been the leader in encouraging organizations to develop businesses in areas where there is a high concentration of primary care to help control their health care costs and provide quality care.

Publications such as *The Patient-Centered Medical Home—A Purchaser Guide* helps businesses encourage their health care plans to support PCMH development.[13] *Patient Centered Medical Home: Performance Metrics for Employers* is a resource of health and productivity metrics that can be used by employers and their supplier partners to gain a comprehensive understanding of the value of health, and establish benchmarks to compare organizations' health and productivity with those of their peers, based on outcomes integral to the PCMH model of care. It includes a description of metric categories used by employers, a business-oriented timeline for understanding those metrics, and 8 detailed case studies that demonstrate the effective use of the medical home in benefit design.[19]

Health Care Reform, PCMH, and Accountable Care Organizations

The reform of the US health care system includes both insurance reform and delivery reform. Delivery reform includes new organizational structures such as accountable care organizations (ACOs), and PCMH's payment system reform includes pay for performance, shared savings models, and other quality incentives; PCMH is a vital route to thriving within new payment models.[21]

Prestige

Having PCMH certification is quickly becoming an important "seal of approval" as more and more institutions are recognizing the importance of PCMH. Practices may proudly display the NCQA seal of a Recognized Physician Practice Connection Patient-Centered Medical Home, and advertise the recognition.

Already Doing the Work

Many primary care practices already meet many of the criteria to be recognized as a PCMH. Such work is that which primary care practices do all the time, and reflects fundamental values of most primary care clinicians. However, doing the work to become formally recognized as a PCMH not only leads to changes that benefit the patients, practice, and staff, but also makes that practice more valuable in the eyes of payors and others. PCMH status will be recognized by affiliated hospitals that are looking for cornerstones of quality care to take the lead in new payment models, such as ACOs.

Education of Residents and Students

Practice sites that are participating in the education of residents and students should earn PCMH certification and should tackle the critical challenge of teaching the next generation of health professionals to function in interprofessional teams.[22] Government agency grants are available to help stimulate these educational endeavors.

BECOMING A PCMH: WHERE TO START?

As with any major undertaking, the process of transforming a practice must go through a series of critical steps: an idea must be proposed and must receive the support of leadership, a transformation plan must be designed and executed, priorities must be set, time must be allotted to the complex process of change, and both human and financial resources must be made available.

Leadership

Many levels of leaders are needed to create a PCMH but first and foremost, the head of a practice or organization, whether it is a Chair, managing partner, or administrator, must be fully engaged and set the tone and course, usually in the face of pushback. Other leaders include those who will organize teams for the day-to-day work: ensuring the practice meets recognition requirements and submitting the application, running quality improvement, executing Plan, Do, Study, Act (PDSA) cycles, retraining staff, performing data collection and analysis, troubleshooting, and cheerleading. The most important quality of these leaders is that they all share the vision of what a practice can and should be.

Time

Transformation takes time. Working groups need time to meet on a regular basis to think, plan, and work toward certification as a PCMH. Redesigning the practice to become a true medical home requires sustained commitment of time, a factor that cannot be emphasized enough. If becoming a PCMH is a priority it must be treated as such; this cannot be done on an ad hoc basis. The application process alone will take at least 6 months and each member can expect to put in easily 100 hours to complete the application process. For the practice redesign team, daily effort will be perpetually required. Many demonstration projects have shown this to be true: a 2-year or even a 3-year project may not allow enough time to change culture or ingrained habits, changes that must occur to improve a practice.[23]

Persistence

Frustration with complex change is inevitable, and change fatigue is a constant threat to progress. Everyone expects immediate results that most likely will not happen. Rather, progress will be slow and methodical, especially if a great deal of change is needed. Time should be dedicated to helping all members of the team understand the change process. Time should also be spent on celebrating each successful small improvement; this is a journey, not a day trip.

Resources

Transformation requires resources. Money may be needed to hire additional staff such as medical assistants, nurses, a case manager, and/or a quality assurance specialist. Investment in essential health information technology (HIT) and hardware is almost inevitably needed.

Loss of clinical income to permit individuals time to work on creating a PCMH is virtually always required. Unfortunately for most practices not involved in a demonstration project or grant, upfront funding is rarely present—yet! As in many quality incentive payment programs, increased revenue comes after making the changes and showing improvements in care. As more payors recognize the improved quality of care and decreased costs resulting from creating PCMH, more upfront investment should become the rule rather than the exception.

As with anything in life that is important, the work is hard but worth the effort. Participants are on a journey to improve their patients' lives as well as their own. The PCMH is the future of health care, and the team must take the lead.

A TEAM APPROACH

After the decision to become a PCMH has been made, the first step is to form a management team to guide strategy, planning, and execution.

The management team, at least for the strategic meetings, should involve the highest leadership available. This leader would be the Department Chair for an academic medical center, who may also want to keep the Dean and others updated. In other organizations, it should include those who are ultimately involved with the finances of the practice. Leaders from many aspects of the health care enterprise are recognizing the value of creating PCMHs and may be willing to provide upfront support for change. Creating more medical homes will ultimately benefit the whole organization, providing greater prestige as well as cost savings and quality care reimbursement.

The management team must include the people in the practice that know the practice well, such as the chief administrator, medical director, and practice and/or operations manager. It may include key nursing personnel and clinicians.

The management team must decide on goals and how to meet those goals, 2 of which are:

- PCMH recognition/certification
- Practice redesign and quality improvement.

Practice size and organization have a major impact on the process of change. An academic medical center with multiple residency programs, a community hospital–based primary care residency without many other residencies, a multigroup practice, or a 1- or 2-doctor practice will obviously have different resources and will confront different problems and issues. All, however, will have many challenges in common, including the most important: each must spend the time and do the work to be successful. Moreover, no matter what size a practice, outside help is virtually always needed, with support for HIT representing a clear priority.

WORKING GROUPS

The management team will also be involved with creating the working groups that will do the actual work of the certification and the transformation processes. It is crucial that both of these working groups must have time available to do their important work.

Certifying Working Group

For the certification working group (CWG), membership should be limited to only a few individuals, but it is absolutely necessary that it includes personnel who know all aspects of the practice and patients. The director of operations and medical director, or their equivalents, usually need to spearhead this work. An electronic medical record

(EMR) or practice management system superuser, as well as a "detail" person (ie, one who is good at doing the actual work of the application), are often vital members of this team. Others can be brought in as needed, such as the HIT or legal personnel, but the core members will need to do the "heavy lifting."

Practice Redesign Working Group

A larger number of individuals can and should be part of the practice redesign working group (RWG), the group that actually does the work of the PCMH. The RWG should be headed by the medical director and director of operations who will do double duty with the CWG. The personnel needed should include leaders in registration, billing, and phone reception, as well as selected nurses, medical assistants, medical recorders, and other clinical personnel. Activist clinicians, including postgraduate year 2 (PGY2) and PGY3 residents (in a residency practice) and HIT superusers, are a must. Again, ad hoc personnel, such as HIT support, can be brought in as needed.

The RWG must accept the commitment to keep abreast of literature and possibly be required to publish and/or present its work at various meetings. Defined regular meeting time, usually weekly, is required.

Focused Work Groups

Smaller groups may be spawned during the ensuing years as improvements are made in the practice. Implementing group visits or tackling a new quality improvement program often require dedicated groups. As improvements in the practice are realized, others may want to offer ideas or become more directly involved. This development is natural as the PCMH matures, and should be encouraged. The entire practice should be involved on some level.

Small practices face unique challenges, and evidence indicates that fewer small practices are engaging in broad practice change, such as introducing electronic records. Several strategies may be particularly important for the 1- or 2-clinician practice. Finding external partners, consultants, and collaborators will usually be needed. Change may need to proceed one step at a time. Finding an external entity such as an insurer, business, group practice, or hospital that is willing to help support change can substantially facilitate real change. Ultimately, any practice that is transforming must follow the same process, providing leadership, time, and resources.

WORKSPACE

Although not a necessity, dedicating a central space to serve as headquarters for transformation and certification efforts is a wise strategy. Necessary materials for the certification process, including application instructions, policies and procedure manuals, and screenshot downloads can be generated and stored in this space. Wall calendars with timelines that provide a visual documentation of needs and progress should be posted here. This headquarters will facilitate steps in this complex process. Careful attention must be given to the Health Insurance Portability and Accountability Act (HIPAA) and Health Information Technology for Economic and Clinical Health (HITECH) protected health information policies to ensure that the headquarters provides adequate protection, including locking the room. In addition, password-protected and/or encrypted computers and USB storage devices are a necessary requirement. A secure, shared drive, if available, makes file sharing safer, easier, and more convenient.

CERTIFYING BODY

Early in the transformation process, the management team will need to select a PCMH recognition or certification program to pursue. Certification is one way that practices can demonstrate that they have met standards for increased access to care, including coordinated and patient-centered care. Certification may result in increased reimbursement from payors, as well as other positive outcomes.

What Criteria Should be Selected to Choose a Certifying Organization?

Although practices may wish to consider ease of application and fit with practice strengths, frankly the chief consideration should be whether a practice payor recognizes a particular recognition program. For example, the NCQA was the first national organization to institute a PCMH recognition program, and several payors and organizations rely on the NCQA to conduct practice evaluation. Checking with insurers in the area to determine which organization they recognize must be done. **Box 1** shows a list of organizations currently providing PCMH certification.

Pay attention to prices/fees and timelines; in many cases, the certifying body will not disclose when things are due or when they are complete.

In February 2011 the 4 primary care physician societies, the AAFP, AAP, ACP, and AOA, provided the guidelines for PCMH recognition and accreditation programs. To help inform practices as to how the competing national programs meet the guidelines, the Medical Group Management Association (MGMA) developed an assessment tool. This document provides a neutral and transparent review of the alternative national programs. If an organization is interested in becoming a PCMH, this tool will help narrow one's assessment of the various programs and focus on the most important elements. This free tool can be found at the MGMA Web site.[24]

STEPS TO PCMH CERTIFICATION

The CWG should start on the application process as soon as possible. It is not necessary to reinvent the wheel; many practices and organizations have gone through the recognition process and have created tools to help organize data or create policies. For example, the PCPCC, ACP Medical Home Builder, Improving Performance in Practice (IPIP), the NCQA workbook, and the Colorado Collaborative workbook are valuable tools to help the practice get started and keep the progress moving.[25] In addition, many state and national PCMH collaboratives are under way. If dollars are available, practice coaches and consultants can be hired to help practices navigate their application.

Box 1
Organizations providing PCMH certification

1. The Accreditation Association for Ambulatory Health Care: 2011 Medical Home Standards

2. The Joint Commission: Primary Care Medical Home 2011 Standards and Elements of Performance (Available July 2011)

3. The National Committee for Quality Assurance: Patient-Centered Medical Home 2011 Standards

4. URAC: Patient Centered Health Care Home (PCHCH) Practice Achievement Version 1.0 (Available June 2011)

5. Blue Cross Blue Shield of Michigan has a program to designate more than 1000 physicians in its PCMH program

Specific steps are necessary to complete a recognition application. Because of its broad national reach, the NCQA application is used here as the template for discussion. This application assigns points to a set of criteria. Some of these are optional, but many are listed as "must haves." Paying attention to the must haves is vital, and reviewing these criteria first makes sense; one may have a tremendous all-around application, but if one misses out on the must haves, the application is negated.

The first item for the CWG to address is to create a timeline; being realistic makes sense, but sticking to the predefined deadlines is a fundamental commitment. An example of a personalized timeline can be found in **Fig. 1**.

The timeline allows the CWG to clearly track interim accomplishments and anticipate subsequent steps. The certification process begins by purchasing or downloading several copies of the certifying criteria and any application materials. Each member of the CWG must become totally familiar with the criteria and how the certifying body expects the practice to prove that the criteria are met.

When all CWG members are satisfied that they understand what is needed, each team member should be assigned a task for which they become the team expert. For example, someone may be assigned the task of creating screen shots of data, some may become expert on the submission process, and others may be assigned to create or update policies. Once the criteria are understood, the CWG must conduct a reasonably thorough practice assessment to determine which criteria are already being met and which need to be addressed. Some items may be met with minor modifications and others may need major practice overhaul. For example, practices that do not own an EMR may need to consider implementing one to attain a higher level of recognition. Practices that have an EMR need to pay attention to the HIT needs and recruit information technology (IT) support staff at the beginning of the process.

This process of taking stock of what a practice already performs well and what it needs to do to reach the application criteria is called a gap analysis; conducting this analysis is essentially a prerequisite to taking any further action. A CWG member is assigned to take the lead in analyzing items that need to be corrected. Close attention must be paid to the timelines: some items require that a policy, procedure, and/or data be in place and tracked for several months. Finding this out several months into the project can postpone the entire application process. An example of a gap-analysis form that one can create for the NCQA application is shown in **Table 3**.

Once the gap analysis has been completed, the CWG can proceed to address practice changes that must be implemented to achieve the target level of recognition. In fact, understanding levels of recognition and aiming for a specific level is the basis for further planning. If the practice will be satisfied in obtaining the lowest level of

Activity	June Week 1 2 3 4	July Week 1 2 3 4	Aug Week 1 2 3 4	Sept Week 1 2 3 4	Oct Week 1 2 3 4	Nov Week 1 2 3 4	Dec Week 1 2 3 4
Confirm practice guidelines							
Conduct application gap analysis							
Write and/or revise policies & procedures							
Gather neccesary data for application							
Patient Centered Medical Home standards 1-6							
Upload data to NCQA application							
Review application							
Payment and submission of application							

Fig. 1. Sample timeline for NCQA application. (*Data from* NCQA 2011 Application, available at: https://inetshop01.pub.ncqa.org/publications/product.asp?dept_id=2&pf_id=30002-150-11 and https://inetshop01.pub.ncqa.org/publications/deptCate.asp?dept_id=2&cateID=300&sort Order=796&mscssid=+300796. Accessed March 10, 2012.)

Table 3
Example of a gap analysis of a primary care office

PCMH Gap Analysis	Criteria Met	Criteria Partially Met	Criteria Not Met	Comments
Standard 1: Enhance Access and Continuity				
Element A: Access during office hours				
Factor 1. Providing same-day appointments	X			
Factor 2. Providing timely clinical advice by telephone during office hours	X			
Factor 3. Providing timely clinical advice by secure electronic during office hours			X	Will not meet
Factor 4. Documenting clinical advice in the medical record		X		Must improve
Element B: After-hours access		X		
Element C: Electronic access		X		
Element D: Continuity		X		
Element E: Medical home responsibilities		X		
Element F: Culturally and linguistically appropriate services (CLAS)		X		
Element G: The practice team		X		
Standard 2: Identify and Manage Patient Populations				

Data from NCQA 2011 Application, available at: https://inetshop01.pub.ncqa.org/publications/product.asp?dept_id=2&pf_id=30002-150-11 and https://inetshop01.pub.ncqa.org/publications/deptCate.asp?dept_id=2&cateID=300&sortOrder=796&mscssid=+300796. Accessed March 10, 2012.

recognition by making just minor improvements, then that plan should be adhered to. If the practice aims for the highest level that will require a lot of work, this must be planned for accordingly. Again, close attention is paid to the "must haves"; assessing the practice against these criteria is the easiest way to ascertain what level is likely to be attainable. **Table 4** shows the requirements for each level of NCQA recognition.

The NCQA application places high value on having policies and procedures in place to satisfy various criteria, but the application always requires practices to "show their work" and to prove that they are following the policy and adhering to the criteria. For example:

- The NCQA requires that the practice have all specified policies and procedures in place for 3 months before submitting an application for PCMH recognition.

Table 4		
Point requirements for each designation level according to NCQA regulations		
Recognition Level	**Points**	**Must-Pass Elements**
Level 1	35–59	6 of 6
Level 2	60–84	6 of 6
Level 3	85–100	6 of 6

Data from NCQA 2011 Application, available at: https://inetshop01.pub.ncqa.org/publications/product.asp?dept_id=2&pf_id=30002-150-11 and https://inetshop01.pub.ncqa.org/publications/deptCate.asp?dept_id=2&cateID=300&sortOrder=796&mscssid=+300796. Accessed March 10, 2012.

- Policies and procedures should be written for the benefit of staff and/or patients at the practice/organization.
- Make policies and procedures specific and measurable. For example, when describing timeframes for response to requests from patients, "immediately" is not a specified timeframe. Replace vague terms with exact numbers of minutes, hours, or days.

The certifying body can ask for more material and may even choose to audit the practice. If an audit uncovers discrepancies from what a practice states it is doing to what they are actually doing, the certifying body may even revoke a decision. **Box 2** lists reasons for which the NCQA may revoke a decision:

Essentially no practice meets every NCQA criteria at the perfect level. Perfection is not required, even for the highest level of recognition. Certain measures can be partially met for 50% credit. Concentrating on the "must haves" is the correct focus.

Carefully label and catalog all data and drafts, and back up your work. You should label any documentation with the Standard, Element, and Factor to which it belongs along with a statement for quick reference. For example, if you document that your practice provides same-day appointments for the 2011 NCQA application, the item should be labeled: *NCQA 2011 PCMH 1 A 1 (provide same-day appointments).* Start to upload data as soon as it is ready; as can be seen from the timeline, these tasks can

---

Box 2
Examples of reasons why NCQA may revoke a designation of PCMH

NCQA May Revoke a PCMH Decision If:

The practice submits false data

The practice misrepresents the credentials of any clinician

The practice misrepresents its PCMH status

Any of the practice's clinicians experiences suspension or revocation of professional licensure

The practice has been placed in receivership or rehabilitation and is being liquidated

State, federal, or other duly authorized regulatory or judicial action restricts or limits the practice's operations

NCQA identifies a significant threat to patient safety or care

Data from NCQA 2011 Application, available at: https://inetshop01.pub.ncqa.org/publications/product.asp?dept_id=2&pf_id=30002-150-11 and https://inetshop01.pub.ncqa.org/publications/deptCate.asp?dept_id=2&cateID=300&sortOrder=796&mscssid=+300796. Accessed March 10, 2012.

be done at the same time. This is hard, time-consuming work but it is worth it, as losing data can derail the entire endeavor. The NCQA and other certifying organizations will provide technical assistance. Do not be afraid to call for help. Take your time at the end for the group to review the application and make any final changes. Make sure all the fees are paid and do not be afraid to call for updates on your status.

PRACTICE REDESIGN

Although earning PCMH recognition is inherently important, recognition does not guarantee that the quality of care being provided is as good as it can be. Improving quality of care, patient experience, and staff satisfaction is the real work of the PCMH, and is far more difficult than the effort needed to become certified. Recognition shows that a practice has the proper systems and protocols in place to address a patient's needs above and beyond the usual way of conducting business. To become a true medical home—to have everyone practice at the top of his or her license and improve the patient quality of care—is more difficult because of the sheer amount of effort and energy involved. To move this needle takes leadership, time, and resources.

The RWG must work in tandem with the CWG throughout and beyond the application process. For small practices, where a few people must perform both functions, working in an iterative fashion to incrementally address care redesign as application sections are completed may be a realistic and sound approach. The RWG must spearhead efforts to redesign the practice and their work will be ongoing, lasting far beyond the certification process. Several programs and organizations can provide assistance with practice redesign, including the PCPCC, Institute for Healthcare Improvement (IHI), TransforMed, and private consultants. The Wagner Chronic Care model has served as the basis for practice redesign in several large learning collaboratives.[26–29]

Obviously, planning for and implementing changes needed to successfully attain PCMH recognition will catalyze practice change, but all successful medical home practices must nurture a culture that is receptive to constant reevaluation and change.

A key method to create change is to follow the PDSA model that is promoted by the IHI and other organizations.[30] A description of a PDSA model IS SHOWN IN **Box 3**. This model can be used to study and implement virtually any pilot into a practice. An example is included that can be implemented to ensure that all diabetic patients receive a yearly monofilament test. The details of the example are shown in italics.

Practice redesign demands constant engagement and education of the entire staff, and especially the physicians. Securing broad buy-in takes time but is critical to success. Everyone should be involved in the PDSA cycles and in how to improve the practice. Many often think of an office practice as having a front end of operations (registration, billing) and the back end (clinical office). A true PCMH functions as though there is no distinction; everyone is included and everyone has an integral role in patient care.

There is nothing without data collection. The old axiom that there is no movement without measurement is true. The most useful tool to support measurement of quality improvement efforts is a high-functioning EMR. IT support is crucial, and sponsoring organizations must accept quality measurement as a practice priority. If no EMR is available, stand-alone registries in which demographic and clinical data are entered are available to help with data collection and data mining. Examples and critiques of various EMRs, registries, and other health IT applications and vendors can be found in trade publications and specialty organizations.

Box 3
PDSA example

Plan:

1. Document the objective of the cycle: what is being improved?

   a. *Yearly monofilament examinations in diabetic patients*

2. State your predictions: what will be the result(s) if the improvement is effective?

   a. *All diabetic patients will have a yearly monofilament examination*

3. Document the initial plan

   a. Who will be doing the testing?

      i. *Medical assistants*

   b. What patients are being selected? (select a small subset)

      i. *All diabetic patients who arrive for a visit during the month will have a monofilament examination performed*

   c. Where will this be done?

      i. *In the examination room*

   d. When will the test occur: specific day or days?

      i. *Every day for 1 month*

   e. How and what will they do? Briefly state the change being implemented

      i. *All medical assistants will receive in-service training on the importance of diabetic foot examinations*

      ii. *All medical assistants will receive in-service training on how to properly perform the monofilament examination and document those results in the EMR*

      iii. *The medical assistants will perform the monofilament test when they room the patient. They will explain to the patient what they are doing, help the patient remove shoes and stockings, and document the results in real time for the clinician to review*

      iv. *A policy/procedure will be written to govern the above action and to be used as a standing order: medical assistants will perform monofilament testing on all diabetic patients and the clinician will review the documentation and attest that it was done*

Do:

1. Complete the test/test completed

   a. *Medical assistants will identify the patients and complete the test per policy/procedure*

2. Document any problems and/ or unexpected observations

   b. *Medical assistants and/or their supervisors will document any problems, including timing and work flow issues. For example: "I was unable to do the test because the clinician wanted to see the patient before I was able to do the monofilament examination"*

3. Begin to analyze your outcome data: essentially…what happened and /or how did the test flow?

   c. *The group will analyze the basic data (how many diabetic patients arrived, how many of those had monofilaments done?), as well as workflow and other issues that surfaced during the "Do" phase of the exercise.*

(continued on next page)

Box 3
(continued)

Study:

1. Complete the analysis of the test outcomes and data

2. Compare how things went: compare your predictions with the actual outcomes

3. Summarize learning

Act:

1. What changes will you make based on the outcomes of your first test of change?

   a. *For example, mandate that medical assistants complete their duties before clinicians see a patient and instruct all on that mandate.*

   b. *Start to refine patient population: do monofilament only on those diabetic patients who have not had one in the last year*

2. Develop/or revise the Plan for next cycle

   a. *Medical assistants will review the diabetic patients' charts to see if a monofilament test has been done within the last year: if not, they will perform the test and document the results, If the test was done, the medical assistant will make a notation in the EMR that it was done within the year and document the result, if known*

   b. *All clinicians will be advised that a monofilament test must be performed by the medical assistant before their own examination*

Several strategies can be used to select practice quality improvement priorities, beginning with determining if local insurers are providing quality incentive dollars and addressing quality items that are being measured. These additional dollars can then be reinvested in the practice to fuel further practice improvement. Many regional and national quality improvement initiatives define quality items that must be measured and reported. Some commonly used quality improvement measures are linked to diabetes care (eg, hemoglobin A_{1c} [HbA_{1c}] >9% or <7%, blood pressure [BP] <140/90 mm Hg or <130/80 mm Hg, low-density lipoprotein [LDL] <130 mg/dL or <100 mg/dL). Other diabetic measures include retinal examinations, foot examinations, and examinations for kidney disease.

Immunization rates and cancer screening rates are also important and commonly used measures. High-priority items that improve health and match the priorities of practice stakeholders should be chosen.

One must make sure that all data are vetted for accuracy; data integrity is a high priority both to improve patient care and for reporting purposes.

- Data integrity examples:
  - HbA_{1c}: if a patient has not had one in a year, it should be counted as >9
    - One way that data may reflect there is an issue is that process measures do not correspond to outcome measures, that is, you have 120 diabetic patients, 40 of whom have actual A_{1c} >9, and 100 A_{1c}s in the last year, which means that your data should reflect that 60/120 patients, or 50%, should be >9. If you are only counting the actual A_{1c} >9, your data will be 40/120 or 33%, much lower than it really is
  - LDL:
    - The percentage of patients whose LDL is <100 should not be greater than the percentage of patients whose LDL is <130
    - BP: both systolic and diastolic BP must be under ceiling

- If your EMR is a patient-centric, who did the last BP check and was it re-checked? Change to pick up only your BP check.
- BP: as in LDL above, you should not have more patients with a BP of <130/80 than patients with a BP of <140/90 mm Hg.

Other ways to improve the practice is to share data with all providers, including residents. Concentrate on those patients who are far away from the goal (HbA$_{1c}$ >9, BP >140/90, and so forth).

Practice transformation and earning recognition as a PCMH can be a daunting task. The process is a long journey, requiring the support, dedication, and commitment of the entire practice team, and everyone has a vital role in improving the care of patients

---

Box 4
PCMH how-to checklist

1. Perform an SWOT (Strengths, Weaknesses, Opportunities, Threats) analysis of your practice to determine pros and cons of seeking transformation and certification as a PCMH.

2. Organize a steering committee that includes key authority figures in your practice/institution to seek support, buy-in, and guidance.

3. Devote time and realistically plan for the ongoing commitment to practice transformation.

4. Create a management team, which will guide strategy, planning, and execution of the process and set goals.

5. Develop a CWG and a practice RWG. Arrange for group members to have protected time to fully participate.

6. Create a workspace dedicated to the certification process.

7. Research those agencies that provide certification and identify the one that best fits your practice needs and goals.

8. Organize all items that are necessary for the application process, thoroughly review the application requirements, and institute any changes that need to be in place before beginning the application process.

   a. Pay special attention to "must haves" required by your certifying organization of choice.

   b. Perform a gap analysis of your practice to see where you are and what you need to do to improve.

   c. Create a timeline for the entire application process, and stick to it!

9. Consider seeking grant opportunities or collaborative initiatives that may offer some financial and process support.

10. Consider hiring consultants to do a practice assessment before developing changes to your practice.

11. Get ready for the journey of change.

    a. Be ready for the pushback and change fatigue.

    b. Perform continuous quality improvement initiatives and PDSA models, and involve every member of the team.

    c. Seek constant feedback from patients, team members, learners, and community.

    d. Address the difficulties and barriers.

    e. Celebrate the victories and achievements.

12. Reap the benefits.

Table 5
Useful web sites and other resources

Resource	Link/Web Site Address
MacColl Institute: Chronic Care Model	http://www.improvingchroniccare.org/index.php?p=The_MacColl_Institute&s=93
American Diabetic Association: ADA	http://professional.diabetes.org/
Self Management Toolkit	http://www.selfmanagementtoolkit.ca/
ACP: Diabetes Portal	http://diabetes.acponline.org/clinician/index.html
NCQA	http://www.ncqa.org/
IPIP QI Teamspace	http://ipip.qiteamspace.com/
Pennsylvania Academy of Family Physicians	http://www.pafp.com/
American Academy of Family Physicians	http://www.aafp.org/online/en/home/membership/initiatives/pcmh.html?intcmp=10004-ca-20
IHI.org	
AHRQ PCMH Resource center	http://www.pcmh.ahrq.gov/portal/server.pt/community/pcmh_home/1483/what_is_pcmh_
American Academy of Pediatrics:	http://aappolicy.aappublications.org/policy_statement/index.dtl#M
American College of Physicians	http://www.acponline.org/advocacy/?hp
American Osteopathic Association	http://www.osteopathic.org
The Patient Centered Medical Home Guidelines: A Tool to Compare National Programs	http://www.mgma.com/Store/ProductDetails.aspx?id=1366580

and efficiency of the office. The work to become a formally recognized PCMH leads to changes that benefit patients, practice, and staff, and will lead to increased reimbursement for quality measures. Once a practice commits to venturing on the journey, it must be sure to have key elements in place: leadership, time, persistence, and resources. Setting clear goals and a strict timeline will help the practice move through the process more smoothly.

Box 4 and **Table 5** provides a summary checklist of the steps involved in the process, as well as several resources that may be helpful in developing and implementing changes in the practice.

REFERENCES

1. Berenson RA, Devers KJ, Burton RA. Will the patient-centered medical home transform the delivery of health care? Timely analysis of immediate health policy issues. Urban Institute/Robert Wood Johnson Foundation; 2011. Available at: http://www.urban.org/retirement_policy. Accessed June 25, 2011.
2. Starfield B, Shi L. The medical home, access to care, and insurance: a review of evidence. Pediatrics 2004;113(Suppl 5):1493–8.
3. Starfield B, Shi L, Macinko J, et al. Contribution of primary care to health systems and health. Milbank Q 2005;83(3):457–502.
4. Grumbach K, Grundy P. Outcomes of implementing patient centered medical home interventions: a review of the evidence from prospective evaluation studies

in the United States. Patient-Centered Primary Care Collaborative. November 16, 2010. Available at: www.pcpcc.net. Accessed June 25, 2011.

5. AHRQ PCMH Resource Center. PCMH (home page). Available at: http://pcmh. ahrq.gov/portal/server.pt/community/pcmh__home/1483/pcmh_home_v2. Accessed March 10, 2012.

6. Standards of Child Health Care. Council on Pediatric Practice (US). Evanston (IL): American Academy of Pediatrics; 1967.

7. Medical Home Initiatives for Children With Special Needs Project Advisory Committee. The medical home. Pediatrics 2002;110:184–6.

8. The Future of Family Medicine. A collaborative project of the family medicine community. Ann Fam Med 2004;2(Suppl 1):S3–32.

9. American College of Physicians. The advanced medical home: a patient-centered, physician-guided model of health care. Philadelphia: American College of Physicians; 2005. Position Paper (Available from America College of Physicians, 190 N. Independence Mall West, Philadelphia, PA 19106.).

10. American Academy of Family Physicians (AAFP), American Academy of Pediatrics (AAP), American College of Physicians (ACP), American Osteopathic Association (AOA). Joint principles of the patient-centered medical home. March 2007. Available at: http://www.acponline.org/pressroom/pcmh.htm. Accessed June 25, 2011.

11. Center for Medicare and Medicaid Innovation. Comprehensive primary care initiative and advanced primary care demonstration. Available at: http://innovations. cms.gov. Accessed June 26, 2011.

12. Fisher ES. Building a medical neighborhood for the medical home. N Engl J Med 2008;359:1202–5.

13. The patient centered medical home—a purchaser's guide. Patient-Centered Primary Care Collaborative; 2008. Available at: www.pcpcc.net. Accessed June 26, 2011.

14. Gilfillan RJ, Tomcavage J, Rosenthal MB, et al. Value and the medical home: effects of transformed primary care. Am J Manag Care 2010;16(8):607–14.

15. Reid RJ, Coleman K, Johnson EA, et al. The Group Health medical home at year 2: cost savings, higher patient satisfaction, and less burnout for providers. Health Aff (Millwood) 2010;29(5):835–43.

16. Genesys HealthWorks integrates primary care with health navigator to improve health, reduce costs. Institute for Healthcare Improvement. Available at: http://www.ihi.org/NR/rdonlyres/2A19EFDB-FB9D-4882-9E23-D4845DC541D8/ 0TripleAimGenesysHealthSystemSummaryofSuccessJul09.pdf. Accessed June 26, 2011.

17. Health Partners uses "BestCare" practices to improve care and outcomes, reduce costs. Institute for Healthcare Improvement. Available at: http:// www.ihi.org/NR/rdonlyres/7150DBEF-3853-4390-BBAF-30ACDCA648F5/0/ IHITripleAimHealthPartnersSummaryofSuccessJul09.pdf. Accessed June 25, 2011.

18. Available at: www.IBX.com. Accessed June 26, 2011.

19. Sherman B, Parry T, Hanson J. Patient centered medical home-performance metrics for employers. Washington, DC: Patient-Centered Primary Care Collaborative; 2011.

20. Fisher E, Wennberg D, Stukel T, et al. The implications of regional variations in Medicare spending. Part 1: the content, quality, and accessibility of care. Ann Intern Med 2003;138:273–87.

21. Public Law 111-148. 111th Congress. An Act Entitled The Patient Protection and Affordable Care Act: March 23, 2010. (HR 3590).

22. Ensuring an effective physician workforce for America. recommendations for an accountable graduate medical education system. Proceedings of a Conference, chaired by Michael M.E. Johns, MD; October 2010, Atlanta (Georgia). Available at: www.macyfoundation.org. Accessed August 20, 2011.
23. Nutting P, Miller W, Crabtree B, et al. Initial lessons from the first national demonstration project on practice transformation to a patient-centered medical home. Ann Fam Med 2009;7(3):254–60.
24. Patient Centered Medical Home Guidelines: A tool to compare national programs. Available at: http://www.mgma.com/Store/ProductDetails.aspx?id=1366580. Accessed June 26, 2011.
25. CCGC's Workbook for NCQA's Physician Practice Connections®—Patient-Centered Medical Home™. Available at: www.healthteamworks.biz/pdf/./final_ppc_pcmh_workbook_v3.pd. Accessed August 20, 2011.
26. Wagner EH. Chronic disease management: what will it take to improve care for chronic illness? Eff Clin Pract 1998;1:2–4.
27. Wagner EH, Austin BT, Davis C, et al. Improving chronic illness care: translating evidence into action. Health Aff (Millwood) 2001;20:64–78.
28. Bodenheimer T, Wagner EH, Grumbach K. Improving primary care for patients with chronic illness. JAMA 2002;288:1775–9.
29. Bodenheimer T, Wagner EH, Grumbach K. Improving primary care for patients with chronic illness, the chronic care model, part 2. JAMA 2002;288:1909–14.
30. Available at: http://www.IHI.org. Accessed June 26, 2011.

Effective Strategies for Behavior Change

Mary Thoesen Coleman, MD, PhD[a,b,]*, Ryan H. Pasternak, MD, MPH[c]

KEYWORDS

- Behavior • Motivational interviewing • Practice • Behavioral intervention
- Disease management • Chronic illness

KEY POINTS

- Behavioral change strategies are used to modify behaviors that lead to chronic illness as well as to change behaviors that improve disease management. Strategies that are most effective in both prevention and management of chronic disease consider factors such as age, ethnicity, community, and technology.
- Most strategies derive their components from application of the health belief model, the theory of reasoned action/theory of planned behavior, transtheoretical model, and social cognitive theory.
- Many tools such as the readiness ruler and personalized action plan form are available to assist health care teams to facilitate healthy behavior change. Primary care providers can support behavior changes by providing venues for peer interventions and family meetings and by making new partnerships with community organizations.

Half of all deaths are caused by modifiable behavioral factors.[1] It is therefore no accident that 5 of 10 health indicators selected by Healthy People 2010[2] are related to behavior: tobacco use, physical activity, obesity, substance use, and sexual behavior. Primary care physicians and their health care team can partner with patients to select behavioral change strategies that are most appropriate for the patient and their individual circumstances. Behavioral change strategies are used to modify behaviors that lead to chronic illness as well as to change or maintain behaviors to improve wellness promotion and disease management. Effective implementation of behavior change practices in the clinical setting require clinicians and staff to take a broad

The authors have nothing to disclose.
[a] Department of Family Medicine, Louisiana State University School of Medicine, 1542 Tulane Avenue, New Orleans, LA 70112, USA; [b] Community Health, LSUHSC Office of the Dean, c/o Emma Korruth, 2020 Gravier Street, Room 526, New Orleans, LA 70112, USA; [c] Adolescent Medicine, Department of Pediatrics, Louisiana State University Health Science Center, c/o Tiffany Palmer, 200 Henry Clay Avenue, New Orleans, LA 70118, USA
* Community Health, Office of the Dean, c/o Emma Korruth, 2020 Gravier Street, Room 526, New Orleans, LA 70112.
E-mail address: mcolem@lsuhsc.edu

public health perspective, recognizing that even small or modest changes of individual behavior (eg, 5%–10% behavior change/quit rate) have a significant impact when implemented broadly across patient populations.[3] Often, the strategies that are most effective in both prevention and management take into consideration factors such as age, ethnicity, family, peers, community, culture, and use of technology. Interventions that combine multiple strategies and are tailored to an individual or specific population may work best.

MODELS OF HEALTH BEHAVIOR CHANGE

Behavioral change theory, including the transtheoretical model, stages of change, reasoned action and planned behavior, health belief, and social cognitive and social learning theory, underlie the use of strategies for behavior change in the primary care office for both prevention and management of chronic illness.

Transtheoretical Model and Stages of Change

The transtheoretical model of behavior change conceptualizes an individual's readiness to change as 1 of 5 stages of change constructs: precontemplation, contemplation, preparation, action, and maintenance. Interventions should account for the patient's current stage of change. For example, if a person indicates that they are not ready to quit smoking, prescribing medications to assist in quitting is an inappropriate action. A more appropriate intervention might be providing assurances that the provider is available to discuss interventions when the patient is ready or providing material on why the patient might want to quit smoking. The transtheoretical model (**Table 1**) was first used to describe tobacco use cessation behavior.[4] Since that time it has been most closely associated with motivational interviewing (MI), which has proved effective in addressing multiple health behaviors, including diet and nutrition.[5]

Table 1 Stages of change and appropriate interventions		
Stage of Change	**Patient Perspectives**	**Other Models/Interventions**
Precontemplation	Not thinking about/interested in change Feeling of no control over behavior Denial of risk to self	MI Health belief model
Contemplation	Considering benefit versus cost of behavior	MI Health belief model
Preparation	Examining options for change Experimenting with minor changes	Cognitive behavioral therapy (CBT) MI
Action	Actively making changes up to 6 mo	CBT MI 12-Step programs
Maintenance	Continuing behavior change more than 6 months	CBT 12-Step programs
Relapse	Return to old behavior (normal part of change process) Demoralization	MI 12-Step programs

Data from Miller W, Rollnick S. Motivational interviewing: preparing people to change addictive behavior. 1st edition. New York: Guilford Press; 1991; and Zimmerman GL, Olsen CG, Bosworth MF. A 'stages of change' approach to helping patients change behavior. Am Fam Physician 2000; 61(5):1409–16.

Theory of Reasoned Action and Theory of Planned Behavior

The theory of reasoned action (TRA) and theory of planned behavior (TPB) suggest that behavior change is determined by the intention to perform a behavior. Individuals consider the consequences of the behavior before change. In TRA, behavior is influenced by an individual's attitude and perceptions of social norms toward a specific behavior. In practice, the provider may want to explore how a patient believes their family and peers will view a change in behavior before suggesting an intervention that does not take into account how the behavior change might affect the patient's day-to-day interactions with them. In TPB, an extension of TRA, a third determinant of behavior change is the perceived behavioral control, or how much control the individual perceives they have over the opportunities, resources, and skills to make the change.[6] The TPB has been used to describe smoking cessation, healthy eating, and exercise, with perceived control being a major predictor of behaviors in circumstances in which volitional control is reduced.[7–9]

Health Belief Model

In the health belief model, an individual makes changes in behaviors based on their perception of the severity of the potential illness, susceptibility to the illness, benefits of changing behavior to prevent or reduce effect of illness, and obstacles to the recommended behavior change. To help a patient make behavior changes, the provider may find it helpful to ask the patient questions such as "How do you think having this diagnosis will change your daily activities? What do you think would help you to make better food choices? What do you think is your greatest challenge?" The individual's confidence in their ability to perform the behaviors needed and cues, including awareness of the condition and actions to prevent or reduce impact, then influence their behavior.[10]

Social Cognitive and Social Learning Theory

According to social cognitive theory, a person's behavior is a result of the reciprocal interaction of personal, behavioral, and environmental factors. A person's thoughts affect behavior and may elicit certain responses from the environment. Although a person's behavior may affect the environment, the environment affects the way a person thinks and feels. This situation is described as the concept of reciprocal determinism.[3] In social learning theory, motivation to make behavioral changes involves 2 forces: a conviction that the behavior change is important and a sense of self-efficacy or confidence in one's ability to carry out the change.[3] The provider applies these theories when they engage in a discussion with a patient about their goals, ask the patient for a plan on how they might make the plan work in their own environment, and ask the patient about how likely they are to be successful in their plan, then work with the patient to adjust the plan so the patient views the likelihood of achieving the goal as high. **Table 2**, adapted from Whitlock and colleagues,[11] provides a summary of the most commonly cited behavior change models, theories, and constructs.

STRATEGIES/TOOLS FOR DISEASE PREVENTION AND HEALTH PROMOTION
MI and Motivational Enhancement Therapy

Although originally developed to address substance use disorders,[12] MI has now been tested across a wide range of target behavior changes. It has been found to be effective both in reducing maladaptive behaviors (eg, problem drinking, gambling, drug abuse) and in promoting adaptive health behavior change (eg, exercise, diet,

Table 2
Most commonly cited behavior change models, theories, and constructs: focus and key concepts

Level Addressed	Theory/Model	Focus	Key Concepts
Theories that address how individual factors such as knowledge, attitudes, beliefs, previous experience, and personality influence behavioral choices	Health belief model	People's perceptions of the threat of a health problem and appraisal of behavior recommended to prevent or manage problem	Perceived susceptibility Perceived severity Perceived benefits of action Perceived barriers to action Cues to action Self-efficacy
	TRA/TPB	People are rational beings whose intention to perform a behavior strongly relates to its performance through beliefs, attitudes, subjective norms, and perceived behavioral control	Behavioral intention Subjective norms Attitudes Perceived behavioral control
	Stages of change/transtheoretical model	Readiness to change or attempt to change a health behavior varies among individuals and within an individual over time. Relapse is a common occurrence and part of the normal process of change	Precontemplation Contemplation Preparation Action Maintenance Relapse
Theories that address processes between the individual and primary groups that provide social identity, support, and role definition	Social cognitive theory/social learning theory	Behavior is explained by dynamic interaction among personal factors, environmental influences, and behavior	Observational learning Reciprocal determinism Outcome expectancy Behavioral capacity Self-efficacy Reinforcement
	Community organization/building	Processes by which community groups are helped to identify and address common problems or goals	Participation and relevance Empowerment Community competence Issue selection

Data from Whitlock EP, Orleans CT, Pender N, et al. Evaluating primary care behavioral counseling interventions: an evidence-based approach. Am J Prev Med 2002;22:267–84.

medication, and visit adherence).[13] The clinical style and apparent mechanisms of change in MI seem to be related to generalizable processes of human behavior and are not limited to specific target problems.[14] Various forms or adaptations for delivering this intervention style have been shown to affect effectiveness, and effectiveness may also vary by audience, with several studies showing greater benefit for minority groups.[13,15]

A cornerstone of MI is that providers use an empathic style of interviewing to enable the patient's own verbalization of reasons for change or change talk. It is also important to avoid or roll with resistance rather than being confrontational as the facilitator of change.[12,14] For example, if a patient states that it is impossible for him to avoid being around other people who smoke, rather than challenge the patient on this statement or offer solutions to how the patient could possibly avoid others who smoke, the provider would acknowledge the difficulty and wait until the patient himself offers a possible solution. Verbalization by the patient results in an increased readiness, an essential component of behavior change, and may help the patient to identify any discrepancies between their current behaviors and their wellness goals.[14]

For clinicians, understanding how to approach a patient through the technique of MI is essential. The FRAMES mnemonic (feedback on personal impairment or risk, emphasis on personal responsibility, clearly given advice to make a change, offering a menu of options for change, empathy as a counseling style, and support of self-efficacy) is useful and frequently used in teaching and practicing MI/ motivational enhancement therapy.[16,17] In addition, working with the patient to identify any discrepancies between their current behavior and goals is an objective when using this counseling style.[17] For example, a provider using the FRAMES method might give nonjudgmental feedback with statements such as: "Drinking a 6 pack of beer a day is more than most of my patients drink and it is not a healthy choice." A statement to encourage responsibility might be: "It is up to you what you do about how much you drink, but I will help." An example of giving advice might be: "I suggest that you consider cutting back on the amount of alcohol you consume." A provider offers a menu of options on how to change behavior: "You might want to join AA, take medication to make alcohol consumption unpleasant, or join a social club that keeps you distracted and occupied." An example of an empathic statement is: "I understand how difficult making this change may be, but I am concerned about your health." A statement that shows faith in an individual's self-efficacy might be phrased: "I believe that you can make a positive change."

5 As

The 5 As method, based on stages of change theory, incorporates principles of MI to address behavior change and has been applied successfully to never, current, and former users of tobacco products.[18] When applying the 5 As method to change of behavior around tobacco use, all persons encountering health care are asked if they have ever or currently use tobacco. Never users enter discussion around primary prevention; former users focus on relapse prevention; and current users are met with advice to quit and an assessment of their willingness to quit. Those unwilling to quit, or precontemplative, are provided with information or factors to promote motivation toward quitting but only proceed to assistance with quitting if they become motivated. Motivated persons are assisted with developing a quit plan and follow-up is arranged. Relapsing patients are met with advice to quit during the next encounter. A diagram of this method is included in **Fig. 1**.[18] Implementing the 5 As protocol for smokers encountered in primary care offices doubles the quit rate (4%–10%) compared with unassisted quit attempts (2%–3%).[3,19] A variation of the 5 As method

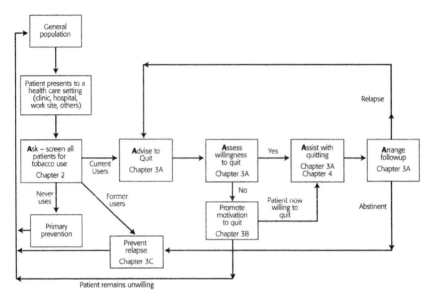

Fig. 1. 5 As model for treatment of tobacco use and dependence. Labels/boxes describe patient in various stages of clinical workflow from general population, to becoming a patient, to entry into each of the 5 As algorithm and through algorithm depending on patient responses to provider steps (As) and patient goals/behaviors. Arrows indicate clinical workflow for patient through each step in the algorithm. "Never uses" refers to patients that have never used tobacco (or engaged in specific behavior). "Current users" denotes patients who have told provider they currently use tobacco and so forth. "Former users" relates to those who had used in past but are not currently using tobacco. "Yes/No" reflect answers to provider questions about tobacco use behaviors. "Relapse" refers to patient returning to use of tobacco or other unhealthy behavior being addressed. "Abstinent" refers to patient avoidance of unhealthy behavior (tobacco use). "Patient remains unwilling" refers to patients unwilling to quit despite having been provided with motivation to quit. "Patient now willing to quit" refers to those patients who have renewed interest in quitting after being provided with additional motivation to do so. (*From* Fiore M, United States Tobacco Use and Dependence Guideline Panel, Treating tobacco use and dependence: 2008 update. Clinical practice guideline. Rockville [MD]: US Department of Health and Human Services, Public Health Service; 2008. xvii. p. 34 [this figure is in the public domain]).

has been proposed by the US Public Health and Canadian Task Force on Preventive Health Care, in which "ask" is replaced with "assess" for existence of specific negative health behaviors and "agree" has been added to elicit provider-patient collaboration on acceptable treatment goals and plan.[11]

Readiness Ruler

Use of a readiness ruler or line is another simple initial technique, to assess patient's readiness for health behavior change.[20] The clinician may draw, or have a patient imagine, a line on which the far left denotes "not interested in/not ready for change (quitting etc.)" and the far right denotes "ready to change (quit) now," or numbers 1 to 10 with similar labels at both ends. The clinician then asks the patient to mark where they believe they are on the line or provide a number between 1 and 10. If the patient does not choose 1 or the far left, they are asked "Why not a lower number like…?" or "Why not further to the left side…?" and are required to verbalize some level of readiness for change. An example of this method and additional questions are provided in

Fig. 2.[20] The clinician may also ask why the patient is not ready, or more ready, for change; identifying barriers to change or perceived positive factors associated with the unhealthy/risky behaviors is a key portion of this assessment.[21,22]

Action Planning

Goal setting and action planning are believed to help with behavior change (**Fig. 3**).[23] My Action Plan (see **Fig. 3**) is a tool that can be used in the office to facilitate conversations

Changing Behavior for Your Health

1. On the line below, mark where you are now on this line that measures change in behavior. Are you not prepared to change, already changing or someplace in the middle?

Not prepared to change   Already changing

2. Answer the questions below that apply to you.

If your mark is on the left side of the line:
How will you know when it's time to think about changing?
What signals will tell you to start thinking about changing?
What qualities in yourself are important to you?
What connection is there between those qualities and "not considering a change"?

If your mark is somewhere in the middle:
Why did you put your mark there and not further to the left?
What might make you put your mark a little further to the right?
What are the good things about the way you're currently trying to change?
What are the not-so-good things?
What would be the good result of changing?
What are the barriers to changing?

If your mark is on the right side of the line:
Pick one of the barriers to change and list some things that could help you overcome this barrier.
Pick one of those things that could help and decide to do it by _____ (write in a specific date).

If you've taken a serious step in making a change:
What made you decide on that particular step?
What has worked in taking this step?
What helped it work?
What could help it work even better?
What else would help?
Can you break that helpful step down into smaller pieces?
Pick one of those pieces and decide to do it by _____ (write in a specific date).

If you're changing and trying to maintain that change:
Congratulations! What's helping you?
What else would help?
What are your high-risk situations?

If you've "fallen off the wagon":
What worked for a while?
Don't kick yourself--long-term change almost always takes a few cycles.
What did you learn from the experience that will help you when you give it another try?

3. The following are stages people go through in making important changes in their health behaviors. All the stages are important. We learn from each stage.
We go *from* "not thinking about it" *to* "weighing the pros and cons" *to* "making little changes and figuring out how to deal with the real hard parts" *to* "doing it!" *to* "making it part of our lives."
Many people "fall off the wagon"and go through all the stages several times before the change really lasts.

Fig. 2. Changing behavior for your health. The readiness to change ruler can be used with patients contemplating any desirable behavior, such as smoking cessation, losing weight, exercise or substance-abuse cessation. The horizontal line represents a readiness ruler. Each section describes potential questions a provider could ask based on a patient's level of readiness as shown by marking the ruler. (*From* Zimmerman GL, Olsen CG, Bosworth MF. A 'stages of change' approach to helping patients change behavior. Am Fam Physician 2000;61(5):1409–16. Available at: http://www.aafp.org/afp/2000/0301/p1409.html. Accessed June 13, 2011; with permission.)

MY ACTION PLAN

DATE: _____

I _____ and _____
                    (name)   (name of clinician)

have agreed that to improve my health I will:

1. Choose one of the activities below:	2. Choose your confidence level:

2. Choose your confidence level:
This is how sure I am that I will be able to do my action plan:

_____Work on something that's bothering me:

_____

10   VERY SURE

5   SOMEWHAT SURE

0   NOT SURE AT ALL

_____Stay more physically active!

3. Complete this box for the chosen activity:

What:_____

_____

_____Take my medications.

How much:_____

When:_____

_____Improve my food choices.

_____

How often:_____

_____Reduce my stress.

_____
(Signature)

_____Cut down on smoking.

_____
(Signature of clinician)

Fig. 3. My Action Plan. The action plan is a signed agreement between clinician and patient on a behavior change plan to improve health. The first column is a list of activities from which a patient is asked to choose to change behavior. The second column is used to detail the plan (what, how much, when, how often). In addition, the patient is asked to rate their confidence on a ladder scale between 1 and 10. There are lines for signatures of both patient and clinician. (*From* Center for Excellence in Primary Care; available at: http://developmentalmedicine.ucsf.edu/pdf/actionPlan/EnglishActionPlan.pdf; with permission.)

with patients around behavioral changes that they might want to make to improve their health. The provider and patient agree to a plan based on the patient's choice about what they wish to work on, such as physical activity, diet, medication adherence, tobacco, stress, or anything that is important to the patient. The patient is asked to describe a possible plan: what they will change, how, when, and how often. The provider asks the patient to rate their confidence in successfully completing the plan on a scale of 1 to 10. If the patient rates confidence at less than 7, the provider asks the patient what changes to the plan would raise their confidence level to a rating of 7. Once the provider and patient are confident in the patient being able to implement the plan (rating of 7 or greater), they record the plan details on the action plan form and sign in agreement. The provider and their health care team follow up with the patient within a reasonable time to encourage the patient to adhere to the plan or adjust it as needed.

Family, Caregiver, and Peer Support

Many individuals with chronic illness find themselves alone to manage a complex set of factors to begin and maintain behavior change. Family and peer support have been shown to be critical to sustained behavior change and health management. Family, caregivers, and peers can assist in applying prevention or disease management plans through goal setting, skill building, practice and rehearsal of behaviors, trouble shooting, and problem solving. Peers can also provide emotional support by encouraging use of new skills, dealing with stress, and being available to listen. Peers can serve as liaisons to the health care system and as activators for seeking and receiving quality regular care. Peers can often provide support as needed and over extended timeframes.[24]

Research on the effectiveness of peer support in changing behaviors is still in its early stages. Celentano and colleagues[25] reported effective reductions in human immunodeficiency virus (HIV) infection using male military recruits as peer educators. Peer-to-peer influence in several studies[26–28] has depended on the specific audience, and improved effectiveness has been reported within specific ethnic groups. A 6-week peer-led community-based diabetes self-management program effectively changed healthy eating behaviors, reading of food labels, and patient-physician communication.[29] Heisler and colleagues[30] compared nurse care management with reciprocal peer support in a randomized controlled trial with 244 veterans with diabetes. The 2 groups did not differ in blood pressure, medication adherence, or diabetes-specific distress, but the peer intervention group had decreased hemoglobin A1c at 6 months and reported better social support. For primary care physicians, group visits in the office for individuals with chronic illness may be a feasible venue to bring peers together.

Family-based therapy has proved efficacious for some chronic diseases and seems essential for complex behavioral-based disorders like anorexia nervosa and for obesity.[31,32] In disordered eating related to both anorexia nervosa and obesity, randomized trials have shown improved long-term outcomes with family-based therapy compared with patient/child-centered treatment or nonspecific control groups.[32–34] Family-focused interventions that taught parents and adolescents how to work as a team to manage diabetes were effective in preventing deterioration in glycemic control.[35–37] In a randomized control trial,[38] a family-based domiciliary intervention program to increase physical activity using trained facilitators to introduce a range of self-regulatory skills, including goal setting in at-risk groups, was no more effective than an advice leaflet for promotion of physical activity.[38]

Community-based Support

For more details on community-based support, see the article elsewhere in this issue. Community-based interventions are receiving increasing attention as community and cultural factors have been shown to affect health-related behaviors. Evidence for community collaboration as an effective strategy for improving chronic illness care is growing. Primary care clinicians can provide patients with information about community programs, provide referrals, and encourage participation, as well as participate themselves in some community programs. The work of Davis-Smith and colleagues,[39] which focuses on African American church communities in central Georgia, shows how a partnership with a church community can result in positive behavior change for diabetic patients. All adult members of the church were screened for diabetes risk; a 6-session group intervention was offered to those with prediabetes. The leadership of the church was committed. Focus groups of church members guided the process. Risk assessment was publicized in the church bulletin and performed during church services. Health professionals presented information at group sessions and participants were supported with phone calls, letters, and session reminders. After 12 months of follow-up, participants in this program had significant weight reduction, lowered fasting blood sugars, and improved blood pressure.

Community interventions can provide a means to effectively structure programs with culturally sensitive attributes.[40] Based on the importance that many Latinos place on controlling disease and using strategies derived from self-efficacy theory, Spanish-speaking individuals were offered a 6-week peer-led program on self-management of diabetes and chronic heart or lung disease.[29] Compared with a control group, the intervention group showed improvements in health behaviors and self-efficacy as well as fewer emergency visits, outcomes that were maintained 1 year later.[29] Gary and colleagues[40] compared an intensive 24-month community-based intervention for African American diabetic patients in which nurse case managers and community health workers made home visits and provided culturally tailored intervention action plans that considered health knowledge and beliefs and provider support with a minimal intervention telephone program that prompted individuals to be involved in their own care. The culturally sensitive, intense intervention resulted in improved diabetic control and a reduction in emergency visits for 235 African American diabetic patients compared with 253 control patients.

Many community interventions use a health facilitator/educator model. A large randomized intervention trial testing the *Be Proud! Be Responsible!* program showed that community-based organizations could successfully bring about sexual behavior change, including condom use, in African American adolescents. The curriculum involves group discussions, videos, games, brainstorming, experiential exercises, and skill-building activities.[41]

BEHAVIOR CHANGE STRATEGIES FOR DISEASE PREVENTION
Tobacco/Substance Use

As the predominant cause of early morbidity and mortality in the United States,[42] tobacco use must be addressed. Disease prevention strategies targeting tobacco use in all patients are a priority. Targeted, brief interventions using MI by clinicians in outpatient office settings have been shown to be effective in increasing quit rates and are cost-effective.[43,44] The 2008 *Public Health Service Guidelines: Treating Tobacco Use and Dependence* uses scientific review of more than 8700 articles to explicitly detail well-graded recommendations for addressing tobacco use in an office and other settings.[18] For brief interventions of less than 10 minutes, the Guidelines recommend the 5 As method described earlier. The amount of face-to-face time spent counseling with more time per session, more intensity, or more sessions increases quit rates.[18,43] Sessions of greater than 10 minutes showed doubling of quit rates compared with no face-to-face contact.[18] Stead and colleagues[43] reported brief counseling of less than 20 minutes to be effective (relative risk [RR] 1.66) compared with usual care, whereas more intensive counseling, time greater than 20 minutes or with additional patient education showed an even greater effect (RR 1.81).[43] These changes reflect an increased quit rate of 4% to 6% over typical unassisted rates of 2% to 3%.[43] The increased quit rates derived from brief interventions have significant public health impact when applied consistently to all tobacco users.

In the Guidelines,[18] studies of adolescent tobacco use were limited and mixed in both their techniques (including MI and cognitive behavioral therapy) and results. Overall the 7 studies included in the meta-analysis for adolescent tobacco use reported improved long-term abstinence rates with brief counseling interventions

(11.6%) compared with usual care (6.7%).[18] Screening, brief intervention, and referral to treatment (SBIRT) programs have been used effectively for mild to moderate alcohol abuse internationally and endorsed by most major medical organizations.[45,46] The US Preventive Services Task Force data present good evidence to provide screening and brief ($\leq$15 minutes) counseling to adults with mild to moderate drinking. The counseling styles recommended include MI with FRAMES and 5 As, as discussed earlier,[47] which achieved an absolute risk reduction of 7% to 14% (net reduction in drinking) at 6 and 12 months, respectively.

More recently, SBIRT has been shown to be effective for drug abuse as well.[48] In 1 large trial with more than 100,000 people, almost 23% screened positive for a spectrum of substance use.[48] Most were recommended for a brief intervention (15.9%). Of those reporting drug use at baseline and referred to brief intervention, rates of drug use at 6-month follow-up were 67.7% less ($P<.001$) and heavy alcohol use was 38.6% less ($P<.001$). Of persons recommended for brief treatment or specialty center referral, self-reported improvements were found for general health ($P<.001$), mental health ($P<.001$), criminal behavior ($P<.001$), and other outcomes.[48] These findings strongly support the use of SBIRT using brief MI techniques in clinical settings.

Nutrition

Poor diet and physical inactivity are looming to surpass tobacco use as the most common causes of death in the United States.[1] Over the last 2 decades, the prevalence of obesity has continued to increase in the United States, with significant increases in men, children, and adolescents.[27,49] In a 1997 meta-analysis of 10 trials that assessed the effectiveness of advice by general practitioners to modify dietary behavior, Ashenden and colleagues[50] found variable results across several provider-directed interventions for nutrition improvement. These interventions consisted primarily of offering advice to modify dietary behavior, sometimes offered only as part of general lifestyle advice.[50] Kristal and colleagues[51] reported significant increase in fruit and vegetable serving consumption and reduction in fat intake in 1205 adults in a health maintenance organization using a tailored self-help intervention that consisted of a computer-generated personalized letter, a motivational phone call, self-help manual, a package of supplementary materials, computer-generated behavioral feedback based on a self-administered food frequency questionnaire, and newsletters. In a meta-analysis of 87 studies involving adults provided nutrition counseling by a dietician, nurse, or physician, Spahn and colleagues[5] concluded that interventions, which combined behavioral theory and cognitive behavioral theory, were effective in improving nutrition-related behavior. The investigators reported that few studies specifically assessed the transtheoretical model of change, but studies that evaluated MI or MI combined with cognitive behavioral therapy reported significant improvements in dietary behavior.[5] Outcomes included decreased body fat, weight loss, and improvement in lipid profiles.

For children with eating disorders, such as anorexia nervosa, family therapy has been shown to be the most effective, long-term intervention.[31,52,53] For overweight and obese children, additional research is still needed. Two recent office-based studies addressing pediatric overweight and obesity used interventions delivered by primary care providers.[54,55] In the study by McCallum and colleagues,[54] the intervention included 4 in-office consultations with a general practitioner, targeting nutrition, physical activity, and sedentary behavior, whereas the control group received standard care; outcome measures were evaluated at 9 and 15 months and the adjusted mean difference in body mass index (BMI; calculated as weight in kilograms divided by the square of height in meters) was −0.2 kg/m^2 (95% confidence interval [CI], −0.6

to 0.1; $P = .25$) at 9 months and -0.0 kg/m^2 (95% CI, -0.5 to 0.5; $P = 1.00$) at 15 months. Schwartz and colleagues[55] used pediatricians and registered dieticians with MI training to provide MI sessions directed toward parents of 91 overweight children. These sessions were described as "minimal" for 1 MI session by a pediatrician or "intensive" for 1 session each by a pediatrician and dietician.[55] At 6 months' follow-up, there was a nonsignificant ($P = .85$) decrease of -0.6, -1.9, and -2.6 BMI percentiles in the control, minimal, and intensive groups, respectively, with an attrition rate of 50% for the intensive group.[55] Each of these studies reported some improvements in diet behavior and physical activity by parental self-report.[54,55] However, there was no improvement seen for BMI or weight-related outcome measures. Additional theory-based research must be performed to address pediatric and adolescent obesity, perhaps adapting effective substance abuse interventions for use in pediatric, adolescent, and adult obesity prevention.[56,57]

Physical Activity

Health care providers may wish to modify the level of physical activity in their patients with chronic illness. Patients with chronic obstructive pulmonary disease were randomly assigned to 1 of 5 groups to determine adherence to a walking program: cognitive behavior modification, behavior modification alone, cognitive component alone, attention, and no treatment. After 12 weeks, patients who underwent cognitive behavior intervention reported in their diaries significantly more walking time than control groups.[58] Suggestions for effective use of the stage of change model for physical activity are found in the *National Guideline Clearinghouse (Exercise Promotion: Walking in Elders)*[59] and *National Guideline Clearinghouse (Physical Activity and Public Health)*[60] and are summarized here. In the precontemplation phase, a provider can: (1) increase awareness by asking patients to keep a diary of their activity level, (2) point out how their behavior influences their health and serves as a model to their children and grandchildren, (3) clarify the effect of sedentary behavior on mood, (4) focus on short-term benefits of physical activity such as sleeping better, (4) link benefits of being physically active to valued activities, and (5) discuss how exercise may contribute to increases in quality of life, such as living independently and avoiding falls.

For patients in the contemplative phase, providers can address ambivalence by: (1) discussing how to overcome barriers to exercise, (2) enhancing self-confidence by using motivating messages such as "You are doing great," (3) delineating socially desirable options such as walking to church or taking the stairs, (4) offering options such as stretching, range-of-motion, and weight-bearing exercises, (5) familiarizing the patient with community resources such as senior centers, parks, and clubs, and (6) assisting them with choice of appropriate apparel for exercise.

For those patients who are prepared to begin exercise in the near future, the provider's tasks are to: (1) provide safety information and appropriate parameters of time and distance for walking, (2) encourage monitoring of progress, (3) establish short-term goals, (4) encourage patients to share intentions with others, (5) advocate exercise as enjoyable, (6) foster family and friend support, (7) offer strategies to overcome pain, fatigue, mobility, and sensory impairments, and (8) help patients deal with temporary unpleasantness associated with exercise by recommending medications before exercise, using ice for painful areas, wearing appropriate socks and shoes, and walking with assistive devices if at risk for falls.

The provider can assist the patient in the action phase who has recently begun exercising regularly by: (1) giving positive constructive feedback, (2) helping the patient increase speed, distance, or time, (3) participating in long-term goal setting, (4) identifying potential circumstances for relapse, (5) encouraging group activity, (6) visiting patients' homes or using phone call conversations to monitor progress, and (6) encouraging self-rewards such as new shoes, new audiotape, or short tips for successes.

For patients in the maintenance phase, whom the provider wishes to assist in maintaining their level of physical activity, the provider can tailor interventions to: (1) provide positive reinforcement, (2) showcase their behavior for others as role models, (3) remind the patients how to make exercise fun and entertaining (use of music, exercising with friends), (4) encourage family support, and (5) prevent discouragement by setting realistic goals.

When patients relapse in their physical activity program, providers can (1) assess stage of relapse by determining conditions when patients were active, (2) learn from patients what worked for them in the past in overcoming barriers, and (3) offer alternatives to barriers such as overcoming inclement weather by exercising in a mall, at home, or in a gym.

Sexual Behavior

Prevention of risky sexual behavior and reduction of sexually transmitted infections (STIs), including HIV, requires multiple approaches tailored to various patient populations, transmission routes, and communities.[28,61] STIs predominately affect adolescents and young adults, and within this population, peer-to-peer influence and behavior has been shown to promote disease prevention and risk reduction.[25,62] Celentano and colleagues[63] used military peer educators within Thai military groups to influence STI prevention practices, including correct and consistent condom use, reduction of alcohol use, brothel patronage, and sexual negotiation skills. Military companies were assigned to 1 of 3 groups, with 450 men in the intervention group, 681 in the diffusion group at the same base in separate barracks from intervention participants, and 414 in distant bases as controls. Baseline HIV testing, risk-reduction counseling, and behavioral interviews were conducted during basic training and every 6 months thereafter. The volunteer peer educators (including squad leaders, paramedics, and chaplains) delivered intervention for 15 months, and men were followed up at 6-month intervals for 2 years. Incident STIs were 7 times less frequent among the intervention groups than controls (RR, 0.15; 95% CI, 0.04–0.55), after adjusting for baseline risk factors ($P<.005$). There was no diffusion of the intervention to adjacent barracks. The intervention decreased incident HIV by 50% in the intervention group.

Approaches tailored to at-risk populations have been shown to be effective particularly among African Americans and Latino adolescents.[28,64] In a meta-analysis of behavioral interventions to reduce HIV transmission, Vergidis and Falagas[28] reported that in 35 randomized controlled trials targeting heterosexual African Americans only, the risk of unprotected sex was reduced, with greater efficacy found for interventions that included peer education. For Latinos, these effects were larger in interventions with segmentation by the same gender. Crosby and colleagues[64] reported reduction of incident STIs (50.4% vs 31.9%; $P = .002$) and increased condom use at last intercourse (72.4% vs 53.9%; $P = .008$) compared with a standard of care control group using a brief in-clinic intervention designed to increase correct and consistent condom use, which was delivered by a lay health educator to young African American men with recent STI. The intervention was tailored to the specific condom use concerns and risk behaviors of each participant. Young men in the intervention group also reported fewer sexual partners (mean 2.06 vs 4.15; $P<.001$) and fewer acts of unprotected sex (mean 12.3 vs 29.4; $P = .045$) compared with controls.[64]

BEHAVIOR CHANGE STRATEGIES FOR CHRONIC DISEASE MANAGEMENT

In addition to addressing health promotion and prevention behaviors related to tobacco/substance use, nutrition and physical activity and sexual behavior, the primary care provider must assist the chronically ill patient in adopting beneficial behaviors related directly to the management of their chronic condition(s). Examples of optimal management strategies include proper medication use and adherence for all disease states, self-monitoring of blood glucose (SMBG) and foot health in diabetes, and monitoring of weight and diet in congestive heart failure.

Appropriate Medication Use and Adherence

Achieving appropriate adherence to prescribed medications is a goal for management of most chronic conditions. In 1 study in 78 outpatients with chronic obstructive pulmonary disease (COPD), Dolce and colleagues[19] found that 54% of patients were underusing medications, 50% overusing medications, and 31% were not using inhalers with proper technique. In 2010, Lareau and Yawn[65] developed a customized strategy to assist nonadherence or improper use of COPD inhaler therapy, grounded in social cognitive theory and the health belief model. In this study, the investigators recommend once-daily medication for patients who understand and agree with therapy (erratic adherence) but who do not keep up with the regimen because of forgetting, busy schedule, or lack of attention to detail. The investigators suggest written instructions for patients with unwitting nonadherence who believe that they are adherent when they are not. Such patients may have cultural or language barriers, making it a challenge to understand how to take medications or the reason for taking the medication. For patients who knowingly do not adhere to medication regimens (witting nonadherence), the recommended strategies include patient education and counseling around pertinent concerns such as toxicity, tolerance, and health beliefs, as well as negotiation of therapy and linking therapy to patient-centered goals.

Effective strategies, based on social cognitive theory, that have been shown to improve medication adherence in elderly patients include simplification of treatment regimens and decreasing the number and frequency of pills, which also minimizes the risk of adverse drug reactions.[66] Behavioral strategies that take into account declining cognitive and physical functioning of elderly individuals can also promote adherence.[67] For example, instructions aimed at medication taking (use of a chart, dispenser tray, calendar, color-coded bottles, special packaging of medications, telephone or mail prompts, and environmental cues within the home such as taking medications with morning coffee, during a television program, or associated with a certain activity), rather than instructions aimed at a health behavior goal, can increase medication adherence.

In a review of randomized controlled trials of long-term interventions to improve adherence behavior related to prescribed medication and treatment outcomes, 26 of 58 trials reported improved adherence but only 18 studies improved patient outcomes.[68] Simply warning patients about adverse effects of medications did not affect adherence. Effective interventions were often multifaceted, involving combinations of elements such as information provision, reminders, self-monitoring, reinforcement, counseling, family therapy, psychological therapy, crisis intervention, telephone follow-up, and supportive care.[68]

McQuaid and colleagues[69] found that adherence to medication regimens in children was only 48% of prescribed medications. Neither knowledge of the disease nor responsibility for management resulted in better adherence. Smith and Shuchman[70] also reported nonadherence to treatment recommendations in one-third of adolescents with a chronic illness, citing psychiatric illness, psychological factors, family issues, and lack of adolescent involvement in decision making as factors. A review of interventions to enhance medication adherence in children and adolescents with chronic illness[71] suggested that education alone was insufficient and a behavioral component may increase efficacy. Behavioral interventions included a variety of approaches, including monitoring and goal setting, providing rewards for medication adherence, contingency contracting, problem solving, and linking medication taking with routines. Text messaging has been used with diabetic teens to increase self-efficacy and self-reported adherence.[72]

Diabetes

For more details on diabetes, see the article elsewhere in this issue. Many health behaviors in chronic illness are disease-specific. For example, disease management of diabetes uniquely requires SMBG and foot care. In a review of 6 randomized controlled trials that studied the effectiveness of SMBG on hemoglobin A1c levels in noninsulin using type 2 diabetic patients, Welschen and colleagues[73] concluded that patients using SMBG, compared with control groups, decreased hemoglobin A1c levels significantly by 0.39, a difference expected to translate to an approximate 14% reduced risk of microvascular complications.[73] Polonsky and colleagues[74] reported better hemoglobin A1c outcomes using a structured primary care SMBG intervention for noninsulin-treated diabetic patients. In an application of theories of reasoned action and planned behavior, patients were trained to record meal sizes, energy levels, and SMBG experiences and plot a 7-point preprandial and postprandial SMBG profile on 3 consecutive days before a scheduled study visit. Training included proper use of the Accu-Chek system (Roche Diagnostics, Indianapolis, IN, USA) and how to recognize and respond to problematic glycemic results. Physicians systematically reviewed data at follow-up visits.[74]

Fisher and Glasgow[24] contend that interventions to increase SMBG are more effective if they address both behavioral interventions to teach self-care and emotional interventions to address problems such as depression. In a recent online survey of diabetic patients, Fisher and colleagues[75] found that survey participants who scored low on information about SMBG, motivation, and behavioral skills also scored low on self-reported frequency of SMBG. Automated phone calls with nurse follow-up,[76] provision of a blood glucose owner's manual,[77] use of a stages of change approach,[78] and MI[79] have been effective in increasing SMBG and often result in decreasing hemoglobin A1c. Piette[80] makes the point that interactive behavior change technology, such as personal digital assistants (PDAs), automated telephone calls, Web sites, and touch-screen kiosks, can support patient self-management, but cautions against a "series of e-mails from an insurance company" encouraging patients to eat more vegetables and fruits. Piette suggests that interactive behavior change technology is more effective when linked with primary care.[80] For example, providers use information from automated phone calls or e-mails to follow-up with patients and determine care plans.

According to planned behavior theory, behavior change is a function of patient perception of control over circumstances to make a change. Newer combinations of technology may provide patients with a locus of control by providing them with the ability to make immediate treatment adjustments based on blood sugar results. Lim and colleagues[81] conducted a 6-month study of 154 elderly diabetic patients, 51 with ubiquitous health care service, a clinical decision support system using a wired telephone-connected glucometer plus mobile phone that delivered text messages, 51 using SMBG, and 52 in a control group. Training on the system averaged 2 to 3 hours but participants challenged by the glucometer or system were given additional training until comfortable. The target frequency of glucose testing was more than 8 times per week, which was met 81.2%, 68.5%, and 31.2% in ubiquitous health care, SMBG, and control groups, respectively (P<.01). A total of 144 patients completed the study and those in the ubiquitous health service significantly decreased fasting and postprandial glucose values, body weight, BMI, and low-density lipoprotein-cholesterol.[81]

Evidence-based effective behavioral strategies related to foot care as part of diabetes disease management are limited. At least 1 small qualitative study[82] identified that patients had beliefs about foot complications and foot self-care practices that could potentially increase, rather than decrease, the risk of ulceration. Educational interventions that tailor the education to individual patients based on needs and risk factors and community-based education on self-management to supplement standard medical practice may make a difference.[83] In a review of 5 randomized controlled studies, Dorresteijn and colleagues[84] did not find sufficient evidence that even multifaceted interventions (involving at least 2 different levels of care: the patient, the provider, or the health care structure) reduced the incidence of foot ulcerations.

Congestive Heart Failure

For more details on congestive heart failure, see the article elsewhere in this issue. Behaviors that must be addressed in the disease management of congestive heart failure include regular weight monitoring, adjustment of dietary salt intake, adherence to medications, and appropriately calibrated physical activity. Patient engagement in these behaviors can reduce hospital readmissions. Copeland and colleagues[85] compared the effects of a telephone intervention by nursing using MI in 458 Veterans Administration patients with congestive heart failure versus a control group. The intervention program successfully improved weight monitoring and exercise, but readmission rates to the hospital were no different and the costs for the intervention were higher. In another program that offered patients with heart failure education regarding daily weight monitoring, diuretic dose adjustment, and symptom recognition with reinforcement strategies (picture-based educational materials, a digital scale, and scheduled follow-up phone calls), more patients reported monitoring daily weights after 12 months; the intervention group had a lower rate of hospitalization or death but there were no differences in heart failure-related quality of life.[86]

Paradis and colleagues[87] piloted a nursing intervention based on a combination of the transtheoretical model and MI that addressed self-care (fluid restriction, low-salt diet, daily weight measurement, exercise, and medication) and self-management (symptom recognition and evaluation, treatment initiation and evaluation). Based on a behavior the patient chooses to improve, the nurse follows a 3-encounter protocol using an ALEGrO algorithm (algorithm to evaluate the stages of change and the conviction and confidence level) (**Fig. 4**), which briefly assesses the stage of change and confidence level followed by a list of potential interventions specific to the stage and level. Suggestions for appropriate conversation starters include "Describe the changes in your life associated with this health problem." In precontemplation, a nurse might "create a doubt in the patient's mind." If the patient is at the precontemplative stage, a nurse might choose from 10 interventions to "discuss the advantages of changing the behavior." For patients in the preparation stage, examples of 12 interventions are available to "discuss strategies, alternatives, and relapse prevention." If patients are in the action stage, 6 possible interventions such as "Ask the patient if he faces problems regarding the new behavior" are provided. Results of the study suggested that this approach has potential for improving self-care behaviors at little cost, with nurses requiring only 2 days of training to perform the necessary intervention techniques.

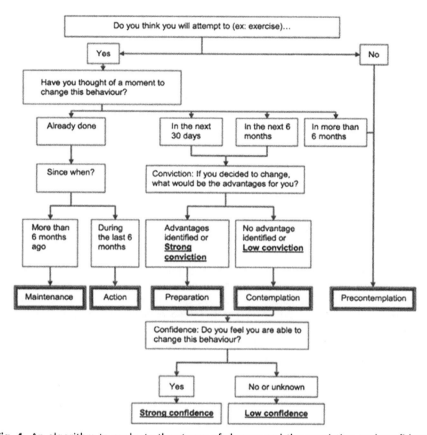

Fig. 4. An algorithm to evaluate the stages of change and the conviction and confidence level (ALEGrO). This algorithm is an attempt to identify a patient's level of readiness for change as well as their confidence and conviction to identify the most appropriate interventions. Top box contains a question asked of a patient to determine interest in changing a behavior. Yes or No boxes indicate patient's response. The No box identifies the patient as in precontemplative phase. The Yes box is followed by asking the patient about timing of change. (Have you thought of a moment to change this behavior?) A patient response of "Already done" calls for further questioning about timing "Since when?" If more than 6 months has passed since the behavior change, the patient is considered to be in maintenance phase (maintenance box). If the change has occurred within the last 6 months, the patient is considered to be in action phase (action box). If the patient response to the timing of change question is a plan to change behavior in more than 6 months, the patient is in precontemplative phase (precontemplation box). If the patient plans to change behavior within the next 6 months, the patient's conviction is determined by asking about advantages of the behavior change. If the patient is not able to identify advantages or there is low conviction (no advantage identified or low conviction box), the patient is in contemplative phase (contemplation box). If the advantages are identified or the patient indicates strong conviction (advantages identified or strong conviction box), the patient is in preparative phase (preparation box). For patients in either contemplative or preparative phases, confidence is assessed by asking "Do you feel you are able to change this behavior?" A "Yes" response indicates strong confidence. A "No" response indicates low confidence. (*From* Paradis V, Cossett S, Frasure-Smith N. The efficacy of a motivational nursing intervention based on the stages of change on self-care in heart failure patients. J Cardiovasc Nurs 2010;25(2):135; with permission.)

The use of e-mail to provide reminders to patients about desired behaviors can prompt healthy changes. A basic e-mail intervention in which home health nurses received e-mail reminders about heart failure-specific recommendations was less expensive than an augmented intervention, although both interventions yielded positive changes in self-care management indicators such as daily weights.[88]

Asthma

For more details about asthma, see the article elsewhere in this issue. In asthma, tailoring treatment plans to individual patients may influence their ability to make behavior change. Haughney and colleagues[89] conducted a discrete choice experiment (9 pairs of choices) to determine relative importance to patients of 6 aspects of asthma management (gaining relief of asthma symptoms, dose of inhaled steroid, personalized asthma plan, number of routinely used inhalers, location of crisis management, and response to deterioration). These investigators found that simpler treatment regimens and fewer inhalers were the most important considerations, even more than symptom control without compromise.

In a study by Janson and colleagues,[90] 3 30-minute sessions of individualized self-management education delivered by certified asthma educators were compared with self-monitoring alone. The self-management education included asthma facts and medication actions, personalized verbal and graphic interpretation of spirometry, peak flow trends, techniques of using metered dose inhalers, and allergen skin testing and strategies for control of environmental exposures. Education included how to monitor peak flows and identify traffic light zones with differing action plans for green, yellow, and red. The intervention group had more symptom-free days, experienced less nighttime awakenings, and decreased rescue ß-agonist use. The intervention group believed that their asthma was better controlled and reported better inhaler techniques and reduced exposure to outside allergens and indoor dust.

CONSIDERATIONS FOR SPECIAL POPULATIONS
Children/Adolescents

Appropriate behavioral interventions often depend on the age of the individual. When trying to help change behavior in children and adolescents with chronic illness or risky behaviors, the health care provider must adapt applications of theory and practice to the developmental level of the patient, comorbidity of the illness, degree of family involvement, and other social or environmental supports.

For younger children, parental influence and support may be required for effective change. In a 10-year prospective randomized controlled study by Epstein and colleagues,[32] obese 6-year-old to 12-year-old children and their parents were randomized to 3 groups for reinforcement of weight loss and behavior change after all were provided with diet, exercise, and behavior management training. The combined child and parent group, which reinforced both parent and child behavior change and weight loss, showed significantly greater decreases in percent overweight for children at 5 and 10 years after intervention (-11.2% and -7.5%, respectively) compared with children in the control group, who were rewarded only for attendance (+7.9% and +14.3%, respectively). The child-only group showed no significant difference to the combined intervention or control group.

Peer-to-peer and family-based therapy interventions may be particularly appropriate for changing adolescent behavior. In addition to the effectiveness of peer interventions for STI/HIV prevention and individual MI interventions for tobacco and substance abuse,[25,26] teen peer interventions are useful in managing asthma. A cluster randomized controlled trial reported that student volunteers trained as asthma peer leaders improved quality of life and decreased school absences.[91]

Other recent studies have explored the use of technology to enhance adolescent behavior change. Use of computer-assisted MI for tobacco use showed improved abstinence over 2 years (odds ratio [OR] 2.42) for current smokers but was nonsignificant for nonsmokers (OR 1.25).[26] Confidentiality and disclosure of health behaviors are of great concern for adolescents and affect use of services.[92,93] In the Healthy Teen Project,[94] when adolescents used PDAs compared with paper or face-to-face interviewing to disclose health behaviors, there was an increase in percentage of visits that included discussion/counseling on fruit/vegetable intake (60.4% vs 41.7%; $P =$ .03), tobacco use (54.9% vs 40.0%; $P = $ .07), and alcohol use (53.9% vs 38.0%; $P = $ .05).[94] In addition, perceived confidentiality was higher (83.7% vs 61.5%; $P = $ .002) and adolescents who used PDA screening were more satisfied with the visit (87.8% vs 63.1%; $P<.001$).[94] Use of technology may be the first step to adolescent disclosure of risky behaviors in the office setting, where providers can then engage and counsel patients in behavior change.

Elderly Individuals

Seventy-five percent of those older than 65 years have at least 1 chronic condition and about half have at least 2 chronic illnesses. Many of these illnesses lead to disabilities that make self-care more difficult. In addition, cognitive decline can adversely affect the patient's ability to remember. Murdaugh and Insel[67] summarized strategies that help elderly individuals to make behavior change related to both medication adherence and other lifestyle changes, including: (1) tailoring educational interventions to the individual based on a detailed medication history, (2) using multidisciplinary teams to manage high complexity of care, (3) promoting behavioral strategies that address difficulties with memory, (4) scheduling ongoing visits with a consistent provider rather than visits as needed to minimize polypharmacy and to monitor physical and cognitive changes that could impair adherence, (5) providing caregiver education and support, and (6) using show-and-tell techniques to teach desired behavior.

George and colleagues[95] reviewed 8 studies for their effect on medication adherence in elderly patients and found that combinations of educational and behavioral strategies were most effective. Attendance at a 17-hour chronic disease self-management program taught by lay people in community settings such as senior centers, churches, libraries, and hospitals has also been shown to improve functional ability and a broader set of health behaviors as well as decrease disability. Participants are instructed in control of symptoms of chronic illness using relaxation techniques, dietary modification, sleep hygiene, and correct use of medication. They also are given information on communications with health care providers, sexual relations, advance directives, nutrition, and pain management.[96]

In elderly people, consideration should be given to their physiologic baseline status before encouraging increased physical activity. Evaluating an older person's balance might be prudent before encouraging physical activity that may increase risk for falls and injury. Tools such as the balance scale[97] can assess balance, and the Borg scale[98] can assess an individual's perception of exertion, an indicator that correlates with the heart rate during activity. Recommendations can then be based on the patient's readiness. Older adults who engage in exercise mostly walk. Bennet and Winters-Stone[99] describe that brief provider can start older adults walking and cite evidence that, if advice is followed up by reminders, patients often maintain activity. Use of pedometers is a tool that can help older patients gauge the intensity of walking that is beneficial (3000 steps per half hour). A minimum speed of 1.22 m/s is needed to cross streets safely.[100]

SUMMARY

Behavior change strategies derive most of their components from application of the health belief model, the TRA/TPB, the transtheoretical model, and social cognitive theory. Brief interventions, such as the 5 As method, make it easier to address stages of change and incorporate principles of MI. Many tools such as the readiness ruler and action plan form are available to the health care team to facilitate healthy behavior change discussions. Providing group visits during which peers can interact and support each other as well as family visits during which children and parents learn to work as teams may facilitate behavior changes. Providers have a greater chance of being effective when they consider the special circumstances of populations such as elderly and young people. Primary care providers can also assist patients by engaging them in community programs that have been proved to improve healthy behaviors.

REFERENCES

1. Mokdad AH, Marks JS, Stroup DF, et al. Actual causes of death in the United States, 2000. JAMA 2004;291(10):1238–45.
2. Healthy behaviors: addressing chronic disease at its roots. Issue Brief (Grantmakers Health) 2004;19:1–39.
3. Baranowski T, Perry CL, Parcel GS. How individuals, environments, and health behavior interact. In: Glanz K, Rimer BK, Lewis FM, editors. Health behavior and health education: theory, research, and practice. 3rd edition. San Francisco (CA): Jossey-Bass; 2002. p. 168.
4. Prochaska JO, DiClemente CC. Stages and processes of self-change of smoking: toward an integrative model of change. J Consult Clin Psychol 1983; 51(3):390–5.
5. Spahn JM, Reeves RS, Keim KS, et al. State of the evidence regarding behavior change theories and strategies in nutrition counseling to facilitate health and food behavior change. J Am Diet Assoc 2010;110(6):879–91.
6. Montano DE, Kasprzyk D. The theory of reasoned action and the theory of planned behavior. In: Glanz K, Rimer BK, Lewis FM, editors. Health behavior and health education: theory, research, and practice. 3rd edition. San Francisco (CA): Jossey-Bass; 2002. p. 67–8.
7. Norman P, Conner M, Bell R. The theory of planned behavior and smoking cessation. Health Psychol 1999;18(1):89–94.
8. Conner M, Norman P, Bell R. The theory of planned behavior and healthy eating. Health Psychol 2002;21(2):194–201.
9. Norman PC, Conner M, Bell R. The theory of planned behaviour and exercise: evidence for the moderating role of past behavior. Br J Health Psychol 2010; 5(3):249–61.
10. Janz NK, Champion VL, Stretcher VJ. The health belief model. In: Glanz K, Rimer BK, Lewis FM, editors. Health behavior and health education: theory, research, and practice. 3rd edition. San Francisco (CA): Jossey-Bass; 2002. p. 47–50.
11. Whitlock EP, Orleans CT, Pender N, et al. Evaluating primary care behavioral counseling interventions: an evidence-based approach. In: Force USPST, ed. Am J Prev Med 2002;22:267–84.

12. Miller W, Rollnick S. Motivational interviewing: preparing people to change addictive behavior. 1st edition. New York: Guilford Press; 1991.
13. Burke BL, Arkowitz H, Menchola M. The efficacy of motivational interviewing: a meta-analysis of controlled clinical trials. J Consult Clin Psychol 2003;71(5):843–61.
14. Miller WR, Rose GS. Toward a theory of motivational interviewing. Am Psychol 2009;64(6):527–37.
15. Hettema J, Steele J, Miller WR. Motivational interviewing. Annu Rev Clin Psychol 2005;1:91–111.
16. Simkin DR. Adolescent substance use disorders and comorbidity. Pediatr Clin North Am 2002;49(2):463–77.
17. Miller WR, Rollnick S. Motivational interviewing: preparing people for change. 2nd edition. New York: Guilford Press; 2002.
18. Fiore M. United States. Tobacco Use and Dependence Guideline Panel. Treating tobacco use and dependence: 2008 update. 2008 update ed. Rockville (MD): US Department of Health and Human Services, Public Health Service; 2008.
19. Dolce JJ, Crisp C, Manzella B, et al. Medication adherence patterns in chronic obstructive pulmonary disease. Chest 1991;99(4):837–41.
20. Zimmerman GL, Olsen CG, Bosworth MF. A 'stages of change' approach to helping patients change behavior. Am Fam Physician 2000;61(5):1409–16.
21. Hesse M. The Readiness Ruler as a measure of readiness to change poly-drug use in drug abusers. Harm Reduct J 2006;3:3.
22. Berg-Smith SM, Stevens VJ, Brown KM, et al. A brief motivational intervention to improve dietary adherence in adolescents. The Dietary Intervention Study in Children (DISC) Research Group. Health Educ Res 1999;14(3):399–410.
23. Bodenheimer T, Davis C, Holman H. Helping patients adopt healthier behaviors. Clin Diabetes 2007;25(2):66–70.
24. Boothroyd RI, Fisher EB. Peers for progress: promoting peer support for health around the world. Fam Pract 2010;27(Suppl 1):i62–8.
25. Celentano DD, Nelson KE, Lyles CM, et al. Decreasing incidence of HIV and sexually transmitted diseases in young Thai men: evidence for success of the HIV/AIDS control and prevention program. AIDS 1998;12(5):F29–36.
26. Hollis JF, Polen MR, Whitlock EP, et al. Teen reach: outcomes from a randomized, controlled trial of a tobacco reduction program for teens seen in primary medical care. Pediatrics 2005;115(4):981–9.
27. Ogden CL, Carroll MD, Curtin LR, et al. Prevalence of overweight and obesity in the United States, 1999-2004. JAMA 2006;295(13):1549–55.
28. Vergidis PI, Falagas ME. Meta-analyses on behavioral interventions to reduce the risk of transmission of HIV. Infect Dis Clin North Am 2009;23(2):309–14.
29. Lorig K, Ritter PL, Villa FJ, et al. Community-based peer-led diabetes self-management: a randomized trial. Diabetes Educ 2009;35(4):641–51.
30. Heisler M, Vijan S, Makki F, et al. Diabetes control with reciprocal peer support versus nurse care management: a randomized trial. Ann Intern Med 2010; 153(8):507–15.
31. Eisler I, Dare C, Russell GF, et al. Family and individual therapy in anorexia nervosa. A 5-year follow-up. Arch Gen Psychiatry 1997;54(11):1025–30.
32. Epstein LH, Valoski A, Wing RR, et al. Ten-year follow-up of behavioral, family-based treatment for obese children. JAMA 1990;264(19):2519–23.
33. Eisler I. Family-based treatment increases full remission at 1-year follow-up compared with adolescent-focused individual therapy in adolescents with anorexia nervosa. Evid Based Ment Health 2011;14(1):27.

34. Lock J, Le Grange D, Agras WS, et al. Randomized clinical trial comparing family-based treatment with adolescent-focused individual therapy for adolescents with anorexia nervosa. Arch Gen Psychiatry 2010;67(10):1025–32.
35. Anderson BJ, Brackett J, Ho J, et al. An office-based intervention to maintain parent-adolescent teamwork in diabetes management. Impact on parent involvement, family conflict, and subsequent glycemic control. Diabetes Care 1999;22(5):713–21.
36. Laffel LM, Vangsness L, Connell A, et al. Impact of ambulatory, family-focused teamwork intervention on glycemic control in youth with type 1 diabetes. J Pediatr 2003;142(4):409–16.
37. Murphy HR, Wadham C, Rayman G, et al. Integrating pediatric diabetes education into routine clinical care: the Families, Adolescents and Children's Teamwork Study (FACTS). Diabetes Care 2006;29(5):1177.
38. Kinmonth AL, Wareham NJ, Hardeman W, et al. Efficacy of a theory-based behavioural intervention to increase physical activity in an at-risk group in primary care (ProActive UK): a randomised trial. Lancet 2008;371(9606):41–8.
39. Davis-Smith YM, Boltri JM, Seale JP, et al. Implementing a diabetes prevention program in a rural African-American church. J Natl Med Assoc 2007;99(4):440–6.
40. Gary TL, Batts-Turner M, Yeh HC, et al. The effects of a nurse case manager and a community health worker team on diabetic control, emergency department visits, and hospitalizations among urban African Americans with type 2 diabetes mellitus: a randomized controlled trial. Arch Intern Med 2009;169(19):1788–94.
41. Jemmott J, Jemmott L, Fong G, et al. Effectiveness of an HIV/STD risk-reduction intervention for adolescents when implemented by community-based organizations: a cluster-randomized controlled trial. Am J Public Health 2008;100(4):720–6.
42. Annual smoking-attributable mortality, years of potential life lost, and productivity losses–United States, 1997-2001. MMWR Morb Mortal Wkly Rep 2005;54(25):625–8.
43. Stead LF, Bergson G, Lancaster T. Physician advice for smoking cessation. Cochrane Database Syst Rev 2008;2:CD000165.
44. Solberg LI, Maciosek MV, Edwards NM, et al. Repeated tobacco-use screening and intervention in clinical practice: health impact and cost effectiveness. Am J Prev Med 2006;31(1):62–71.
45. Babor T, Higgins-Biddle J. Brief interventions for hazardous and harmful drinking: a manual for use in primary care. Department of Mental Health and Substance Dependence WHO; 2001.
46. United States Preventive Services Task Force. Screening and behavioral counseling interventions in primary care to reduce alcohol misuse: recommendation statement. Ann Intern Med 2004;140(7):554–6.
47. United States Preventive Services Task Force. Screening and behavioral counseling interventions in primary care to reduce alcohol misuse: recommendation statement. Am Fam Physician 2004;70(2):353–8.
48. Madras BK, Compton WM, Avula D, et al. Screening, brief interventions, referral to treatment (SBIRT) for illicit drug and alcohol use at multiple healthcare sites: comparison at intake and 6 months later. Drug Alcohol Depend 2009;99(1–3):280–95.
49. Hedley AA, Ogden CL, Johnson CL, et al. Prevalence of overweight and obesity among US children, adolescents, and adults, 1999-2002. JAMA 2004;291(23):2847–50.

50. Ashenden R, Silagy C, Weller D. A systematic review of the effectiveness of promoting lifestyle change in general practice. Fam Pract 1997;14(2):160–76.

51. Kristal AR, Curry SJ, Shattuck AL, et al. A randomized trial of a tailored, self-help dietary intervention: the Puget Sound Eating Patterns study. Prev Med 2000; 31(4):380–9.

52. Robin AL, Siegel PT, Moye AW, et al. A controlled comparison of family versus individual therapy for adolescents with anorexia nervosa. J Am Acad Child Adolesc Psychiatry 1999;38(12):1482–9.

53. Lemmon CR, Josephson AM. Family therapy for eating disorders. Child Adolesc Psychiatr Clin North Am 2001;10(3):519–42, viii.

54. McCallum Z, Wake M, Gerner B, et al. Outcome data from the LEAP (Live, Eat and Play) trial: a randomized controlled trial of a primary care intervention for childhood overweight/mild obesity. Int J Obes (Lond) 2007;31(4):630–6.

55. Schwartz RP, Hamre R, Dietz WH, et al. Office-based motivational interviewing to prevent childhood obesity: a feasibility study. Arch Pediatr Adolesc Med 2007;161(5):495–501.

56. Bild D, Daniels SR, Donato S, et al. Working group report on future research directions in childhood obesity prevention and treatment. Bethesda (MD): National Heart Lung Blood Institute, National Institutes of Health; 2007.

57. Pentz MA. Understanding and preventing risks for obesity. In: DiClemente RJ, Crosby RA, Santelli JS, editors. Adolescent health: understanding and preventing risk behaviors. 1st edition. San Francisco (CA): Jossey-Bass; 2009. p. 147, 164 p.157,158.

58. Kaplan R. Adherence for patients with chronic obstructive pulmonary disease. In: Shumaker SA, Ockene JK, Riekert KA, editors. Handbook of health behavior change. 3rd edition. New York (NY): Springer; 2009. p. 617.

59. Exercise Promotion: Walking in Elders. 2007. Available at: http://www.guideline.gov/content.aspx?id=10948. Accessed October 30, 2011.

60. Physical activity and public health: updated recommendation for adults from the American College of Sports Medicine and the American Heart Association. 2008. Available at: http://www.guideline.gov/content.aspx?id=11688. Accessed October 30, 2011.

61. Sales JM, Milhausen RR, Diclemente RJ. A decade in review: building on the experiences of past adolescent STI/HIV interventions to optimise future prevention efforts. Sex Transm Infect 2006;82(6):431–6.

62. Latkin CA, Donnell D, Metzger D, et al. The efficacy of a network intervention to reduce HIV risk behaviors among drug users and risk partners in Chiang Mai, Thailand and Philadelphia, USA. Soc Sci Med 2009;68(4):740–8.

63. Celentano DD, Bond KC, Lyles CM, et al. Preventive intervention to reduce sexually transmitted infections: a field trial in the Royal Thai Army. Arch Intern Med 2000;160(4):535–40.

64. Crosby R, DiClemente RJ, Charnigo R, et al. A brief, clinic-based, safer sex intervention for heterosexual African American men newly diagnosed with an STD: a randomized controlled trial. Am J Public Health 2009;99(Suppl 1):S96–103.

65. Lareau SC, Yawn BP. Improving adherence with inhaler therapy in COPD. Int J Chron Obstruct Pulmon Dis 2010;5:401–6.

66. Frishman WH. Importance of medication adherence in cardiovascular disease and the value of once-daily treatment regimens. Cardiol Rev 2007;15(5):257–63.

67. Murdaugh C, Insel K. Problems with adherence in the elderly. In: Shumaker SA, Ockene JK, Riekert KA, editors. Handbook of health behavior change. 3rd edition. New York: Springer; 2009. p. 499–518.

68. Haynes RB, Yao X, Degani A, et al. Interventions to enhance medication adherence. Cochrane Database Syst Rev 2005;4:CD000011.
69. McQuaid EL, Kopel SJ, Klein RB, et al. Medication adherence in pediatric asthma: reasoning, responsibility, and behavior. J Pediatr Psychol 2003;28(5): 323–33.
70. Smith BA, Shuchman M. Problem of nonadherence in chronically ill adolescents: strategies for assessment and intervention. Curr Opin Pediatr 2005; 17(5):613–8.
71. Dean AJ, Walters J, Hall A. A systematic review of interventions to enhance medication adherence in children and adolescents with chronic illness. Arch Dis Child 2010;95(9):717–23.
72. Franklin VL, Waller A, Pagliari C, et al. A randomized controlled trial of Sweet Talk, a text-messaging system to support young people with diabetes. Diabet Med 2006;23(12):1332–8.
73. Welschen LM, Bloemendal E, Nijpels G, et al. Self-monitoring of blood glucose in patients with type 2 diabetes who are not using insulin: a systematic review. Diabetes Care 2005;28(6):1510–7.
74. Polonsky WH, Fisher L, Schikman CH, et al. Structured self-monitoring of blood glucose significantly reduces A1C levels in poorly controlled, noninsulin-treated type 2 diabetes: results from the Structured Testing Program study. Diabetes Care 2011;34(2):262–7.
75. Fisher WA, Kohut T, Schachner H, et al. Understanding self-monitoring of blood glucose among individuals with type 1 and type 2 diabetes: an information-motivation-behavioral skills analysis. Diabetes Educ 2011;37(1):85–94.
76. Piette JD. Enhancing support via interactive technologies. Curr Diab Rep 2002; 2(2):160–5.
77. Moreland EC, Volkening LK, Lawlor MT, et al. Use of a blood glucose monitoring manual to enhance monitoring adherence in adults with diabetes: a randomized controlled trial. Arch Intern Med 2006;166(6):689–95.
78. Jones H, Edwards L, Vallis TM, et al. Changes in diabetes self-care behaviors make a difference in glycemic control: the Diabetes Stages of Change (DiSC) study. Diabetes Care 2003;26(3):732–7.
79. Knight KM, McGowan L, Dickens C, et al. A systematic review of motivational interviewing in physical health care settings. Br J Health Psychol 2006;11(Pt 2): 319–32.
80. Piette JD. Interactive behavior change technology to support diabetes self-management: where do we stand? Diabetes Care 2007;30(10):2425–32.
81. Lim S, Kang SM, Shin H, et al. Improved glycemic control without hypoglycemia in elderly diabetic patients using the ubiquitous healthcare service, a new medical information system. Diabetes Care 2011;34(2):308–13.
82. Gale L, Vedhara K, Searle A, et al. Patients' perspectives on foot complications in type 2 diabetes: a qualitative study. Br J Gen Pract 2008;58(553):555–63.
83. Canadian Agency for Drugs and Technologies in Health. Rapid response report: summary of abstracts. Educational strategies for prevention of diabetic foot complications: clinical evidence and guidelines. Available at: http://cadth.ca/media/pdf/htis/feb-2011/K0317Diabetic_Foot_Complications_final.pdf. Accessed April 10, 2012.
84. Dorresteijn JA, Kriegsman DM, Valk GD. Complex interventions for preventing diabetic foot ulceration. Cochrane Database Syst Rev 2010;1:CD007610.
85. Copeland LA, Berg GD, Johnson DM, et al. An intervention for VA patients with congestive heart failure. Am J Manag Care 2010;16(3):158–65.

86. DeWalt DA, Malone RM, Bryant ME, et al. A heart failure self-management program for patients of all literacy levels: a randomized, controlled trial [ISRCTN11535170]. BMC Health Serv Res 2006;6:30.

87. Paradis V, Cossette S, Frasure-Smith N, et al. The efficacy of a motivational nursing intervention based on the stages of change on self-care in heart failure patients. J Cardiovasc Nurs 2010;25(2):130–41.

88. Feldman PH, Murtaugh CM, Pezzin LE, et al. Just-in-time evidence-based e-mail "reminders" in home health care: impact on patient outcomes. Health Serv Res 2005;40(3):865–85.

89. Haughney J, Fletcher M, Wolfe S, et al. Features of asthma management: quantifying the patient perspective. BMC Pulm Med 2007;7:16.

90. Janson SL, McGrath KW, Covington JK, et al. Individualized asthma self-management improves medication adherence and markers of asthma control. J Allergy Clin Immunol 2009;123(4):840–6.

91. Shah S, Peat JK, Mazurski EJ, et al. Effect of peer led programme for asthma education in adolescents: cluster randomised controlled trial. BMJ 2001; 322(7286):583–5.

92. Ford CA, Millstein SG, Halpern-Felsher BL, et al. Influence of physician confidentiality assurances on adolescents' willingness to disclose information and seek future health care. A randomized controlled trial. JAMA 1997;278(12): 1029–34.

93. Ford C, English A, Sigman G. Confidential health care for adolescents: position paper for the society for adolescent medicine. J Adolesc Health 2004;35(2): 160–7.

94. Olson AL, Gaffney CA, Hedberg VA, et al. Use of inexpensive technology to enhance adolescent health screening and counseling. Arch Pediatr Adolesc Med 2009;163(2):172–7.

95. George J, Elliott RA, Stewart DC. A systematic review of interventions to improve medication taking in elderly patients prescribed multiple medications. Drugs Aging 2008;25(4):307–24.

96. AHRQ. Preventing Disability in the Elderly With Chronic Disease. Research in Action 2002(3). Available at: http://www.ahrq.gov/research/elderdis.htm. Accessed April 10, 2012.

97. Berg K. Measuring balance in the elderly: preliminary development of an instrument. Physiotherapy Canada 1989;41(6):304–11.

98. Borg G. Borg's perceived exertion and pain scales. Champaign (IL): Human Kinetics; 1998.

99. Bennett J, Winters-Stone K. Motivating older adults to exercise: what works? Age Ageing 2011;40(2):148–9.

100. Langlois J, Keyl P, Guralnik J, et al. Characteristics of older pedestrians who have difficulty crossing the street. Am J Public Health 1997;87(3):393–7.

Self-Management Education and Support in Chronic Disease Management

Patrick T. McGowan, PhD[a,b],*

KEYWORDS

- Chronic conditions • Self-management support • The 5 As
- Community self-management programs • High-risk patients

KEY POINTS

- The difficulty of providing effective care for patients with chronic health conditions with additional challenges (eg, health literacy, homelessness, obesity, and unhealthy lifestyles) in an acute care setting.
- Self-management support strategies (ie, ways to assist patients to develop knowledge, skills and confidence) can influence patient behavior and be incorporated into office care.
- Evidence-based self-management support strategies and techniques enhance the efficiency and effectiveness of patient care.
- In addition to usual office care, health care professionals need to incorporate self-management support to influence patients' behavior and do whatever is possible to maximize the use and effectiveness of community services.

This information describes the rationale for incorporating SMS strategies into office practice. Health care professionals will know:

- The concept of self-management support.
- Communication techniques that encourage patients to express their most important concerns.
- How to obtain agreement with the patient to set the boundary for the visit.
- How to use strategies that coincide with the patient's readiness to address a behavior.
- Ways to get patients to make goals and action plans.
- How to teach patients a problem-solving process they can use in their lives.
- Evidence-based community self-management program.

The author has nothing to disclose.
[a] Centre on Aging, University of Victoria, Victoria, British Columbia, Canada; [b] Ladner Office, University of Victoria, Suite 210, 4907 Chisholm Street, Delta, British Columbia V4K 2K6, Canada
* Ladner Office, University of Victoria, Suite 210, 4907 Chisholm Street, Delta, British Columbia V4K 2K6, Canada.
E-mail address: pmcgowan@uvic.ca

In the current environment, it is likely that most patients are seeking assistance to manage chronic health problems, which is to be expected in light of current health, government, and media reports on the prevalence and increasing incidence of chronic conditions. As of 2009, almost half of all American adults were living with a chronic condition, and nearly 30% had 2 or more chronic conditions[1]; chronic diseases such as heart disease, cancer, hypertension, stroke, and diabetes accounted for 80% of all deaths.[2] Among patients living with 1 or more chronic conditions, nearly 25% report at least 1 activity limitation, such as difficulty walking.[1] Caring for patients with chronic diseases comprises more than 75% of health care costs and patients with chronic disease make up a disproportionate percentage of all physician office visits.[1] Despite the growing prevalence of chronic disease, evidence suggests that 30% to 80% of patients' expectations are not met in routine primary care visits[3] and there is diminishing satisfaction with the way the care is coordinated.[4,5]

Factors contributing to the increased incidence of chronic disease include the aging of the population as well as high rates of obesity, smoking, poor nutrition, decreased physical activity, and poor access to primary care.[6] For example, obesity increases the risk of developing chronic conditions such as diabetes and heart disease, and the rate of obesity in adults has doubled in the last 20 years.[6] In addition, more than one-third of all adults do not meet recommendations for aerobic physical activity and only 24% of adults report eating 5 or more servings of fruits and vegetables per day.[7] Several of the factors that contribute to the high incidence of chronic disease are modifiable lifestyle factors that serve as the target for chronic disease prevention and management.

People with multiple chronic conditions often require multiple health care providers and caregivers, which are rarely coordinated with one another.[1] In consumer surveys, more than half of patients with serious chronic conditions reported seeing 3 or more different physicians[8] and often received conflicting advice.[9] In providing care, a 2001 survey[1] of physicians reported that they were less satisfied providing care for people with chronic conditions than for all patients, and reported that coordinating care for people with chronic conditions was particularly difficult. Many thought that their training had not adequately prepared them to provide appropriate care, specifically to (1) coordinate in-home and community services, (2) educate patients with chronic conditions, (3) manage the psychological and social aspects of chronic care, (4) provide effective nutritional guidance, and (5) manage chronic pain. Many also thought that there was poor coordination between themselves and the myriad of nonmedical services, which led to unnecessary service use. Another consequence of poor coordination was that patients often received conflicting advice from different providers.[1]

Effective health care delivery requires thinking beyond specific disease management to the coordination of medical care and assistive services across care settings and among multiple providers. By reenvisioning health care delivery, the Chronic Care Model provides a multidimensional solution to this complex situation at the organizational, health care system, community, and individual levels.[10] SMS is one of the essential elements in this model and involves collaboratively helping patients to develop skills and confidence in their ability to manage.

SELF-MANAGEMENT SUPPORT

In recent years, the main task of managing a chronic health condition has been shifting to the patient, but considerable responsibility still remains with clinicians, who can use their expertise to inform, activate, and assist patients to self-manage. Primary care practices that have worked well with the management of acute conditions are having mixed success with helping patients to successfully manage their chronic conditions. For several chronic conditions, a large number of patients remain in poor control despite excellent evidence guiding management and treatment. For example, in the United States, two-thirds of persons with diabetes[11] and half of persons with hypertension[12] are inadequately controlled. In addition, evidence suggests that patient outcomes are mediated through patients' sense of empowerment, engagement, and behavior after they leave the medical setting; therefore, targeting patients' health beliefs and behaviors may be a more effective strategy for improving patient health and quality of life.

Definition of Self-Management Support

Self-management support (SMS) has emerged as a resource to assist patients, families, and caregivers in this changing environment. Although SMS has been defined in various ways, there seems to be a growing consensus on how it is understood. It is generally conceived as having an intervention comprising techniques, tools, and programs to help patients choose and maintain healthy behaviors. It is also seen as a fundamental transformation of the patient-caregiver relationship into a collaborative partnership.[13] When SMS is referred to as an outcome it usually describes a set of patient attitudes, skills, and behaviors. For example, the patient engaged in SMS would (1) have knowledge of the condition and/or its management; (2) adopt a care plan agreed and negotiated in partnership with health professionals; (3) actively share in decision making with health professionals; (4) monitor and manage signs and symptoms of the condition; (5) manage the impact of the condition on physical, emotional, occupational, and social functioning; (6) adopt lifestyles that address risk factors and promote health by focusing on prevention and early intervention; and (7) have access to and confidence in the patient's ability to use support services.[14]

SMS versus patient education

SMS differs from patient education in several ways. Patient education usually involves clinicians providing disease-specific information, teaching specific disease-related skills (eg, how to monitor glucose levels and how to use asthma medication), and contingency planning (ie, what to do if a situation occurs). SMS focuses more on teaching skills that can be generalized and that patients can use to manage their own health conditions independently. Self-management skills include learning how to solve problems, finding and using community resources effectively, working with the health care team, and learning how to initiate new health promotion behaviors. The major differences between patient education and self-management education have been clearly delineated[15]: (1) patient education provides information and teaches technical disease-related skills, whereas self-management teaches skills on how to act on problems; (2) problems covered in patient education are widespread common problems related to a specific disease, whereas the problems covered in self-management education are identified by the patient; (3) patient education is disease specific and offers information and technical skills related to the disease, whereas self-management provides problem-solving skills that are relevant to the consequences of chronic conditions in general; (4) patient education is based on the underlying theory that disease-specific knowledge creates behavior change, which in turn produces better outcomes, whereas self-management education is based on the theory that greater patient confidence in their capacity to make life-improving changes yields better clinical outcomes; (5) the goal of traditional patient education is compliance, whereas the goal in self-management education is increased self-efficacy and improved clinical outcomes; and (6) in traditional patient education, the health professional is the educator, but, in self-management, the educators may be health professionals, peer leaders, or other patients.

Both types of education are useful in assisting patients to achieve the best quality of life and independence. Although necessary, disease-specific patient education is generally not sufficient for people to manage a lifetime of chronic disease care.[16–18] With diabetes, a literature review found that information alone was not sufficient to improve clinical outcomes and greater patient knowledge did not correlate with improved glycemic control.[19] In another major review (Cochrane),[20] patient education alone did not improve health outcomes in patients with asthma. The evidence makes a strong case that the best type of education for patients experiencing chronic conditions should be multifaceted and include (1) disease-specific education, (2) general management skills (eg, problem solving, finding and using resources, working with the health care team); (3) use of strategies that increase patients' confidence (ie, self-efficacy) in their ability to engage in behaviors needed to manage their conditions on a daily basis; and (4) adequate peer role models and support networks that help in the initiation and maintenance of the desired behavioral changes.

INCORPORATING SMS INTO PRACTICE

SMS can take place in several ways: on an individual basis, between the clinician and the patient, family member, or peer; in disease-specific group education programs; in group settings led by either peer leaders or clinicians; and through interactive technology, such as online group self-management programs and text messaging. It can also take place in a variety of settings, the most popular being the clinicians' offices as increasing emphasis is being focused on using behavioral techniques during routine clinic visits.

SMS is a set of behavioral strategies clinicians can use to encourage patients to engage in managing their health conditions. Comprehensive general practice guidelines for working with high-risk patients including the homeless, refugees, and persons with low health literacy have been developed.[21–23] As shown in **Fig. 1**, specific tools

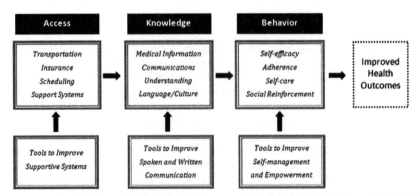

Fig. 1. Factors necessary to improve health outcomes and tools to help. (*From* DeWalt DA, Callahan LF, Hawk VH, et al. Health literacy universal precautions toolkit. Prepared by North Carolina Network Consortium, The Cecil G. Sheps Center for Health Services Research, The University of North Carolina at Chapel Hill, under Contract No. HHSA290200710014. AHRQ publication no. 10-0045-EF. Rockville (MD). Agency for Healthcare Research and Quality; 2010. p. 4.)

that clinicians can use with patients to help them improve supportive systems,[21] communication, self-management, and empowerment are described later.

A model that has provided structure to the interaction between health professionals and patients is the 5 As.[24] Several professional associations, such as the American Medical Association,[25] The Lifescripts Consortium,[26] and The Registered Nurses Association of Ontario,[27] have used the 5As construct as the basis for evidence-based best practice guidelines in providing SMS to adults with chronic health conditions.[13] This construct has also been used in caring for children experiencing chronic health conditions.[28] The 5 As are: assess, advise, agree, assist, and arrange. This construct has been applied to primary care interventions for a variety of behaviors[29–31] because the goal of the 5 As is to develop a personalized, collaborative action plan that includes specific behavioral goals and a specific plan for overcoming barriers and reaching those goals. There are several behavioral-oriented techniques within the 5 As construct that are interrelated but not necessarily sequential, and superior results will occur if a combination of techniques is used, especially for complex cases.[32] Comprehensive general practice guidelines for working with high-risk patients including the homeless, refugees, and persons with low health literacy are also available.[21–23] Specific strategies and techniques included in the 5 As construct increase patients' knowledge, skills, and confidence.

Establishing Rapport and Setting the Visit Agenda

Establishing a rapport with the patient and setting the visit agenda with the patient are key steps in SMS. Studies have shown that visits are most productive when clinicians take time to build rapport, listen actively, answer questions using lay terms, and focus on 2 or 3 key agenda items.[33–35] One way to help with building rapport with a patient is to encourage the patient to bring a partner or friend to visits; this person can help to provide additional support, assist with communication, and help with development of an appropriate, actionable care plan. Setting a visit agenda can be challenging because providers and patients often have differing ideas for the visit. The patients' perspective on illness usually revolves around patients' concerns, which include having clear explanations about the cause of the illness, and this sets expectations for the interaction. This often differs from the physicians' disease and diagnosis perspective in that it originates from a context based on personal, family, and cultural beliefs of which the health care provider may not be aware.[36] A provider may want to acknowledge his/her own agenda and then elicit the patient's and family member's goals for the visit. For example, a provider may say something like, "Good afternoon George, we have 15 minutes together today. I need to talk about your medicines, what do you want to talk to me about?" This technique provides an opportunity for both the clinician and patient to deal with their most important concerns. The clinician initiates the conversation, sets appointment boundaries (ie, "We have 15 minutes together"), and then sets out a sample agenda item. Because patients' first-voiced concern is often not the most pressing one,[37,38] providers can assist patients to prioritize their most immediate and important problem by asking, "What else is happening?" or, "Please tell me more about that…" Repeating this question 2 or 3 times may be required before the main problem surfaces, the problem that needs to be addressed before the others can be dealt with. This technique provides an opportunity for patients to identify and prioritize their most important concerns.

Screening for Depression

Untreated depression in individuals with comorbid chronic health conditions increases morbidity and mortality and reduces the capacity for self-management.[15] Major depression is a serious major health concern commonly seen in those with chronic conditions[39] and is one of the most common comorbidities associated with chronic illness. It is estimated that up to one-third of individuals with serious medical conditions experience symptoms of depression, and, with a growing elderly population and the associated increase in prevalence of chronic medical conditions, a concomitant increase in the prevalence of depression is anticipated.[40] Cross-sectional correlation studies using self-report surveys and screenings have confirmed that depression affects the ability to self-manage diabetes,[41,42] and a meta-analysis[43] found that, compared with nondepressed patients, depressed patients were 3 times more likely to be noncompliant with medical treatment recommendations. In addition, a population-based study[44] found that the prevalence of functional disability was higher in subjects with chronic conditions and comorbid major depression than in individuals with either chronic conditions or major depression alone. These results suggest that there is a joint effect of depression and chronic conditions on the ability to self-manage. Clinicians need to ensure that appropriate screening for depression occurs and that appropriate referrals and follow-up takes place. Commonly used screening tools are the Patient Health Questionnaire-2 (PHQ-2)[45] and The Geriatric Depression Scale (GDS).[46]

Closing the Loop and Using Ask-Tell-Ask

Studies suggest that patients often leave office visits without getting the information they want,[47,48] feeling overwhelmed and unable to understand the information that was provided.[49,50] To avoid misunderstanding and misinformation, providers can use an effective communication technique known as Ask-Tell-Ask and a related process known as Closing the Loop to ensure that patients understand the information. In a study involving adults with diabetes, using Closing the Loop resulted in improved patient comprehension and diabetes outcomes.[51] For example, to ensure the patient gets the required information, the clinician specifically inquires, "Please tell me what you want to know?" and then provides the relevant information. The clinician can then make sure the patient understands the information by asking, "I've given you a lot of information today, can you explain it back to me so I can be sure that I explained it clearly?" This exchange provides an opportunity to ensure the patient has understood the information and that any misunderstandings are addressed. The Ask-Tell-Ask technique focuses on patients identifying their own health goals, and behaviors that influence these goals, whereas Closing the Loop focuses on understanding.

Developing an Action Plan

A widely used technique to bring about patient behavior change is the action plan. It is used to encourage patients to initiate new behaviors (eg, walking, using soap when washing their hands), to modify existing behaviors (eg, eating, alcohol use, smoking), or to discontinue a behavior (eg, unsafe sex). The purpose of an action plan is to increase self-efficacy,[52] and self-efficacy is associated with healthier behaviors and improved clinical outcomes.[53]

The state of knowledge of the effectiveness of making goals and action plans to improve clinical outcomes is limited because action plans are usually included with other strategies in the intervention.[54] There is evidence suggesting that goal setting and making action plans can result in better diet; increased exercise and weight loss[55]; improved dietary fat, fruit, and vegetable intake[56–58]; healthy behaviors; and better clinical outcomes.[53,59] Research has found that goal setting and action planning seem to be effective across the socioeconomic spectrum.[60]

To assist a patient with developing an individualized action plan, a clinician may ask, "Is there anything you would like to do this week to improve your health?[61]

Clinicians can work with patients to identify a specific goal and to develop a short-term action plan that specifies something the patient wants to accomplish between the current visit and the next visit. A written template is then completed to clearly specify a behavior (eg, to go walking), degree (eg, 10 blocks), time of day (eg, during the afternoon), and number of times between this and the next visit (eg, 4 times). An acronym originating from the US Centers for Disease Control and Prevention commonly used to describe an action plan is SMART goals (specific, measurable, achievable, realistic, and time specific). The clinician then asks patients to indicate their level of confidence, or self-efficacy, in accomplishing the plan, rating their confidence on a scale of 0 to 10. The template is then signed by both parties and the patient takes a copy home after the visit. Following up on whether the patient accomplished the action plan is integral to the success of this process and time should be set aside in the next visit for patients to report back on their progress.

By working with the clinician to develop an action plan, patients choose a behavior that they are motivated to change and, through a goal-setting process, develop an action plan that is highly specific, achievable, and is based theoretically on self-efficacy (ie, the level of confidence that a person has to carry out the behavior). According to Bandura,[62] self-efficacy affects every phase of health behavior change: whether a person considers changing a health behavior; how much a person benefits from the changed behavior; how well a person maintains the change achieved; and how vulnerable a person is to relapse. The action plan must reflect contributions, preferences, and assessment of feasibility by the patient. Research has shown that patients who set specific goals with performance feedback have higher levels of goal achievement and adherence than patients who used informal goal setting or planning without specified goals.[63]

Patients are often overwhelmed by the complexity of managing chronic disease and find it difficult to initiate and maintain behaviors, not knowing how or where to start. The action planning process addresses this difficulty by breaking the behavior into small steps; for example, exercising can be broken into walking a certain distance a specified number of times. Self-efficacy theory is used by asking patients to specify their confidence in achieving the action plan, because the theory postulates that the more confidence the individual has, the greater probability the plan will be achieved. It does not matter what the action plan is about; the intent of the process is to teach the patient how to use the action planning process of accomplishing a task by breaking it into small, achievable steps, which is a well-documented process for developing higher levels of self-efficacy.

Problem Solving

Another core SMS skill is the ability to solve problems.[64–68] This process usually involves problem identification; generation of possible solutions, including the solicitation of suggestions from friends and health care professionals; solution implementation; and the evaluation of results. Clinicians can teach patients this process, whereby a problem is identified, possible solutions are generated, and one of the possible solutions is selected, implemented (often using an action plan), and then evaluated. Effective problem solving is critical for patients with chronic conditions who will most likely be facing health management issues and exacerbations in the course of their lives. The average amount of time patients spend with health professionals is less than 10 hours a year; therefore, patients need to use effective coping skills at home.[69] The use of problem solving has been shown to be effective with depression,[70,71] substance abuse,[70] cancer,[70] and in dietary behaviors.[70,72]

Using Pros and Cons and Motivational Interviewing

Using a decisional balance SMS technique known as Pros and Cons, clinicians can encourage patients to modify behavior when they are confident that the patients could carry out the particular behavior if they wanted to but may not believe that changing the behavior is important. In this process, the clinician asks the patient to list all of the good aspects about the current behavior (eg, alcohol use). The patient's response might include, "It helps me relax; I enjoy drinking with my friends; it takes away my boredom and stress; and I don't have to think about the bad things in my life." The clinician then asks the patient to list all of the not-so-good aspects about this alcohol-use behavior. Responses may include, It's hard on my health; it costs a lot of money; I get in a lot of fights; and I might lose my job and family." The role of clinicians is to guide the process and not enforce their own opinions on the good or bad aspects of the behavior. When patients review the written pros versus cons list, they usually see that there are more not-so-good aspects than good aspects and that the not-so-good aspects are more important. Experiencing this decisional balance is often all that is needed for patients to prepare for making a behavior change. The Pros and Cons method has been shown to be effective in the promotion of cancer[73] and diabetes screening.[74]

Motivational interviewing

While interacting with patients, clinicians have unique opportunities to apply strategies that encourage and motivate patients to make important behavior changes. Motivational interviewing (MI) is a patient-centered, directive method of communication with the goal of enhancing motivation to change behavior by exploring and resolving ambivalence.[75,76] however, with widespread dissemination of this complex technique, it is likely that reinvention has occurred, reflecting practitioners' particular understanding and style, and this reinvention may have further added or removed critical elements. To address these concerns, Miller and Rollnick[77] provided clarity with respect to what MI is and is not, specifically that MI, as detailed by Miller and Rollnick,[77] is a multistep process that (1) incorporates reflective listening to guide resolution of ambivalence about change; (2) is intended to enhance patients' motivation for change (change talk); (3) honors patient autonomy; (4) is a complex clinical skill that requires practice to increase proficiency, rather than a formula to be followed step by step; (5) is a method to elicit solutions from the patient, rather than to provide solutions for them; and (6) is not necessary if the patient is ready for change.

A recent meta-analysis by Rubak[78] evaluated the effectiveness of using MI with patients who had various diseases and found that MI produced significant effects in some areas (body mass index, total blood cholesterol, systolic blood pressure) but not in others (cigarettes smoked per day and A1C levels). Lewin and colleagues[79] recommended that MI be used to counsel patients/families on health behavior change and that MI may be most effective in brief encounters of 15 minutes or less. Several studies show that appropriately trained clinicians can successfully use MI skills with their patients.[78] Miller and Rollnick[77] recognize that most health care professionals learn about MI through self-study or in 1-hour or 2-hour workshops. They state that, although this clinical method is simple, it is not easy to master, requiring repeated practice with feedback and encouragement from knowledgeable guides to facilitate both skill and comfort of use.

There is increasing interest in stepped-care[80,81] approaches for SMS. In these approaches, patients with chronic health conditions are conceptualized at different levels of a pyramid depending on their level of disease and treatment complexity.

Healthier members of the public are at the lower level of the pyramid where prevention and early diagnosis of disease are the priorities. Health literacy is an integral component at this level. At the second level, where patients have some form of chronic illness, the emphasis shifts to self-management, the appropriate administration of medication, and health education. At the third level, patients experiencing complex diseases and requiring complex care are assigned care plans guided by case management and advanced SMS techniques.

Personal Health Records

An additional SMS strategy for clinicians to consider is to encourage patients to use monitoring methods, such as diaries, logs, or personal health records, to keep track of their health conditions, appointments, medications, and various providers. The American Health Information Management Association provides a guide to help patients choose a personal health record.[82] In addition, free user-friendly online personal health records are available from the Web (eg, Web MD PHR, My Health INFO, and Patient Ally). Clinicians could either distribute these or explain how to access them and provide a brief explanation on their use. Research on the value of monitoring methods such as personal health records is limited and has produced mixed results. Although some studies have found that people have high satisfaction with personal health records and think they can help in communicating more effectively with clinicians,[83–86] other studies[87,88] have found that these records were not effective in improving self-management or health-related behaviors. Even though the current evidence is limited and does not fully support the use of personal health record systems,[89] these inexpensive tools may be effective for particularly high-risk patients.

Group Visits

Another technique that is gaining popularity for providing SMS is group visits.[90,91] A common model involves groups of up to 10 patients seen together by the clinician for a 2-hour period. In a previous encounter, the clinician explains the group visit process to each patient and gets their consent to participate in the visit. For the first 20 minutes of the group visit, the clinician consults with each participant to establish their main concerns. Next, the clinician may provide a 20-minute lecture/explanation of a topic raised by several participants. Then, in the group with all participants listening, the clinician may address each participant's primary concern, which allows for vicarious peer learning. Brainstorming and problem solving are used whenever appropriate. At the end, each patient makes an action plan and develops a follow-up method. Group visits have been shown to improve efficiency, encourage and elicit greater adherence and satisfaction, improve health outcomes, and reduce hospitalizations with patients experiencing coronary artery disease[92] and diabetes,[93,94] and with chronically ill older adults.[95,96] A starter kit for conducting group visits is available online from Group Health Cooperative.[97]

Linking Patients to Community Resources

Traditional practices that have worked well with people experiencing acute conditions have limited success with high-risk patients needing to manage chronic conditions for their lifespan.[1,98] Therefore, patient care, particularly for high-risk patients, can be improved and supplemented by involving nonmedical community resources, which can provide numerous services, including transportation, food, shelter, financial assistance, and other public health services that may help to address patient challenges in managing the patient's own health. Because most patient outcomes are achieved through behaviors after they have left the clinical setting,[15] clinicians should direct efforts to providing appropriate community referrals and to ensuring that patients follow through with using these services. For example, research has shown that the probability of participating in a community self-management program increased 18 times when it was recommended by a health professional.[99] Additional practice efforts may be devoted to assisting with transportation problems, making follow-up telephone calls to the patient and community resource, involving a volunteer patient advocate/navigator, and/or making arrangements for involving other social agencies that deal with food, shelter, and basic necessities of life.

The most familiar and common way that evidence-based SMS is delivered in nonmedical community centers is through specially designed programs that emerged during the last decade. These programs include both disease-specific and generalized programs led by lay persons and health professionals.[100–102] A cursory review of recent literature reveals a growth in the development, scope, and evaluation of these programs and includes programs for adults and children with asthma,[103–105] cancer,[106] chronic obstructive pulmonary disease,[107] human immunodeficiency virus,[108] bulimia nervosa,[109] chronic kidney disease,[110] congestive heart disease,[111] dementia,[112] low vision,[113] macular degeneration,[114] depression,[115] and stroke.[116] In addition, the US National Council on Aging has recommended several evidence-based programs including the Chronic Disease Self-Management Program,[101] EnhancedWellness,[117] EnhancedFitness,[118] Active Choices,[119] Active Living Every Day,[120] Strong for Life,[121] A Matter of Balance,[122] Healthy IDEAS,[123] and Prevention & Management of Alcohol Problems in Older Adults: A Brief Intervention.[124] These programs have been shown to be effective across a wide range of settings for people with many different types of disease and for people from different cultures and socioeconomic groups. A comprehensive review on the strengths and weaknesses relating to program settings, using professional or lay leaders, using disease-specific or generic programs, and group or individual programs, has been published by McGowan and Lorig.[125]

These evidence-based self-management programs are being implemented through the US National Council on Aging. The programs provide basic information, teach specific skills, and use strategies to increase patients' confidence in their ability to manage their condition. Specific skills include (1) problem solving (learning to identify

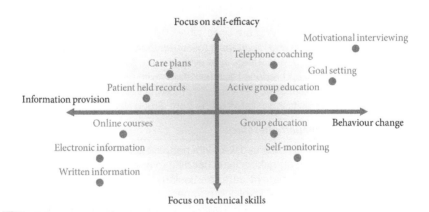

Fig. 2. Continuum strategies to support self-management. (*From* The Health Foundation. Evidence: helping people help themselves. London: The Health Foundation, 2011; with permission. Available at: http://www.health.org.uk/publications/evidence-helping-people-help-themselves/.)

a problem, generate possible solutions, implement a solution, and evaluate the results), (2) decision making (learning how to identify warning signals when caring for their symptoms, having suitable guidelines to follow, and making appropriate choices to manage their symptoms properly), (3) resource use (learning how to find and use resources effectively), (4) patient-provider relationships (learning how to build relationships with health care providers), and (5) taking action (learning how to carry out a specific behavior to achieve a goal, which patients learn to do by making short-term, realistic, and achievable action plans).

SUMMARY

SMS is an opportunity for clinicians to enhance the effectiveness of their medical and clinical expertise and, at the same time, to engage with and encourage patients to participate in managing their own personal care. This support is implemented by developing a coaching relationship with patients that clearly delineates the role and responsibilities of both players. Clinicians can use specific strategies and tools that encourage patients to engage in self-management, including the basic trio of self-management skills that includes goal setting, action planning, and problem solving.[61] In addition to integrating these SMS strategies in the office, clinicians can also directly link patients to evidence-based, community self-management programs.

Throughout the world, a wide range of methods (**Fig. 2**) have been described as supporting self-management interventions and are as varied as handing out leaflets and brochures, telemonitoring, intensive telephone coaching, MI, group and online programs, and structured education. The literature review conducted by The Health Foundation[126] found that not all mechanisms to support self-management had equal outcomes and that some approaches were significantly more effective than others. Interventions focusing on behavior change and supporting self-efficacy were associated with greater change and more sustained levels of behavioral change, clinical benefits, quality of life, and patterns of health care resource use.

The components that have been found to work well to support self-management include involving people in decision making; emphasizing problem solving; developing care plans as a partnership between service users and professionals; setting goals and following up on the extent to which these are achieved over time; promoting healthy lifestyles and educating people about their conditions and how to manage them; motivating people to self-manage using targeted approaches and structured information and support; helping people to monitor their symptoms and know when to take appropriate action; helping people to manage the social, emotional, and physical impacts of their conditions; proactive follow-up; and providing opportunities to share and learn from other service users.[126]

It is not clear how self-management works in the larger health care context. Investigating this process, the recent evaluation of SMS programs conducted by RAND Health[127] suggests a chain of self-management support effect. As patients participate in evidence-based self-management programs and interact with health professionals who use SMS strategies, they become more knowledgeable and skilled and have higher self-efficacy. This process influences their behavior as well as the behavior of their health providers. Patients attain better disease control, leading to improved health outcomes and higher patient satisfaction, which in turn leads to better health care use as well as improved workplace productivity and lower costs. Effective SMS strategies and programs not only involve changes at the clinician-patient level but also require changes at multiple levels: office environment, health system, policy, and environmental supports.[128]

A goal of health care providers is to provide evidence-based medicine; specifically, to use the best available evidence gained from the scientific method in medical decision making. However, for many chronic health conditions, a large proportion of people remain in poor control (eg, with diabetes and hypertension). At present, the US medical system is not structured to assist people in incorporating the advances of evidence-based medicine into their lives, and this is where SMS may show significant benefit. In addition, the physical and social environment in which people live create major challenges, making it difficult for them to make the changes required for disease control. Policy makers at all levels can have an impact in addressing this challenge. The broader goal is to achieve evidence-based health, which can be conceptualized as the synergetic impact of evidence-based medicine, self-management support, and community health services and policy.[129]

REFERENCES

1. Robert Wood Johnson Foundation. Chronic care: making the case for ongoing care. Available at: http://www.rwjf.org/files/research/50968chronic.care.chartbook.pdf. Accessed May 20, 2011.
2. Centers for Disease Control and Prevention. Chronic diseases and health promotion. Available at: http://www.cdc.gov/chronicdisease/overview/index.htm. Accessed June 10, 2011.
3. Kravitz RL. Patients' expectations for medical care: an expanded formulation based on review of the literature. Med Care Res Rev 1996;53(1):3–27.
4. Safran DG. Defining the future of primary care: what can we learn from patients? Ann Intern Med 2003;138:248–55.
5. Schoen C, Osborn R, Squires D, et al. New 2011 survey of patients with complex care needs in eleven countries finds that care is often poorly coordinated. Health Aff (Millwood) 2011;30(12):2437–48.
6. Triple Solution for a healthier America. The impact of chronic diseases on healthcare. Available at: http://www.forahealthieramerica.com/ds/impact-of-chronic-disease.html. Accessed May 20, 2011.
7. BRFSS prevalence and trends data. Atlanta (GA): Centers for Disease Control and Prevention; 2008. Available at: http://apps.nccd.cdc.gov/brfss/page.asp?cat=AC&yr=2007&state=US#AC. Accessed May 20, 2011.
8. The Gallup Organization. Serious chronic illness survey. Washington, DC: The Gallup Organization; 2002.
9. Harris Interactive, Inc. Chronic illness and caregiving. New York (NY): Survey conducted for Partnership for Solutions and Robert Wood Johnson Foundation 2000.
10. Wagner EH. Chronic disease management: what will it take to improve care for chronic illness? Eff Clin Pract 1998;1:2–4.
11. Saydah SH, Fradkin J, Cowie CC. Poor control of risk factors for vascular disease among adults with previously diagnosed diabetes. JAMA 2004;291(3):335–42.
12. Egan BM, Zhao Y, Axon RN. US trends in prevalence, awareness, treatment, and control of hypertension, 1988-2008. JAMA 2010;303:2043–50.
13. Bodenheimer T, MacGregor K, Sharifi C. Helping patients manage their chronic conditions. Oakland (CA): California Healthcare Foundation; 2005.
14. National Health Priority Action Council. Australian Government Department of Health and Ageing, Canberra (Australia). National chronic disease strategy. Available at: http://www.health.gov.au/internet/main/publishing.nsf/content/7E7E9140A3D3A3BCCA257140007AB32B/$File/stratal3.pdf. Accessed June 26, 2011.

15. Bodenheimer H, Lorig K, Holman H, et al. Patient self-management of chronic disease in primary care. JAMA 2002;288(19):2469–75.
16. Newman S, Steed L, Mulligan K. Self-management interventions for chronic illness. Lancet 2004;364(9444):1523–37.
17. Norris SL, Lau J, Smith SJ, et al. Self-management education for adults with type 2 diabetes: a meta-analysis of the effect on glycemic control. Diabetes Care 2002;25(7):1159–71.
18. Krichbaum K, Aarestad V, Buether M. Exploring the connection between self-efficacy and effective diabetes self-management. Diabetes Educ 2003;29(4): 653–62.
19. Norris SL, Engelgau MM, Narayan V. Effectiveness of self-management training in type 2 diabetes: a systematic review of randomized-controlled trials. Diabetes Care 2001;24(3):561–87.
20. Gibson PG, Powell H, Wilson A, et al. Limited (information only) patient education programs for adults with asthma. Cochrane Database Syst Rev 1998;1:CD001005.
21. DeWalt DA, Callahan LF, Hawk VH, et al. Health literacy universal precautions toolkit (Prepared by North Carolina Network Consortium, The Cecil G. Sheps Center for Health Services Research, The University of North Carolina at Chapel Hill, under Contract No. HHSA290200710014.) AHRQ Publication No. 10-0045-EF). Rockville (MD): Agency for Healthcare Research and Quality; 2010.
22. Canadian Public Health Association. Low health literacy and chronic disease prevention and control – perspectives from the health and public health sectors. Available at: http://www.cpha.ca/uploads/portals/h-l/kl_summary_e.pdf. Accessed June 10, 2011.
23. Bonin E, Brehove T, Kline S, et al. Adapting your practice: general recommendations for the care of homeless patients. Nashville: Health Care for the Homeless Clinicians' Network, National Health Care for the Homeless Council. Available at: http://www.nhchc.org/Publications/6.1.04GenHomelessRecsFINAL.pdf. Accessed June 10, 2011.
24. Glynn T, Manley M. How to help your patients stop smoking. A National Cancer Institute manual for physicians. Bethesda (MD): US Department of Health and Human Services; 1989. Report No.: NIH Pub No 89-3064.
25. American Medical Association. Physician resource guide to patient self-management support. Available at: http://www.ama-assn.org/ama1/pub/upload/mm/433/phys_resource_guide.pdf. Accessed January 16, 2011.
26. National Heart Foundation of Australia and Kinect Australia for the Lifescripts Consortium. Lifescripts practice manual: supporting lifestyle risk factor management in general practice. 2005. Available at: http://www.health.gov.au/internet/main/publishing.nsf/Content/23AC9B5E0B9169EECA25775F001A8AC6/$File/manualed1.pdf. Accessed January 16, 2011.
27. Registered Nurses Association of Ontario. Strategies to support self-management in chronic conditions: collaboration with clients. Available at: http://www.rnao.org/Storage/72/6710_SMS_Brochure.pdf. Accessed June 10, 2011.
28. Cincinnati Children's Hospital Medical Centre. Evidence-based care guidelines for chronic care: self-management. Cincinnati (OH): Cincinnati Children's Hospital Medical Centre; 2007.
29. Goldstein MG, DePue J, Kazura A. Models for provider-patient interaction: applications to health behavior change. In: Shumaker SA, Schon EB, Ockene JK, et al, editors. The handbook of health behavior change. New York: Springer; 1998. p. 85–113.

30. Ockene JK, Ockene IS, Quirk ME, et al. Physician training for patient-centered nutrition counselling in a lipid intervention trial. Prev Med 1995;24(6):563–70.

31. Pinto BM, Lynn H, Marcus BH, et al. Physician-based activity counseling: intervention effects on mediators of motivational readiness for physical activity. Ann Behav Med 2001;23(1):2–10.

32. Glasgow RE, Toobert DJ, Barrera M, et al. Assessment of problem-solving: a key to successful diabetes self-management. J Behav Med 2004;27:477–90.

33. Prochaska JO, Velicer WF, Rossi JS, et al. Stages of change and decisional balance for twelve problem behaviors. Health Psychol 1994;13:39–46.

34. Hettema J, Steele J, Miller WR. Motivational interviewing. Annu Rev Clin Psychol 2005;1:91–111.

35. Amrhein PC, Miller WR, Yahne CE, et al. Client commitment language during motivational interviewing predicts drug use outcomes. J Consult Clin Psychol 2003;71:862–78.

36. Lang F, Floyd MR, Beine KL, et al. Sequenced questioning to elicit the patient's perspective on illness: effects on information disclosure, patient satisfaction, and time expenditure. Fam Med 2002;34(5):325–30.

37. Barsky AJ. Hidden reasons some patients visit doctors. Ann Intern Med 1981; 94:492–8.

38. Burack RC, Carpenter RR. The predictive value of the presenting complaint. J Fam Pract 1983;16:749–54.

39. Chapman A, Gratz K. The borderline personality disorder survival guide. Oakland (CA): New Harbinger; 2007.

40. Moussavi S, Chatterji E, Verdes A, et al. Depression, chronic disease and decrements in health: results from the World Health Surveys. Lancet 2007;370(9590): 851–8.

41. Park H, Hong Y, Lee H, et al. Individuals with type 2 diabetes and depressive symptoms exhibited lower adherence with self-care. J Clin Epidemiol 2004;57: 978–84.

42. Lerman I, Lozano L, Villa AR, et al. Psychosocial factors associated with poor diabetes self-care management in a specialized center in Mexico City. Biomed Pharmacother 2004;58(10):566–70.

43. DiMatteo MR, Lepper HS, Croghan TW. Depression is a risk factor for noncompliance with medical treatment: meta-analysis of the effects of anxiety and depression on patient adherence. Arch Intern Med 2000;160(14):2101–7.

44. Schmitz N, Wang J, Malla A, et al. Joint effect of depression and chronic conditions on disability: results from a population-based study. Psychosom Med 2007;69:332–8.

45. Kroenke K, Spitzer RL, Williams JB. The Patient Health Questionnaire 2: validity of a two-item depression screener. Med Care 2003;4(11):1284–92.

46. Yesavage JA, Brink TL, Rose TL, et al. Development and validation of a geriatric depression screening scale: a preliminary report. J Psychiatr Res 1982–1983; 17(1):37–49.

47. Iliffe S, Lenihan P, Orrell M, et al. The development of a short instrument to identify common unmet needs in older people in general practice. Br J Gen Pract 2004;54:914–8.

48. Smith F, Orrell M. Does the patient-centred approach help identify the needs of older people attending primary care? Age Ageing 2007;36:628–31.

49. Heisler M, Bouknight RR, Hayward A, et al. The relative importance of physician communication, participatory decision making, and patient understanding in diabetes self-management. J Gen Intern Med 2002;17(4):243–52.

50. Gallagher R. How to improve our patients' health literacy. BCMJ 2008;50(9): 525–6.
51. Schillinger D, Piette J, Grumbach K, et al. Closing the Loop. Physician communication with diabetic patients who have low health literacy. Arch Intern Med 2003;163:83–90.
52. Bodenheimer T, Davis C, Holman H. Helping patients adopt healthier behaviors. Clin Diabetes 2007;25(2):66–70.
53. Marks R, Allegrante JP, Lorig K. A review and synthesis of research evidence for self-efficacy enhancing interventions for reducing chronic disability: implications for health education practice (part 1). Health Promot Pract 2005;6(1):37–43.
54. Bodenheimer T, Handley MA. Goal-setting for behaviour change in primary care: an exploration and status report. Patient Educ Couns 2009;76(2): 174–80.
55. Ammerman A, Pignone M, Fernandez L, et al. Counselling to promote a healthy diet. Systematic evidence review (prepared by the Research Triangle Institute/ University of North Carolina under Contract No 290-97-0011). Rockville (MD): Agency for Healthcare Research and Quality; 2002. Available at: http://www. ahrz.gov/downloads/pub/prevent/pdfser/dietser.pdf. Accessed June 10, 2011.
56. Cullen KW, Baranowski T, Smith SP. Using goal setting as a strategy for dietary behaviour change. J Am Diet Assoc 2001;101(5):562–6.
57. Pignone MP, Ammerman A, Fernandez L, et al. Counseling to promote a healthy diet in adults: a summary of the evidence for the U.S. Preventive Services Task Force. Am J Prev Med 2003;24(1):75–92.
58. Shilts MK, Horowitz M, Townsend MS. Goal setting as a strategy for dietary and physical activity behaviour change: a review of the literature. Am J Health Promot 2004;19:81–3.
59. Lippke S, Wiedemann AU, Ziegelmann JP, et al. Self-efficacy moderates the mediation of intentions into behavior via plans. Am J Health Behav 2009; 33(5):521–9.
60. Handley M, MacGregor K, Schillinger D, et al. Using action plans to help primary care patients adopt healthy behaviors: a descriptive study. J Am Board Fam Med 2006;19(3):224–31.
61. Bodenheimer T, Grumbach K. Improving primary care: strategies and tools for a better practice. New York: McGraw-Hill; 2007.
62. Bandura A. Social foundations of thought and action: a social cognitive theory. Englewood Cliffs (NJ): Prentice Hall; 1986.
63. Strecher VJ, Seijts GH, Kok G, et al. Goal setting as a strategy for health behavior change. Health Educ Q 1995;22:190–200.
64. Funnell MM, Brown TL, Childs BP. National standards for diabetes self-management education. Diabetes Educ 2008;31(S1):97–104.
65. Glasgow RE, Funnell MM, Bonomi AE, et al. Self-management aspects of the improving chronic illness breakthrough series: implementation with diabetes and heart failure teams. Ann Behav Med 2002;24:80–7.
66. Glasgow RE, Davis CL, Funnell MM, et al. Implementing practical interventions to support chronic illness self-management. Jt Comm J Qual Saf 2003;29(11):563–74.
67. Lorig KR, Holman H. Self-management education: history, definition, outcomes, and mechanisms. Ann Behav Med 2003;26(1):1–7.
68. Whitlock EP, Orleans T, Pender N. Evaluating primary are behavioral counseling interventions: an evidence-based approach. Am J Prev Med 2002;22(4):267–84.
69. Anderson RM, Funnell MM. Patient empowerment: myths and misconceptions. Patient Educ Couns 2010;79:277–82.

70. Malouff JM, Thorsteinsson EB, Schutte NS. The efficacy of problem solving therapy in reducing mental and physical health problems: a meta-analysis. Clin Psychol Rev 2007;27:46–57.
71. Bell AC, D'Zurilla TJ. Problem-solving therapy for depression: a meta-analysis. Clin Psychol Rev 2009;29(4):348–53.
72. Hill-Briggs F, Gemmell L. Problem solving in diabetes self-management and control: a systematic review of the literature. Diabetes Educ 2007;33(6): 1032–52.
73. Strong C, Liang W. Relationships between decisional balance and stage of adopting mammography and Pap testing among Chinese American women. Cancer Epidemiol 2009;33(5):374–80.
74. Kellar I, Sutton S, Griffin S, et al. Evaluation of an informed choice intervention for type 2 diabetes screening. Patient Educ Couns 2008;72(2):232–8.
75. Miller WR, Rollnick S. Motivational interviewing: preparing people for change. 2nd edition. New York: Guilford Press; 2002.
76. The motivational interviewing page. Available at: http://www.motivationalinterview. org. Accessed June 10, 2011.
77. Miller MR, Rollnick S. Ten things that motivational interviewing is not. Behav Cogn Psychother 2009;37(2):129–40.
78. Rubak S, Sandbaek A, Lauritzen T, et al. Motivational interviewing: a systematic review and meta-analysis. Br J Gen Pract 2005;55(513):305–12.
79. Lewin SA, Skea ZC, Entwistle V, et al. Interventions for providers to promote patient-centred approach in clinical consultations. Cochrane Database Syst Rev 2001;(4):CD003267. DOI: 10.1002/14651858.CD003267.
80. Glasgow R. A practical model of diabetes management and education. Diabetes Care 1995;18:117–26.
81. Von Korff M, Tiemens B. Individualized stepped care of chronic illness. West J Med 2000;172:133–7.
82. AHIMA Personal Health Record Practice Council. Helping consumers select PHRs: questions and considerations for navigating an emerging market. J AHIMA 2006; 77(10):50–6.
83. Sherger JE. Primary care needs a new model of office practice. BMJ 2005;330: E358–9.
84. Tang PC, Lansky D. The missing link: bridging the patient-provider health information gap. Health Aff (Millwood) 2005;24:1290–5.
85. Tang PC, Black W, Buchanan J, et al. PAMFOnline: integrating ehealth with an electronic medical record system. AMIA Annu Symp Proc 2003;2003:644–8.
86. Wald JS, Middleton B, Bloom A, et al. A patient-controlled journal for an electronic medical record: issues and challenges. Stud Health Technol Inform 2004;107(Pt 2):1166–70.
87. Newell SA, Sanson-Fisher R, Girgis A, et al. Can personal health record booklets improve cancer screening behaviors? Am J Prev Med 2002;22(1):15–22.
88. Grant RW, Wald JS, Schnipper JL, et al. Practice-linked online personal health records for type 2 diabetes mellitus: a randomized controlled trial. Arch Intern Med 2008;168(16):1776–82.
89. Tang PC, Ash JS, Bates DW, et al. Personal health records: definitions, benefits, and strategies for overcoming barriers to adoption. J Am Med Inform Assoc 2006;13(2):121–6.
90. Scott JC, Conner DA, Venohr I, et al. Effectiveness of a group outpatient visit model for chronically ill older health maintenance organization members. J Am Geriatr Soc 2004;52:1463–70.

91. Noffsinger EB, Scott JC. Understanding today's group visit models. Group Pract J 2000;49(2):48–58.
92. Masley S, Phillips S, Copeland JR. Group office visits change dietary habits of patients with coronary artery disease –the dietary intervention and evaluation trail (D.I.E.T.). J Fam Pract 2001;50(3):235–9.
93. Trento M, Passera P, Tomalino M, et al. Group visits improve metabolic control in type 2 diabetes: a 2-year follow up. Diabetes Care 2001;24:995–1000.
94. Sadur CN, Moline N, Costa M, et al. Diabetes management in a health maintenance organization. Diabetes Care 1999;22:2011–7.
95. Coleman EA, Eilertsen TB, Kramer AM, et al. Reducing emergency visits in older adults with chronic illness. A randomized, controlled trial of group visits. Eff Clin Pract 2001;4:49–57.
96. Beck A, Scott J, Williams P, et al. A randomized trial of group outpatient visits for chronically ill older HMO members: the cooperative health care clinic. J Am Geriatr Soc 1997;45:543–9.
97. Group Health Cooperative. Group visit starter kit. Available at: http://www.umassmed.edu/uploadedFiles/diabetes/resources/GroupVisitPlannerStarterKit.pdf. Accessed January 16, 2012.
98. Accessed June 5, 2011. Health Council of Canada. Stepping it up: moving the focus from health care in Canada to a healthier Canada. Available at: http://www.healthcouncilcanada.ca/docs/rpts/2010/promo/HCCpromoDec2010.pdf. Accessed January 16, 2012.
99. Murphy L, Theis K, Brady T, et al. A health care provider's recommendation is the most influential factor in taking an arthritis self-management course: a national perspective from the arthritis conditions and health effects survey. Arthritis Rheum 2009;56(9):S307–8.
100. Lorig K, Lubeck D, Kraines RG, et al. Outcomes of self-help education for patients with arthritis. Arthritis Rheum 1985;28(6):680–5.
101. Lorig KR, Sobel DS, Stewart AL, et al. Evidence suggesting that a chronic disease self-management program can improve health status while reducing hospitalization. Med Care 1999;37:5–14.
102. Barlow J, Wright C, Sheasby J, et al. Self-management approaches for people with chronic conditions: a review. Patient Educ Couns 2002;48(2):177–87.
103. Vazqueza I, Romero-Fraisa E, Blanco-Apariciob M, et al. Psychological and self-management factors in near-fatal asthma. J Psychosom Res 2010;68(2):175–81.
104. Espinoza-Palma T, Zamorano A, Arancibia F, et al. Effectiveness of asthma education with and without a self-management plan in hospitalized children. J Asthma 2009;46(9):906–10.
105. Guevara JP, Wolf FM, Grum CM, et al. Effects of educational interventions for self-management of asthma in children and adolescents: systematic review and meta-analysis. BMJ 2003;326(7402):1308–9.
106. Van Weert E, Hoekstra-Weebers JE, May AM, et al. The development of an evidence-based physical self-management rehabilitation programme for cancer survivors. Patient Educ Couns 2008;7(12):169–90.
107. Bourbeau J, Nault D, Dang-Tan T. Self-management and behaviour modification in COPD. Patient Educ Couns 2004;52(3):271–7.
108. Gifford AL, Groessl EJ. Chronic disease self-management and adherence to HIV medications. J Acquir Immune Defic Syndr 2002;31(53):S163–6.
109. Carrard I, Rouget P, Fernandez-Aranda F, et al. Evaluation and deployment of evidence based patient self-management support program for bulimia nervosa. Int J Med Inform 2006;75(1):101–9.

110. Thomas-Hawkins C, Zazworksky D. Self-management of chronic kidney disease. Am J Nurs 2005;105(10):40–8.

111. Baker DW, Asch SM, Keesey JW, et al. Differences in education, knowledge, self-management activities, and health outcomes for patients with heart failure cared for under the chronic disease model: the improving chronic illness care evaluation. J Card Fail 2005;11(6):405–13.

112. Mountain G. Self-management for people with early dementia: an exploration of concepts and supporting evidence. Dementia 2006;5(3):429–46.

113. Rees G, Saw CL, Lamoureux EL, et al. Self-management programs for adults with low vision: needs and challenges. Patient Educ Couns 2007;69(1):39–46.

114. Brody BL, Roch-Levecq AC, Thomas RG, et al. Self-management of age-related macular degeneration at the 6-month follow up: a randomized controlled trial. Arch Ophthalmol 2005;123(1):46–53.

115. Bachman J, Swenson S, Reardon ME, et al. Patient self-management in the primary care treatment of depression. Adm Policy Ment Health 2006;33(1):76–85.

116. Jones F. Strategies to enhance chronic disease self-management: how can we apply this to stroke? Disabil Rehabil 2006;28(13–14):841–7.

117. Phelan EA, Williams B, Leveille S, et al. Outcomes of a community-based dissemination of the health enhancement program. J Am Geriatr Soc 2002; 50(9):1519–24.

118. Ackermann RT, Cheadle A, Sandhu N, et al. Community exercise program use and changes in healthcare costs for older adults. Am J Prev Med 2003;25(3): 232–7.

119. Castro CM, King AC. Telephone-assisted counselling for physical activity. Exerc Sport Sci Rev 2002;30(2):64–8.

120. Wilcox S, Dowda M, Griffin SF, et al. Results of the first year of Active for Life: translation of two evidence-based physical activity programs for older adults into community settings. J Am Public Health 2006;96(7):1201–9.

121. Etkin CD, Prohaska TR, Harris BA, et al. Feasibility of implementing the Strong for Life program in community settings. Gerontologist 2006;46(2):284–92.

122. Tennsdedt S, Howland J, Lachman M, et al. A randomized controlled trial of a group intervention to reduce fear of falling and associated activity restriction in older adults. J Gerontol 1998;54(6):384–92.

123. Ciechanowski P, Wagner EH, Schmaling KB, et al. Community-integrated home-based depression treatment in older adults: a randomized controlled trial. JAMA 2004;291(13):1569–77.

124. Barry KL, Blow FC. Management of alcohol problems in older adults: screening and brief intervention implementation manual. Available at: http://www.healthyaging programs.org/content.asp?sectionid=71&ElementID=338. Accessed June 5, 2011.

125. McGowan P, Lorig K. The delivery of self-management interventions. In: Newman S, Steed L, Mulligan K, editors. Chronic physical illness: self-management and behavioural interventions. Berkshire (England): Open University Press, McGraw-Hill; 2008. p. 78–97.

126. De Silva D. Helping people help themselves: a review of the evidence considering whether it is worthwhile to support self-management. Available at: http://www.health. org.uk/public/cms/75/76/313/2434/Helping%20people%20help%20themselves% 20publication.pdf?realName=03JXkw.pdf. Accessed May 25, 2011.

127. Patient self-management support programs: an evaluation. Final contract report. AHRQ Publication No. 08-0011. Rockville (MD): Agency for Healthcare Research and Quality; 2007. Available at: http://www.ahrq.gov/qual/ptmgmt/. Accessed June 5, 2011.

128. Battersby M, Von Korff M, Schaefer J, et al. Twelve evidence-based principles for implementing self-management support in primary care. Jt Comm J Qual Patient Saf 2010;36(12):561–70.
129. Moskowitz D, Bodenheimer T. Moving from evidence-based medicine to evidence-based health. J Gen Intern Med 2010;26(6):658–60.

Health Information Technology

Transforming Chronic Disease Management and Care Transitions

Shaline Rao, MD[a,*], Craig Brammer, BA[a], Aaron McKethan, PhD[a],
Melinda B. Buntin, PhD[b]

KEYWORDS

- Health information technology • Electronic health records • Meaningful use
- Care transitions • Chronic disease management

KEY POINTS

- Adoption and use of health information technology (HIT) is a key effort in improving care delivery, reducing costs of health care, and improving the quality of health care in an era in which 90 million Americans suffer from chronic disease and nearly 7 out of every 10 deaths can be attributed to the impact of a chronic disease.
- Early evidence of cost and quality benefits from electronic health record (EHR) use suggest that HIT will play a significant role in transforming primary care practices and chronic disease management in the coming years.
- EHRs and HIT can be used effectively to manage chronic diseases, HIT can facilitate communication and reduce efforts related to transitions in care, and HIT can improve patient safety by increasing the available information to all providers and to the patient as well, improving disease management and safety simultaneously.

New technology is critical to the progress and success of medicine. When Rene Laennec developed the stethoscope, he revolutionized the ability to use physical examination to improve diagnostic accuracy. Alexander Fleming discovered penicillin, preventing countless deaths from the complications of infection. Providers have long embraced technologic changes in all forms, taking advantage of medical and nonmedical developments to ensure their patients' health. Examples include the electrocardiogram, magnetic resonance imaging, and telephone-based note dictation services.[1] The newest frontier of technology that is affecting the practice of medicine is HIT. HIT refers to the

The authors have no disclosures.
[a] Office of the National Coordinator for Health Information Technology, US Department of Health and Human Services, 200 Independence Avenue SW, Suite 729-D, Washington, DC 20201, USA; [b] Division of Health and Human Resources, Congressional Budget Office, Ford House Office Building, 4th Floor Second and D Streets, SW, Washington, DC 20515-6925, USA
* Corresponding author.
E-mail address: shaline.rao@columbia.edu

Prim Care Clin Office Pract 39 (2012) 327–344
doi:10.1016/j.pop.2012.03.006   **primarycare.theclinics.com**
0095-4543/12/$ – see front matter © 2012 Elsevier Inc. All rights reserved.

technologies that allow a provider to capture patient information electronically through EHRs, share this information among providers through a secure health information exchange network, improve medication adherence and safety with electronic prescribing, and to engage patients and families using patient portals and telehealth capabilities.[2] HIT has the potential to improve the quality of care delivered, reduce the costs associated with delivering health care, and engage patients and families in innovative ways.[3]

Provider rates of adopting EHR systems, use of electronic prescribing, and participation in efforts to exchange information regionally have increased steadily in the last 10 years.[4,5] Although hospitals and large health systems have led the way in this movement, primary care practices and community-based practitioners are increasingly embracing EHR and other technology solutions to improve the quality of care they deliver. EHRs, electronic prescribing, secure information exchange, and telehealth are a few of the ways that HIT expands beyond the basic purpose of capturing a patient history electronically, especially for patients with complex or chronic disease, for which these tools have the potential to improve patient care by drawing on information tailored to the patient and to improve coordination among providers as these patients move through multiple sites of care.

Chronic diseases result in significant economic, health, and quality-of-life burdens for individuals, families, and communities. More than 90 million Americans suffer from chronic disease, and chronic disease leads to 7 out of every 10 deaths.[6] As the population continues to age and medical advances reduce mortality from chronic diseases, there will be an increase in the numbers of patients living with 1 or more chronic diseases, a need to improve the care these patients receive, and a need to lower the costs associated with caring for them. Health IT is a key effort to ensure achievement of these goals.

The United States Federal Government took note of early investments and the resulting savings and quality improvements enabled by EHRs[7] and created the Office of the National Coordinator for Health IT in 2004. More recently, legislators have encouraged increased adoption of HIT with the Health Information Technology for Economic and Clinical Health (HITECH) Act, a provision of the American Recovery and Reinvestment Act of 2009. With the investment of federal funds into HIT and the growing interest between providers and patients to use HIT to improve health care, HIT innovations are likely to play a significant role in primary care practices and chronic disease management in the coming years.

This article discusses the role of HIT in transforming primary care management of chronic disease. Recent federal efforts to improve adoption of EHRs are described, as well as the role HIT can play in managing complex chronic disease, the role of HIT in patient engagement, how HIT can transform health care transitions, and the future directions of HIT and chronic disease management.

BACKGROUND: FEDERAL LEGISLATION

To accelerate the use of HIT and EHRs, Congress passed the HITECH Act. HITECH committed between $14 billion and $27 billion in incentive payments to hospitals and individual providers for adopting and effectively using a certified EHR during the course of care.[8] Certified products ensure that newly adopted EHRs have the functionalities necessary to affect cost, quality, and patient engagement. The legislation also expanded the Office of the National Coordinator through several programs created to guide physicians, hospitals, and other health care providers as they adopt EHRs and become meaningful users.

For primary care providers, the meaningful use of an EHR can result in payments from the Center for Medicare and Medicaid Services to defray the costs associated with incorporating an EHR into practices.[8] To become a meaningful user of EHRs, there are core functionalities that must be present in the EHRs used, and core measures that must be met. As detailed in the *New England Journal of Medicine* and on the Office of the National Coordinator's Web site, these core objectives and measures represent stage 1 of the meaningful use program.[8,9] In the next few years, these objectives will become more focused on quality and outcome rather than on process and data capture. For example, data capture includes ensuring that a record system tracks single point data, such as age, gender, baseline blood pressure, and recent hemoglobin A1C test results. Capturing this type of data is the first step to better management of patients and is the information-gathering phase of HIT adoption. As HIT systems become more sophisticated and more complete over time, providers will be encouraged to transition from simple data capture to data analysis, such as identifying individual blood pressure trends and ensuring that they meet guidelines, as well as tracking a provider's patient panel to determine whether, on average, their diabetic patients' A1C levels are on target. Adopting and effectively using an EHR takes time and patience, and the federal legislative parameters are designed to accommodate the growing pains of a primary care practice adopting and using an EHR.

To improve the experience of those who are newly adding EHRs systems, the Regional Extension Center Program was built out of the HITECH legislation. Congress allotted $667 million in 2009 to 2010 to create centers across the United States designed to help practices choose, implement, and meaningfully use EHRs in all practice sizes and environments.[10] Currently, primary care physicians are target priority providers for the extension centers. Using lessons learned from early adopters and local champions in the health care community, the extension centers will streamline the adoption and integration process, allowing providers to take advantage of the capabilities like clinical decision support tools, registry development tools, and electronic prescribing built into EHRs, specifically improving their ability to manage patients with complex and chronic disease. An interested provider wanting to partner with and use resources for HIT provided by their regional extension center can identify the closest center using the Office of the National Coordinator Web site.[11]

HIT AND CHRONIC DISEASE MANAGEMENT

HIT, and specifically EHRs, electronic prescribing, information exchange networks, and patient-facing portals, can play a crucial role in improving the outcomes and management of chronic diseases like cardiovascular disease and diabetes. Many models of chronic disease management have been proposed, all targeting similar goals. In the Kaiser model, chronic disease management refers to the need for the following services from primary care providers and their partners[12]:

- Disease management for people who need regular follow-up care and are at high risk
- Supporting self-care for people with a chronic disease who are at low risk of complications and hospitalization
- Case and transition management for people with complex needs who are high-intensity users of unplanned secondary care.

From the primary care provider perspective, HIT and EHRs touch on and enhance each of these key steps involved in chronic disease management. HIT, including

EHRs, is designed to improve the costs associated with chronic disease, assist in the management of the high-risk individual, track and improve quality measures, and empower patients and family.

Managing the High-Risk Individual

Individuals with 1 or more chronic diseases are at high risk for hospitalization, adverse drug events, and poor outcomes. Chronic disease management in the office, therefore, involves identifying and meeting patients' needs and controlling the disease to avoid hospitalization and disease progression. Effective care of these patients requires timely ordering of screening tests and preventative health visits, routine monitoring, availability to answer questions for the patient, management of medications to optimize disease control, and a multidisciplinary, evidence-based approach to applying care. The requisite knowledge, options for medications, and evidence-based best practices for each chronic disease are increasing and pose a significant challenge for each practitioner to apply efficiently to each individual patient.

EHRs can take a customized approach to each patient and support the provider in tracking, coordinating, and managing necessary tasks. EHRs have many capabilities, known among technology developers as functionalities, and they represent the features within an EHR that help clinicians and patients manage disease. One example is the clinical decision support systems, which can trigger alerts for screening tests and overdue care, help schedule follow-up appointments, and facilitate ordering of appropriate tests and specialist referrals.[13] Reminders for cardiovascular and diabetic care have been shown in a randomized control trial of 8500 patients in 17 health systems to improve rates of receiving recommended care.[14] Guidelines for care can be mapped onto individual patients based on their recent laboratory data and visit history, allowing the latest guidelines to be acknowledged and addressed at each visit. A recent retrospective study of 23,000 patients with clinical decision support used in EHRs to screen patients for cardiovascular risk factors revealed that automated selection of patients in need of antiplatelet and lipid-lowering therapy targeted similar rates of at-risk individuals in the study population more rapidly but with equal accuracy to manual review by a physician, suggesting that HIT can save time for providers but still accurately identify the at-risk patients.[15] Collecting information into an electronic system and enhancing this system with secure information exchange has been shown to reduce admissions to the hospital from the emergency room and, in one study from Vanderbilt, resulted in $1 million cost reduction per year in their study hospitals, through decreased testing and decreased hospitalizations when patient information was readily available.[16]

Ensuring Patient Safety

Patient safety in chronic disease can also be improved via EHR functionalities, specifically using electronic prescribing, drug interaction alerts, allergy documentation prompts, and alerts to notify providers of missed opportunities for medications.[17] A randomized study of warfarin interactions, a medicine frequently used for atrial fibrillation, showed a reduction in warfarin interactions using EHRs to screen and alert providers.[18] This study involved 9900 patients with about one-third on interacting prescriptions (warfarin plus another medication). Initiation of an EHR in all study centers with interaction alerts shows a decrease in interacting prescriptions; however, the total interactions did not decrease to zero. A recent survey of providers at the Veterans Affairs (VA) affiliated with the University of California, Los Angeles (UCLA) showed that providers perceived electronic documentation of allergies and current medications as important in preventing drug interactions and polypharmacy, but only some providers found the drug interaction alert helpful, especially those who were practicing subspecialty care.[19] Reducing adverse drug reactions, improving adherence to medication guidelines, and improving preventative health all have the potential to improve chronic disease outcomes and reduce the costs associated with chronic disease, but the evidence is still growing as technologies develop around provider and patient needs.[20–22] One limitation of drug interaction alerts is that many types of interactions exist, and there is no literature yet on the best way to stratify alerts or effective ways to prevent overalerting.

Improving Communication

Another driver of cost and quality-of-life infringement in the outpatient community is the need to bring patients to the office for simple requests or to share routine information. Managing a chronic disease can be overwhelming for a patient, and being unable to reach a known provider or unable to find information often prompts a patient to seek care at an emergency department, urgent care, or to come to the clinic for more frequent appointments.[23] EHRs have the capacity to improve communication using secure messaging and data exchange. Secure messaging has been shown to accommodate a variety of communication needs, including patient-provider conversations on patient portals, reminders for medications and scheduled visits using mobile devices or patient portals, provider-provider discussions via e-mail or a secure portal, and communication of results using similar avenues. Data and information exchange allows information from hospitals, specialty clinics, laboratories, and radiology centers to securely send data to a patient's record. Providers and patients then have information more readily available, and unnecessary studies and delays are avoided. A recent meta-analysis by the University of Minnesota on literature pertaining to secure exchange showed that improved access to information improved efficiency but that the availability of exchange was limited by privacy concerns, leading to inconclusive data around cost savings and quality improvement.[24,25] Chronic disease management requires not only preventing onset of disease but also finding cost-effective ways to deliver care. HIT and EHRs aid in coordinating care and creating new venues for information sharing so that costs associated with unnecessary or delayed testing, adverse drug events, and unnecessary visits are all reduced.[7] In addition to providing clinicians with the opportunity to better manage the complexities of chronic disease, HIT investments also offer ways to reduce the costs of delivering this care.

Reducing Cost

Facilitating the care of high-risk individuals, improving patient safety, and improving communication have their own independent merits, but these HIT efforts also reflect opportunities for cost savings. The patient-centered medical home (PCMH) is a model that incorporates HIT into its care coordination model, and HIT related cost savings have been shown. One pilot study of PCMH efforts by Group Health Cooperative in Washington showed a 29% decrease in emergency visits and an 11% reduction in ambulatory care sensitive admissions. This result was achieved using longer patient visits as well as increased telephone visits, virtual/e-mail visits, patient portals, and scheduled provider time for electronic care coordination and outreach. Net cost savings were about $17 per person, which is a trend toward net savings but, in this small study, not yet statistically significant.[26] Intermountain Health Group implemented a PCMH model that required the use of EHRs specifically to enable providers to improve their management of chronic disease and care coordination. Their study evaluated patients in a PCMH model versus controls not in a PCMH. They showed improved quality with an absolute reduction in mortality of 3.4% as well as showing that they had cost savings averaging $640 per patient per year, up to $1650 for higher risk patients.[27] EHR use was integral to achieving these savings, adding to the body of evidence that HIT serves as an important tool in achieving better quality outcomes for equal, and even lower, costs.

Improving Chronic Disease Management: Quality Measures and Population Health

As EHRs become more widely implemented, the data available about patients and provider practice patterns will grow. A core piece of the medical home and patient-centered care is using clinical data to improve care delivery.[28] To do this effectively, targets and measures must be in place to identify where patients and providers are achieving standard of care and where they are failing. The previously mentioned functionalities can identify whether individual patients are meeting national standards; for example, whether a patient has received age-appropriate cholesterol screening and influenza or other standard vaccinations, or whether a patient with diabetes has an A1C level at target. Communicable diseases have been tracked using surveillance data, registries, and other large data sources for many years. This model is now applicable to chronic disease. Cardiologists have begun to develop disease registries to study population trends and to identify areas of need.[29] The American College of Cardiology and the American Heart Association, both professional societies that establish guidelines for cardiovascular care, collaborated to form the PINNACLE (Practice Innovation and Clinical Excellence) program, which uses a registry of more than 14,000 patients to track adherence to performance measures. This registry includes such measures as β-blocker and statin use in patients with known coronary disease. The successes of the PINNACLE program prompted disease registry and panel management to be built into certified EHR products. EHRs bring the power of registries and panel-level management to all providers. Examples of how individual or groups of providers can use registry functions and other tools to improve quality are shown in **Table 1**, and include tracking the number of patients with diabetes with A1C levels at goal, the number of patients with hypertension with documented blood pressures at goal, or screening a panel of eligible patients for the pneumococcal vaccine. These registry and panel management tools facilitate quality improvement efforts and ensure that guideline and evidence-based care can be delivered. Early on, providers may find the impact only at the practice level, but, as data exchange increases among diverse electronic systems, these data can be use to create community-wide or even statewide registries and networks of information.

As data are entered into the EHRs, each individual primary care provider can look across his or her patients to see whether they are achieving their targets. When surveyed, many providers think that they are 100% compliant with aspirin use for cardiovascular risk reduction, that their diabetics are largely under control, and that their patients have been adequately screened for age-appropriate immunizations.[30] Panel management functionalities allow providers and their staff to quickly identify those in need of influenza vaccines and send reminders, check which patients have a hemoglobin A1C that is not at target, and ensure follow-up with each patient and triage them using electronic communication, office visits, or hospitalization as needed.[31] Providers can identify whether patients are filling their prescriptions using data from e-prescribing networks, and can follow their own habits for laboratory and radiology use. Integrated health systems that have a pharmacy component may find that tracking prescriptions is easier. Data are limited, but new models of linkages between health system EHRs and retail pharmacies are entering the market. One example is the collaboration of CVS Caremark and MinuteClinic with both Cleveland Clinic in Ohio and Allina Health System in Minnesota to integrate their EHR systems

Table 1
EHR functionalities required for meaningful use and applications for chronic disease management

Functionality	Example	References
Record demographics	Osteoporosis requires education and prevention along with management to reduce highly morbid fractures. Ethnic and gender disparities are known both in the incidence and management of this disease. EHRs improve screening and management of disease, reducing disparities and improving outcomes	Navarro RA, Greene DF, Burchette R, et al. Minimizing disparities in osteoporosis care of minorities with an electronic medical record care plan. Clin Orthop Relat Res 2011;469(7):1931–5
Record vital signs	Documentation of vital signs, specifically blood pressure, has shown improved rates of screening, higher rates of guideline-based medication therapy, and improved outcomes as more patients achieve target blood pressure. Achieving target pressures reduces the incidence of morbidity and mortality associated with hypertension	Kinn JW, Marek JC, O'Toole MF, et al. Effectiveness of the electronic medical record in improving the management of hypertension. J Clin Hypertens (Greenwich) 2001;4(6):415–19
Problem list, medication list, allergy list	Problem lists, medication lists, and allergy lists share vital information about patients, especially those with multiple health issues. Documenting these features improves screening and preventative health and reduces adverse drug events and allergy exposures	Poon EG, Wright A, Simon SR, et al. Relationship between use of electronic health record features and health care quality: results of a statewide survey. Med Care 2010;48(3):203–9
Capture smoking status	Smoking contributes to cardiovascular events and lung cancer. Capturing smoking status increases rates of counseling for cessation interventions and counseled. This is a key step to improving quit rates	McCullough A, Fisher M, Goldstein A, et al. Smoking as a vital sign: prompts to ask and assess increase in cessation counseling. J Am Board Fam Med 2009;22:625–32
Electronic prescribing	Elderly patients often take multiple medications; failure to improve could be caused by nonadherence. EHR and e-prescribing data can aid providers in monitoring whether patients are not responding or not adhering to a desired treatment plan, allowing providers to design an optimal plan with their patients, improving outcomes and reducing cost. Adherence was assessed using pharmacy data, claims data, and, in some cases, electronic pillboxes	(1) Cutler DM, Everett W. Thinking outside the pillbox – medication adherence as a priority for health care reform. N Engl J Med 2010;362(17):1553–5 (2) Gellad WF, Grenard JL, Marcum ZA. A systematic review of barriers to medication adherence in the elderly: looking beyond cost and regimen complexity. Am J Geriatr Pharmacother 2011;9(1):11–23

(continued on next page)

Table 1
(continued)

Functionality	Example	References
CPOE for medications	CPOE systems enhance the ability to screen for necessary treatments and ensure that prescribed treatments adhere to guidelines. Recent efforts to study cardiovascular risk factors used CPOE to accurately assess and improve antiplatelet and lipid-lowering therapy to at-risk patients	Persell SD, Dunne AP, Lloyd-Jones, DM, et al. Electronic health record-based cardiac risk assessment and identification of unmet preventative needs. Med Care 2009;47:418–24
Drug interaction and allergy checks	Chronic disease lends itself to multiple medications, which increases the risk for adverse drug interactions and drug allergies. EHRs have been shown to reduce preventable adverse drug events	(1) Gandhi TK, Seger AC, Overhage JM, et al. Outpatient adverse drug events identified by screening electronic health records. J Patient Saf 2010;6:91–6 (2) Rommers MK, Zegers MH, De Clercq PA, et al. Development of a computerized alert system, ADEAS, to identify patients at risk for an adverse drug event. Qual Saf Health Care 2010;19(6):e35
Information exchange capabilities and data submission capabilities	Information exchange and data submission allow a patient's data from different sites of care to be shared and important information released to public health entities. In chronic disease, redundant testing, imaging, and failure to communicate information in a timely matter impedes good-quality care and raises cost. Robust exchange and submissions capabilities allow all care providers, health care sites, and patients to have easy access to vital information, especially at the point of care	(1) Frisse ME, Holmes RL. Estimated financial savings associated with health information exchange and ambulatory care referral. J Biomed Inform 2007;40(Suppl 6):S27–32 (2) Walker J, Pan E, Johnston D, et al. The value of health care information exchange and interoperability. Health Aff (Millwood) 2005;(Suppl Web Exclusives):W5-10–W5-18
CDS	CDS can improve decision making and patient monitoring, especially for chronic disease. CDS in an EHR has been shown to improve glycemic control and hypertension in diabetics	O'Conner PJ, Sperl-Hillen JM, Rush WA, et al. Impact of electronic health record clinical decision support on diabetes care: a randomized trial. Ann Fam Med 2011;9:12–21. Doi: 10.1370/afm.1196

Drug formulary checks	Medications can be costly, and those with chronic diseases spend considerably more than those not on pharmaceuticals. Failure to adhere to patient formularies and to use generics drives costs and contribute to nonadherence. EHRs can alert providers to nonformulary choices and encourage generics, reducing costs and improving care delivery	Stenner SP, Chen Q, Johnson KB. Impact of generic substitution decision support on electronic prescribing behavior. J Am Med Inform Assoc 2010;17:681–8
Incorporate laboratory results	Incorporating laboratory results in the EHR can improve the time to communicating results, allows more accurate tracking of disease over time, and prevents redundant testing, all of which are important to patients with chronic disease undergoing frequent visits and testing	Singh H, Wilson L, Reis B, et al. Ten strategies to improve management of abnormal test result alerts in the electronic health record. J Patient Saf 2010;6(2):121–3
Generate patient lists for quality improvement	Chronic disease requires frequent follow-up and close monitoring; to identify patients in need of visits, patients lists of conditions like hypertension or diabetes can be targeted, patients encouraged to schedule an appointment, and outcomes can be tracked	Rai A, Prichard P, Hodach R, et al. Using physician-led automated communications to improve patient health. Popul Health Manag 2010;14(4):175–80
Identify patient-specific educational resources	Targeting educational resources to individual patients using EHRs keeps them informed about their specific disease combinations, engages them, and enables them to play an active role in disease management	Jones DW, Peterson ED, Bonow RO, et al. Partnering to reduce risks and improve cardiovascular outcomes. Circulation 2009;119:340–50
Summary of care record for care transitions	Patients with chronic diseases and older age, among other factors, are hospitalized at higher rates, and seek care in a greater number of health sites. Improved communication provides seamless care, and EHRs have been shown to improve communication between sites of care through information exchange and clinical summaries	Kripalani S, LeFevre F, Phillips CO, et al. Deficits in communication and information transfer between hospital-based and primary care physicians: implications for patient safety and continuity of care. JAMA 2007;297:831–41
Record advance directives	End-of-life care remains high cost and it is important that providers and patients discuss goals of care in advance to avoid undesired and costly care delivery. One obstacle is the communication of advance directives. EHRs facilitate documentation of advance directives and appropriate administration of end-of-life care	Lindner SA, Davoren JB, Vollmer A, et al. An electronic medical record intervention increased nursing home advance directive orders and documentation. J Am Geriatr Soc 2007;55:1001–6

(continued on next page)

Table 1
(continued)

Functionality	Example	References
Reminders for preventative and follow-up care	Chronic disease requires the patient to remember more tasks than patient with simpler disease. Reminders have been show to improve providers' rate of counseling patients and improving outcomes against known HEDIS measures	Sequist T, Gandhi T, Karson A, et al. A randomized trial of electronic clinical reminders to improve quality of care for diabetes and coronary artery disease. J Am Med Inform Assoc 2005;12:431–7
Provide patient access to data (personal health records, portals)	Managing chronic disease involves guidance and management from the provider but also active engagement from the patient. To improve outcomes, patients must be active participants in their care as well as having access to their own information. Personal health records and portals are linked to EHRs and provide a patient-facing piece of the EHR. The VA has improved patient engagement using their MyHealtheVet system	Chumbler NR, Haggstrom DA, Saleem J. Implementation of health information technology in Veterans Health Administration to support transformational change. Med Care 2011;49(Suppl):S36–42

Abbreviations: CDS, clinical decision support; CPOE, computer provider order entry; HEDIS, healthcare effectiveness data and information set.

regionally.[32] A few years ago, paper charts were abstracted to identify racial variations in hospital-based adverse events. Black patients were identified as having higher rates of hospital-acquired infections and adverse drug events.[33] EHRs allow these assessments to be made in real time using both administrative and clinical data to ensure that the most accurate picture of patient care is being assessed. Disparities and practice pattern discrepancies can be viewed for outpatient and inpatient care, and communities can target interventions at the demographics of their patient population, creating a higher level of customization than was previously possible. Using the data and analytics in EHRs is critical to identifying best practices and low-cost methods for delivering care. A medical home requires these efforts, and HIT is crucial to developing these new primary care models built around the patient and ensuring the highest quality and most cost-effective care for individuals and communities.

HIT AND SELF-MANAGEMENT SUPPORT

EHRs have functionalities that facilitate management of chronic disease at the point of care in the office, but a chronic disease is primarily managed by the patients when they return to their daily routines. Therefore, patient and family involvement at home is critical to effective chronic disease management. Self-management support programs have been shown to improve systolic blood pressure by 5 mm Hg and result in clinically significant reduction in A1C levels in diabetics.[34] Self-management programs often occur separately from medical care and connecting the two is difficult. With EHRs, information gathered from self-management can be stored and used in decision making. A personal health record or patient portal is a more direct means of engaging patients in self-management. Patient-facing options include stand-alone systems (USB or CD), systems tethered to EHRs (Kaiser), and Web-based services (Google Health). These tools help people access key information about their own health, and in some situations, patients are able to input their data into a secure system that communicates with their EHR and their providers. Group Health and Kaiser have described examples of success with the use of personal health records. These two groups use tethered systems, allowing direct communication between the patient-facing side and the provider side of their EHRs. More recently, the VA hospitals launched MyHealtheVet, a Web-based portal system that allows veterans to do online prescription refills, receive reminders and alerts, and securely message providers.[35] Surveys of patients reveal general satisfaction when they have access to a personal record or portal and largely view the information available to them as helpful and accurate.[36] Electronic access to their data also allows patients to track developments or progress in their care, reporting downward turns in a timely manner. Similarly, treatments or medications not being tolerated can be reported promptly, allowing care to be improved in shorter cycles than currently done.

The Institute of Medicine has prioritized the patient as a "copilot in their care,"[37] and as personal records and portals increase in availability, patients will be better able to understand and manage their conditions,[37] as well as take an active role in sharing information with multiple providers and/or sites of care. As these innovations are rolled out in various communities, it is important to ensure that they are accessible to all patients. Access to these innovations is still a major issue. When invited, as in a single-center study in Texas, 69% of patients enrolled in the patient portal, suggesting a high level of interest among patients. Disparities were noted in uptake, identifying that racial minorities are slower to enroll in a patient portal system.[38] Patient portals can be expensive to launch and often are the last step when launching an EHR system, because providers focus initially on their pieces of the new technology. Limitations to wider use of patient portals include cost of implementation, support services, and integrating a user-friendly system with the provider's EHR system. Currently available tools like Google Health are independent and do not securely or easily interoperate with secure EHR systems. Personal health records and portals have shown evidence of improving patient and family engagement in care, and the next few years will reveal the impact on self-management.

Telehealth

One of the most vexing features of chronic disease management is the inability to monitor information and examine patients between visits. Patients document blood sugars in notebooks, take their blood pressures at home, and have variable amounts of data that can be shared with the provider in between office visits to improve care. Personal health records and portals may provide the opportunity to improve the ability to manage patients at home, because many feature tools with which patients can enter specific information. Other electronic devices are also being designed to create a new avenue for delivering care. Telehealth, a new field of medicine, refers to using remote monitoring devices, mobile technology, wireless and Internet-based services,[39] and videoconference capabilities to improve disease management and communication between patients and providers. The use of videoconference can get clinicians in touch with their patients when they are remote. Wireless technology like smart phone reminders such as the Text4Baby program, which improves adherence for prenatal care, and other applications to manage chronic diseases are increasing. As use of smart phones increases, there will be more data validating the use of many of these applications. Systematic reviews of small studies about remote monitoring devices have shown that patients have a high rate of compliance with using these technologies and report themselves as feeling more engaged and better at managing their health.[40] Small studies have also suggested modest clinical improvements from early investments in home monitoring and telehealth devices. A telehealth enhancement to standard case management was added to heart failure management programs run by Aetna in New Jersey and, although clinical outcomes were unchanged, these patients had increased use of their case manager and a reduced number of hospital days in 6 months. Cost savings were not estimated but fewer hospital days suggests that cost savings may be possible using telehealth to enhance current standards of care.[41] The data are currently insufficient to say whether these efforts are cost-effective and will improve quality in the long term, but many providers and patients are embracing the available tools and are putting them to use.

HIT AND CARE TRANSITIONS

The final area of chronic disease management is emphasizing improvements in care transitions. The term care transitions refers to the movement patients make between health care practitioners and settings as their condition and care needs change during the course of a chronic or acute illness.[42] Patients with chronic diseases, especially multiple comorbidities, find themselves seeking care at their primary care practice, specialty clinics, the emergency department, rehabilitation and nursing home facilities, and in the hospital. Common difficulties in care transitions include failures in performing medication reconciliation, maintaining accurate medication lists, transferring advance directives, communication between providers, appropriate education and instructions for patients, timely follow-up visits, and ability to access key information about patients.[43] The impact of these failures is substantial. For example, a diabetic patient admitted for complications is sent home on a new insulin regimen. If this patient did not receive appropriate documentation of the new doses, timely follow-up to ensure that the new treatment plan is achieving target therapy, and instructions on how to manage the transition from the hospital, there is an increased risk for adverse drug events, readmission to the hospital, and worsening of the condition. In a 2009 study of 11.8 million Medicare beneficiaries, nearly 20% were rehospitalized within 30 days of admission and 34% were readmitted within 90 days for the same diagnosis-related group as reported on Medicare billing forms.[44] Almost 13% of beneficiaries experienced 3 or more provider transfers in a 30-day period.[44] Mishandled transitions compromise patient safety, contribute to unnecessarily high rates of health services use, and expose the chronically ill to lapses in quality.[45]

EHRs and HIT have a significant role to play in reducing the complications of care transitions. The theme present in most care transition failures is the lack of adequate information. The patient, the discharging team, and the receiving team must all be privy to key information to ensure that care is coordinated and that the patient is actively engaged. A large body of evidence suggests that care transitions can be improved with postdischarge follow-up, comprehensive assessments and care planning, interactions between postacute and outpatient providers, coordination of community resources, self-management tools, medication review and management therapies, and integration of these solutions with HIT.[42] Many of the tools highlighted for patient engagement have also been used successfully in facilitating transitions in care. For patients who are discharged to home, interventions such as daily home videophone monitoring or transmission of physiologic measures, self-care instruction, and symptom management tools using patient-facing health records or portals have all contributed to improve outcomes during transitions of care.[46] An Internet-based communication system implemented between long-term care facilities and the emergency room at the Cleveland Clinic showed more effective transfer of key information such as active medication list and improved patient and provider satisfaction.[47]

Reducing adverse drug events and hospital readmissions requires not only engagement from the patient and their families but also improved knowledge sharing between providers. It is imperative that the acute care providers communicate with the outpatient care team and there be similarly effective communication between long-term care facilities and other points of care.[48] An EHR system with a network for health information exchange allows all this information to be readily available during a transition. Medications are more likely to be reconciled when protocols are built into EHRs and clinical summaries and information exchange can be improved.[49] EHRs can efficiently produce clinical summaries, medication and allergy lists, and other documentation for a transfer by paper to a provider without an EHR. To improve the ability to exchange information, the Federal Government has implemented the DIRECT program, a national network to enable secure exchange of key health information, such as summary care records, referrals, discharge summaries, and other clinical documents in support of continuity of care and medication reconciliation. DIRECT protocols are also being built into certified EHR products to ensure that meaningful users are able to connect with and use the DIRECT program and are meant to be applicable to providers using partial or complete EHR systems.[50]

The Patient Navigator system, implemented at Geisinger, is an EHR system that links patients, care managers, and physicians and has been shown to improve care coordination and outcomes, and to reduce costs.[51] It uses an Internet-based laboratory result display and trends results over time for patients to see their own conditions over time. Patients can also receive clinical reminders, schedule appointments, request prescriptions refills from their physician, find educational materials, and send secure e-mail to their providers. This system is integrated with the official EHR system used by the inpatient and outpatient sites of care. Care managers help the patient with discharge planning, follow-up appointments, medication therapy management, and tracking of their condition when at home using the features of the EHR system and remote monitoring devices. This system has resulted in a reduction in readmissions for chronic conditions like heart failure and diabetes, improved patient satisfaction and safety, and improved adherence to treatment plans.[52] Although Geisinger is unique in how it integrates acute care, outpatient care, and payment, the lessons learned from the use of EHRs and HIT to manage chronic disease and transitions of care are important and replicable.

Care transitions represent a major vulnerability in the current US health care system, especially for those with chronic disease who experience these transitions frequently. Transitions leave patients at risk for adverse events, increase the cost of care, and lead to poor-quality outcomes. EHRs and HIT are key investments to improving transitions of care and provide an opportunity to change patient outcomes and quality of life.

CHALLENGES AND FUTURE DIRECTIONS

Some vanguard communities and health systems have invested heavily in EHRs and HIT, but this is largely a new frontier for many providers and hospitals. The early evidence suggests that EHR functionalities and patient engagement strategies have the potential to improve chronic disease management in the primary care practice, at home with the patient, and during transitions of care. Most of the existing evidence for HIT benefits is in large, self-contained systems. Small practices are less likely to have an EHR, and if they do have some functionalities, they are more likely to be partial systems or basic systems.[53] To affect chronic disease as described earlier, complex, integrated EHR systems are needed. Communication between these systems is also important. To improve adoption and use of HIT, especially for smaller practices, the Office of the National Coordinator created the Beacon Community Collaborative and the Regional Extension Center Programs. These programs are designed to identify best practices for using HIT and EHRs to improve health outcomes and reduce costs across a community. The Beacon program awarded $15 million to each of 17 communities to create a shared model of HIT and EHR investments to drive quality improvements and cost efficiencies at the community level.[54] However, these communities have recognized several unresolved issues that many communities looking to adopt EHRs now face, such as how to accurately exchange health information, how to maintain the security of personal health information, and how to sustain costly investments in technology. The Regional Extension Centers assist small practices in implementing HIT, creating a shared resource to mimic the scale of resources available to large, self-contained systems.[10] A final initiative that is underway is the National Health Information Network, which is a federal effort to create an infrastructure by which data from disparate entities can be securely exchanged, including partial EHR systems. This initiative also explores the ways long-term care facilities, pharmacies, and other sites of care can be integrated.[55] These federal efforts represent the first steps to addressing issues that require additional attention to sustain innovations in HIT.

A key dependency in improving care transitions is the secure exchange of information. Adopting an EHR and using it at the point of care and having a personal health record are pieces of the puzzle, but, to ensure safe transitions in care, personal health information must be securely transferred from each site of care. Communities like Indianapolis, Indiana (a Beacon grant recipient) have a sustainable regional health information exchange network,[56] but many communities struggle to exchange data. Even in Indianapolis, where data exchange is robust, a new avenue is being forged with retail pharmacies to enhance data exchange. The Department of Health and Human Services, along with health care leaders across the country, is working to develop standards for privacy and exchange while the technology community works to provide the products that ensure patient safety and privacy. Each state has received a grant through the State Health Information Exchange Program to invest in a secure, state-based exchange network to improve communication in the health care system. The DIRECT program will create the standards and infrastructure to allow authorized providers to securely exchange information, integrating with certified EHR products and the health information exchange networks in each community and state.[57]

In addition to improving the security of patient information and its exchange, communities that invest in HIT must consider sustainability. Geisinger Health System, another Beacon grant recipient, is one of several communities across the nation that has created payment incentives for providers to share in savings that result from quality improvements.[51] They have shown cost savings from the sharing of information, in reduced visits, reduced imaging, and better transitions in care, resulting in lower readmissions for targeted chronic conditions like diabetes. Their model highlights an example of sustainability of HIT. Federal legislation, like the HITECH Act, can also reduce barriers to adoption. In addition, the growing body of evidence for improved patient safety and transitions of care in chronic disease creates a professional obligation to adopt EHRs as a key component of best practice.[58] The next step is a sustainability plan, and that involves restructuring payments to providers and hospitals to incentivize quality improvement and cost efficiency. To better identify payment opportunities for quality, the new Center for Medicare and Medicaid Innovation is investigating opportunities for shared savings models, accountable care organizations (ACOs), PCMH, and bundled or value-based payments to identify where quality can be delivered for lower cost and allow providers to share in those savings.[59] These models have not yet been tested in the diverse communities across the United States. The Center for Medicare and Medicaid Innovation is also coordinating with other federal partners for the Partnership for Patients Initiative,[60] a patient safety campaign that is a public-private partnership to reduce preventable adverse events, especially among those with chronic disease and repeat hospitalizations using HIT investments.

In some cases, the consumers or patients will drive sustainability as they move to adopt new technologies that allow them to better manage their chronic diseases, but it will take collaboration from providers, hospitals, health plans, and the State and Federal Government to ensure that quality improvement and cost efficiency are prioritized and best practices are adopted with regard to EHRs, new health technologies, and the resulting privacy, security, and exchange needs.

SUMMARY

EHRs and HIT have been shown to improve health outcomes, reduce costs, and improve patient self-management, safety, and satisfaction. Health IT plays an integral part in the optimal management of chronic disease. The body of evidence supporting EHRs and HIT is growing as more providers adopt and use health records. The Federal Government has put in place several programs to aid providers in adoption and sustain investments through innovative payment models that reward high-quality and cost-effective care. Health IT and EHRs can be customized to suit the provider and patient preferences, and allow each provider and patient to engage in a collaborative manner. As more people are living with chronic diseases, HIT will play an increasingly important role, transforming primary care and chronic disease management by aligning all stakeholders, with the goals of improving overall population health, improving the patient experience of care, and reducing costs.

REFERENCES

1. Drezner JL. Understanding adoption of new technologies by physicians. MedGenMed 2000;2(1):E16.
2. Available at: http://healthit.hhs.gov. Accessed September 15, 2011.
3. DesRoches CM, Campbell EG, Rao SR, et al. Electronic health records in ambulatory care – a national survey of physicians. N Engl J Med 2008;359(1):50–60.
4. Bazemore A, Burke M, Xierali I. Establishing a baseline: health information technology adoption among family medicine diplomates. J Am Board Fam Med 2011; 24(2):132.
5. Hing E, Hall MJ, Ashman JJ. Use of electronic medical records by ambulatory care providers: United States, 2006. Natl Health Stat Report 2010;22:1–21.
6. Publication No. 08–0084Decision maker brief: chronic disease management. Agency for Healthcare Quality and Research; 2008.
7. Buntin MB, Burke MF, Hoaglin MC, et al. The benefits of health information technology: a review of the recent literature shows predominantly positive results. Health Aff (Millwood) 2011;30(3):464–71.
8. Blumenthal D, Tavenner M. The "meaningful use" regulation for electronic health records. N Engl J Med 2010;363(6):501–4.
9. Available at: http://healthit.hhs.gov. Accessed September 15, 2011.
10. Maxson E, Jain S, Kendall M, et al. The Regional Extension Center Program: helping physicians meaningfully use health information technology. Ann Intern Med 2010;153(10):666–70.
11. Available at: http://healthit.hhs.gov/portal/server.pt/community/hit_extension_program/1495/home/17174. Accessed September 15, 2011.
12. [web site]DMAA definition of disease management. Washington, DC: Disease Management Association of America; 2008. Available at: http://www.dmaa.org/dm_definition.asp. Accessed May 15, 2008.
13. Sequist T, Gandhi T, Karson A, et al. A randomized trial of electronic clinical reminders to improve quality of care for diabetes and coronary artery disease. J Am Med Inform Assoc 2005;12:431–7.
14. Peterson KA, Radosevich DM, O'Connor PJ, et al. Improving diabetes care in practice, findings from the TRANSLATE trial. Diabetes Care 2008;31(12):2238–43.
15. Persell SD, Dunne AP, Lloyd-Jones DM, et al. Electronic health record-based cardiac risk assessment and identification of unmet preventative needs. Med Care 2009;47:418–24.
16. Frisse ME, Johnson KB, Chen Q, et al. The financial impact of health information exchange on emergency department care. J Am Med Inform Assoc 2011. [Epub ahead of print].
17. Nemeth LS, Wessell AM. Improving medication safety in primary care using electronic health records. J Patient Saf 2010;6:238–43.
18. Feldstein AC, Smith DH, Perrin N, et al. Reducing warfarin medication interactions: an interrupted time series evaluation. Arch Intern Med 2006;166(9): 1009–15.
19. Spina JR, Glassman PA, Good CB, et al. Potential safety gaps in order entry and automated drug alerts: a nationwide survey of VA physician self-reported practices. Med Care 2011;49(10):904–10.

20. Gandhi TK, Weingart S, Borus J, et al. Adverse drug events in ambulatory care. N Engl J Med 2003;348:1556–64.
21. Buck MD, Atreja A, Brunker CP, et al. Potentially inappropriate medication prescribing in outpatient practices: prevalence and patient characteristics based on electronic health records. Am J Geriatr Pharmacother 2009;7(2):84–92.
22. Fenton JJ, Cai Y, Weiss NS, et al. Delivery of cancer screening: how important is the preventative health examination? Arch Intern Med 2007;167:580–5.
23. Smith PC, Rodrigo A, Bublitz C, et al. Missing clinical information during primary care visits. JAMA 2005;293:565–71.
24. Walker J, Pan E, Johnston D, et al. The value of health care information exchange and interoperability. Health Aff (Millwood) 2005;(Suppl Web Exclusives): W5-10–W5-18.
25. Fontaine P, Ross S, Zink T, et al. Systematic review of health information exchange in primary care practices. J Am Board Fam Med 2010;23:655–70.
26. Reid RJ, Fishman PA, Larson EB, et al. Patient-centered medical home demonstration: a prospective, quasi-experimental, before and after evaluation. Am J Manag Care 2009;15(9):e71–87.
27. Dorr DA, Wilcox AB, Brunker CP, et al. The effect of technology-supported, multidisease care management on the mortality and hospitalization of seniors. J Am Geriatr Soc 2008;56(12):2195–202. Findings updated for presentation at White House roundtable on Advanced Models of Primary Care, August 10, 2009.
28. Bates DW, Bitton A. The future of health information technology in the patient-centered medical home. Health Aff (Millwood) 2010;29(4):614–21.
29. Chan PS, Oetgen WJ, Buchanan D, et al. Cardiac performance measure compliance in outpatients: the American College of Cardiology and National Cardiovascular Data Registry's Pinnacle Program. J Am Coll Cardiol 2010;56(1):8–14.
30. Erhardt L, Komajda M, Hobbs FD, et al. Cardiologists' awareness and perceptions of guidelines for chronic heart failure. The ADDress your Heart survey. Eur J Heart Fail 2008;10:1020–5.
31. Rai A, Prichard P, Hodach R, et al. Using physician-led automated communications to improve patient health. Popul Health Manag 2010;14(4):175–80.
32. Available at: www.info.cvscaremark.com. Accessed September 1, 2011.
33. Metersky ML, Hunt DR, Kliman R, et al. Racial disparities in the frequency of patient safety events: results from the National Medicare Patient Safety Monitoring System. Med Care 2011;49:504–10.
34. Chodosh J, Morton SC, Shekelle P, et al. Meta-analysis: chronic disease self-management programs for older adults. Ann Intern Med 2005;143:427–38.
35. Chumbler NR, Haggstrom DA, Saleem J. Implementation of health information technology in Veterans Health Administration to support transformation change: telehealth and personal health records. Med Care 2011;49:S36–42.
36. Hassol A, Walker JM, Kidder D, et al. Patient experiences and attitudes about access to a patient electronic health care record and linked web messaging. J Am Med Inform Assoc 2004;11(6):505–13.
37. Institute of Medicine. Crossing the quality chasm: a new health system for the twenty-first century. Washington, DC: National Academies Press; 2001.
38. Goel M, Brown TL, Williams A, et al. Disparities in enrollment and use of an electronic patient portal. J Gen Intern Med 2011. DOI: 10.1007/s11606-011-1728-3.
39. Shah B, Adams M, Peterson E, et al. Secondary prevention risk interventions via telemedicine and tailored patient education (SPRITE): a randomized trial to improve postmyocardial infarction management. Circ Cardiovasc Qual Outcomes 2011;4:235–42.

40. Pare G, Janna M, Sicotte C. Systematic review of home telemonitoring for chronic diseases: the evidence base. J Am Med Inform Assoc 2007;14(3):269–77.
41. Wade MJ, Desai AS, Spettell CM. Telemonitoring with case management for seniors with heart failure. Am J Manag Care 2011;17(3):e71–9.
42. Coleman EA, Boult CE, American Geriatrics Society Health Care Systems Committee. Improving the quality of transitional care for persons with complex care needs. J Am Geriatr Soc 2003;51(4):556–7.
43. Hughes RG, Clancy CM. Improving the complex nature of care transitions. J Nurs Care Qual 2007;22(4):289–92.
44. Jencks SF, Williams MV, Coleman EA. Rehospitalizations among patients in the Medicare fee-for-service program. N Engl J Med 2009;360(14):1418–28.
45. Naylor MD, Aiken LH, Kirtzman ET, et al. The importance of transitional care in achieving health reform. Health Aff (Millwood) 2011;30(4):746–54.
46. Wakefield BJ, Ward MM, Holman JE, et al. Evaluation of home telehealth following hospitalization for heart failure: a randomized trial. Telemed J E Health 2008; 14(8):753–61.
47. Hustey FM, Palmer RM. An internet-based communication network for information transfer during patient transitions from skilled nursing facility to the emergency department. J Am Geriatr Soc 2010;58(6):1148–52.
48. Coleman EA. Falling through the cracks: challenges and opportunities for improving transitional care for persons with continuous complex care needs. J Am Geriatr Soc 2003;51(4):549–55.
49. Nassaralla CL, Naessens JM, Hunt VL, et al. Medication reconciliation in ambulatory care: attempts at improvement. Qual Saf Health Care 2009;18(5):402–7.
50. Available at: http://wiki.directproject.org/. Accessed September 25, 2011.
51. Gilfillan RJ, Tomcavage J, Rosenthal MB, et al. Value and the medical home: effects of transformed primary care. Am J Manag Care 2010;16(8):607–14.
52. Paulus RA, Davis K, Steele GD. Continuous innovation in health care: implications of the Geisinger experience. Health Aff (Millwood) 2008;27(5):1235–45.
53. DesRoches C, Campbell EG, Blumenthal D, et al. Electronic health records in ambulatory care – a national survey of physicians. N Engl J Med 2008;259:50–60.
54. Maxson ER, Jain SH, McKethan AN, et al. Beacon communities aim to use health information technology to transform the delivery of care. Health Aff (Millwood) 2010;29(9):1671–7.
55. Dixon BE, Zafar A, Overhage JM. A framework for evaluating the costs, effort, and value of nationwide health information exchange. J Am Med Inform Assoc 2010; 17(3):295–301.
56. McDonald CJ, Overhage JM, Barnes M, et al. The Indiana network for patient care: a working local health information infrastructure. Health Aff (Millwood) 2005;24(5):1214–20.
57. Office of the National Coordinator, US Dept of Health and Human Services. Available at: http://healthit.hhs.gov/portal/server.pt?open=512&objID=1488&mode=2. Accessed September 15, 2011.
58. Mechanic D. Rethinking medical professionalism the role of information technology and practice innovations. Milbank Q 2008;86(2):327–58.
59. Available at: http://innovations.cms.gov/. Accessed September 30, 2011.
60. Available at: http://www.healthcare.gov/center/programs/partnership/index.html. Accessed September 30, 2011.

Pharmacologic Issues in Management of Chronic Disease

Gina DeSevo, PharmD*, Jacqueline Klootwyk, PharmD, BCPS

KEYWORDS

- Polypharmacy • Inappropriate prescribing • Adherence • Adverse drug events

KEY POINTS

- As the number of medications that patients are prescribed increases, an increase in pharmacologic-related issues and complications may occur, such as polypharmacy, inappropriate prescribing, medication nonadherence and nonpersistence, and adverse drug reactions and events.
- By attempting to reduce polypharmacy, inappropriate prescribing, medication nonadherence and nonpersistence, and adverse drug events, health care professionals will improve patient safety and well-being, and optimize medical management of chronic disease.

More often than not, the management of chronic diseases is coupled with the use of multiple medications. The number of medications that each individual takes is determined by a variety of factors and greatly depends on the patient's underlying conditions, health status, and related health beliefs. Medication use does not only include prescription medications but also involves over-the-counter medications, vitamins, minerals, herbal products, and dietary supplements that are available without a prescription.

Prevalence of medication use in the United States has been well documented. The 2006 Slone Survey, a telephone survey of 2529 ambulatory patients 18 years and older, revealed that 82% of participants had taken at least 1 medication (prescription, over-the-counter, vitamin, mineral, herbal, or supplement) during the week prior, 29% had taken at least 5, and 7% had taken at least 10. The survey also found that 52% had taken at least one prescription medication within the previous week and 12% had taken 5 or more.[1] A survey study of 2976 community-residing adults aged 57 to 85 years reported that 81% of adults used at least 1 prescription medication and 29% used at least 5 prescription medications.[2] In addition, a cross-sectional study

The authors have nothing to disclose.
Department of Pharmacy Practice, Jefferson School of Pharmacy, Thomas Jefferson University, 130 South 9th Street, Suite 1540, Philadelphia, PA 19107, USA
* Corresponding author.
E-mail address: gina.desevo@jefferson.edu

Prim Care Clin Office Pract 39 (2012) 345–362
doi:10.1016/j.pop.2012.03.007
0095-4543/12/$ – see front matter © 2012 Elsevier Inc. All rights reserved.

was completed in 3070 patients aged 75 years and older enrolled in the Ginkgo Evaluation of Memory Study to examine the use of prescription drugs and dietary supplements. This study found that nearly 90% of patients were using at least 1 prescription drug and approximately 60% of patients were using at least 3 prescription drugs. In addition, more than 80% of the cohort patients were using at least 1 dietary supplement and about 50% were using at least 3. The average number of prescription drugs per patient was 3.5 (range 0–18), and the average number of dietary supplements per person was 3.4 (range 0–17).[3]

Management of chronic disease heavily relies on the use of medications. This fact is of great importance because chronic diseases have emerged as the leading cause of morbidity and mortality in the United States.[4] As a result, more medications will be prescribed, which may result in increasing numbers of pharmacologic-related problems and complications, including polypharmacy, inappropriate prescribing (IP), medication nonadherence and nonpersistence, and adverse drug reactions and events.

POLYPHARMACY

Multiple definitions for polypharmacy are used throughout the literature, but it is most often defined in one of two ways. The first relates to an absolute number of medications. This number varies and may range from 2 to 9 medications.[5] A literature review of 16 studies related to polypharmacy found that of 7 studies that defined polypharmacy, 4 defined it as the use of 5 or more medications.[6] This definition can be limiting, as it implies that patients should not be on 5 or more medications when, in fact, patients may require numerous medications for the management of chronic disease. Patients often suffer from multiple chronic diseases, each requiring multiple medications as per guideline recommendations to be adequately treated.

The second definition for polypharmacy involves the use of more medications than are clinically indicated.[5] With this definition, medications without an indication or lacking efficacy for a condition and therapeutic duplications would be considered unnecessary, and therefore labeled as polypharmacy. This definition takes into account medication appropriateness and requires a thorough review of each medication. The incidence and prevalence of polypharmacy thus varies depending on which definition is used. For example, one may look at prevalence of medication use as already described or IP prevalence, discussed in more detail later.

Risk Factors

Polypharmacy has been investigated frequently in the elderly.[5–9] Several risk factors for polypharmacy have been identified and include increased age, white race, increased numbers of health care visits, supplemental insurance, and seeing multiple providers.[5,10] In addition, several characteristics related to health increase the risk for polypharmacy, including overall poorer health status, depression, hypertension, anemia, asthma, angina, diverticulosis, osteoarthritis, gout, diabetes mellitus, and the use of 9 or more medications.[5] In the Kuopio 75+ Study conducted in Finland, investigators evaluated factors associated with polypharmacy (defined as 6–9 drugs) and excessive polypharmacy (defined as 10 or more drugs) in home-dwelling individuals age 75 years and older. Characteristics associated with excessive polypharmacy included age 85 years and older, female gender, and moderate self-reported health (in contrast to good or poor self-reported health). Poor self-reported health and diagnoses of chronic obstructive pulmonary disease, diabetes, depression, heart disease, and pain were all significantly associated with both polypharmacy and excessive polypharmacy.[7] Furthermore, a review completed by Rollason and Vogt[8] identified female sex, increasing age, rural residence, and low education as characteristics that increase the risk of polypharmacy in the elderly. Purchasing over-the-counter medications and borrowing medications from family members and friends may also contribute to polypharmacy.[8] Patients may also receive inappropriate new prescriptions to treat adverse effects of other medications in the belief that the adverse effect is a symptom of a new disease state.[8,9]

Consequences of Polypharmacy

The consequences of polypharmacy are numerous and significant. There is a clear association between polypharmacy and drug-related problems, such as inappropriate drug doses, adverse drug reactions, drug interactions, nonadherence, and omission of drug therapy.[5,6,8] Other reported consequences of polypharmacy include a higher prevalence of geriatric syndromes, increased morbidity and mortality, and increased medical costs.[5] Additional studies have found polypharmacy to be associated with increased hospital admissions, fatal adverse drug events (ADEs), emergency room visits, risk of fractures, dysphagia, malnutrition, mobility impairments, and serious hypoglycemia in patients with insulin-dependent diabetes.[6]

Tools and Interventions to Reduce Polypharmacy

Multiple tools and interventions to reduce polypharmacy have been investigated. Evidence-based strategies include using medication algorithms, performing medication reviews, and providing physician education. Although it may not be feasible to use all of these strategies at each office visit, a combination of approaches may be useful to apply to office patients during the course of their chronic disease.

Medication algorithms

In a cohort study of 70 community-dwelling elderly patients referred for comprehensive geriatric assessments, the Good Palliative-Geriatric Practice algorithm was used to reduce polypharmacy. The algorithm used a series of questions to discuss with the patient and/or guardian/family to help determine whether a drug should be stopped or shifted to a safer or more efficacious option. For example, questions addressed whether the indication was appropriate for the patient's age and if there were any adverse symptoms related to the drug. Based on the algorithm, discontinuation of 311 medications (58% of all medications) was recommended in 64 patients. Two hundred fifty-six of the 311 medications (82%) were successfully discontinued after discussions with the patients, guardians, and physicians. Six of the 256 medications discontinued (2%) were restarted because of symptom reoccurrence. Overall, even after combining nonconsent (patient, guardian/family, and/or physician did not wish to discontinue drug) and failures, 81% of the medications were successfully discontinued. Furthermore, 88% of patients reported a subjective global improvement in health.[11]

Medication reviews

Fillit and colleagues[12] investigated the approach of encouraging members of a Medicare managed care program at high risk of polypharmacy (prescribed 5 or more medications) to participate in a medication review with their physicians. The physicians who participated in the trial were also provided with education on polypharmacy before the reviews. Forty-two percent of the patients surveyed participated in a medication review. Following the review, 20% of the patients reported a medication discontinuation, 29% reported a change in dose, and 17% reported having informed their physician of a new medication. Forty-five percent of the physicians surveyed after the reviews reported making a change in their prescribing.

Involvement of clinical pharmacists in medication reviews has also been evaluated. One longitudinal cohort study involved drug therapy reviews provided by a clinical pharmacist, physician and patient education, and recommendations to physicians and patients to rectify polypharmacy-related issues in outpatients at high risk for polypharmacy (prescribed 5 or more medications for at least 4 months). Two identical interventions were conducted 1 year apart. A sustained decrease in overall polypharmacy events of 72.1% was achieved at 6 months after the second intervention ($P = .001$).[13]

INAPPROPRIATE PRESCRIBING

IP in the management of chronic disease includes both errors of commission and errors of omission. Errors of commission refer to the inappropriate addition of a medication (ie, medications that are generally poorly tolerated or may exacerbate a concomitant disease), often referred to as potentially inappropriate medications (PIM). Errors of omission refer to the underutilization of a medication when one is recommended (ie, medications recommended in their respective disease state guidelines to prevent morbidity and/or mortality). These errors are an area of particular concern in the elderly population, for whom the number of chronic medical conditions and corresponding number of medications increase with age. IP is a growing problem worldwide. It has been shown that 21.3% and 40% of community-dwelling and nursing home patients, respectively, of age 65 years and older are prescribed potentially inappropriate medications.[14] In hospitalized patients, 25% to 35% of patients older than 65 are prescribed a PIM that could potentially affect outpatient medication regimens after discharge.[15,16]

Risk Factors for Inappropriate Prescribing

Risk factors for IP include age older than 85 years, female gender, and polypharmacy.[14-18] In a prospective, observational study of 597 acutely ill elderly patients by Gallagher and colleagues,[15] female patients were significantly more likely to be prescribed a PIM than were male patients, according to both the Beers criteria and Screening Tool of Older Persons' Potentially Inappropriate Prescriptions (STOPP). Polypharmacy, which has been previously described, has been shown to be a risk factor for IP. Patients taking more than 5 medications are 3.3 times more likely to have been prescribed a PIM compared with those taking 5 or fewer medications. In addition, there are numerous new medications approved each year as well as medications with new indications, which further complicates the decision-making process. Tools to reduce IP are discussed in the following sections.

Consequences of Inappropriate Prescribing

IP can be problematic for several reasons. It can lead to ADEs, hospitalizations, increased health care (expenditure) costs, as well as nonadherence and nonpersistence over time.[19] Errors of omission can also lead to the lack of therapeutic benefit, potentially leading to undesired morbidity and mortality.

Adverse drug events

Risk factors for ADEs are numerous and complex. As adults age, there are physiologic changes that make them more prone to adverse drug reactions as well as events. The US Food and Drug Administration (FDA) defines an adverse event as "any undesirable experience associated with the use of a medical product in a patient."[20] An adverse drug reaction has alternatively been defined by the International Conference on Harmonization as "a response to a drug which is noxious and unintended and which occurs at doses normally used in man for prophylaxis, diagnosis, or therapy of disease or for the modification of physiologic function."[21]

ADEs in the elderly are commonly attributable to IP, specifically errors of commission. In those older than 65 years, studies have shown that approximately 6% to 16% of hospital admissions are due to PIMs.[15,16] Furthermore, another study showed that approximately 29% of patients presenting to the emergency department were taking at least one PIM.[22] ADEs not requiring a visit to the emergency department or admission to a hospital may be underreported in these studies. There have been several tools validated to reduce IP and in turn potentially reduce ADEs (see later discussion).

Impact on health care expenditure/cost

Few studies have evaluated the impact on health care costs associated with IP. It has been estimated that the annual costs for a 700-bed teaching hospital are $5.6 million, of which $2.8 million is attributable to all ADEs and preventable ADEs, respectively.[23] In addition, errors of omission may lead to increased morbidity and mortality in patients not receiving medications proved to prevent hospitalizations or death. Some examples include statin use in patients with atherosclerosis, or angiotensin-converting enzyme (ACE) inhibitor use in patients with chronic heart failure (CHF).[17] The cost of adding these life-saving medications has been evaluated in an Irish population. In a study of 600 patients, the 30-day costs were estimated at approximately $13,488, with 1-year costs approximately $157,843.[17]

Tools and Interventions for Inappropriate Prescribing

Evaluating medication appropriateness and IP is a critical part of optimal management of chronic disease, and several tools have been well validated, including the Beers criteria, the Medication Appropriateness Index (MAI), the STOPP, and the Screening Tool to Alert doctors to Right Treatment (START).[16,17,24–28] Various disadvantages have emerged from the Beers criteria and MAI tool, which has led to the recent development of the STOPP and START tools.

Beers criteria

The Beers criteria are the tool most commonly referred to when discussing PIMs. The criteria were first developed in 1991 and have since been updated twice, first in 1997 and most recently in 2003.[25–27] The current Beers criteria contain a list of drugs generally not to be used in elderly patients and separates PIMs into 2 categories: "independent of diagnosis and condition" and by "specific diagnosis and condition."[27] Beers criteria do not include errors of omission. The Beers criteria have been criticized as they do not take patient-specific factors into account and mainly state which medications should not be used. In addition, there are conflicting data regarding the Beers criteria and their ability to reduce ADEs. In a study of 177,504 patients presenting to United States emergency departments, no significant association between the Beers criteria and ADEs was found.[18] On the other hand, there have been a few studies that have found a significant association between PIMs and ADEs according to the Beers criteria.[29–31] A mail survey of 626 Medicare-eligible patients showed that 51.4% were prescribed a PIM and 22% reported experiencing an unwanted adverse effect from a prescribed medication in the past year. In addition, it showed that ADEs were significantly associated with PIMs in comparison with those not prescribed a PIM (odds ratio [OR] 2.14; 95% confidence interval [CI] 1.26–3.65).[31] The Agency for Healthcare

Research and Quality (AHRQ) has modified the 1997 Beers criteria; the new criteria include 33 medications from the Beers list and subdivides them into 3 categories. These categories include 11 medications to "always avoid," 8 medications that are "rarely appropriate," and 14 medications that have "some indications for use" in the elderly population irrespective of dose, frequency of administration, or duration.[28] These criteria were the initial basis for the addition of IP to the 2006 Health Plan Employer Data and Information Set (HEDIS) measures.[32] Since 2006, IP has been included in the HEDIS performance measures for physicians.[33]

Medication appropriateness index

In addition to clinical judgment, appropriate medication use can be measured using the MAI. The MAI is a validated 10-item prescribing questionnaire that addresses indication, effectiveness, dose, duration, correct directions, practical directions, drug-drug-interactions, drug-disease interactions, therapeutic duplication, and cost of treatment.[24] Three items specifically evaluate prescribing of PIMs and polypharmacy (indication, duplication, and effectiveness). Recently, a modified 6-item MAI score, which includes drug-drug-interactions, drug-disease interactions, indication, effectiveness, therapeutic duplication, and appropriate duration, were evaluated and compared with the Beers criteria to determine PIM use and ADEs in elderly patients in a primary care clinic. Whereas Beers criteria pertain only to those older than 65 years, the MAI can be used in any patient to assess the appropriateness of drug regimen. At baseline, 98.7% of patients were taking a PIM according to the modified MAI compared with 48.7% of patients according to the Beers criteria. This result may be attributed to the fact that the MAI uses implicit criteria as opposed to the explicit list contained in the Beers criteria. During a 3-month follow-up, 14.4% of patients experienced an ADE. The modified MAI score was shown to be a significant predictor of ADEs compared with both the standard 10-item MAI and the Beers criteria, neither of which was a predictor of ADEs. The ADE risk increased 13% for every 1 point of the modified MAI score.[34] Although this tool has been validated in both the ambulatory and inpatient settings, it is rarely completed for each patient's medications because of time restraints.[24,35] In addition, this tool does not evaluate errors of omission.

Screening tool of older persons' potentially inappropriate prescriptions

In 2008, 2 IP tools were validated to be used in the elderly population, the STOPP and the START tools. These tools were designed to be used together to look at errors of commission and errors of omission, repectively.[36] In a recent study by Gallagher and colleagues., the combined use of STOPP and START in 400 hospitalized patients was associated with an absolute risk reduction of 35.7% in errors of commission and an absolute risk reduction of 21.2% in errors of omission.[37] An advantage of the STOPP criteria, compared with the Beers criteria, is that the STOPP criteria are organized according to physiologic system and each STOPP criterion is accompanied by an explanation.[16,37]

In a study of 715 hospital admissions of patients 65 years or older, STOPP was shown to identify more PIMs and ADEs than the Beers criteria. In this study, 35% (STOPP) versus 25% (Beers criteria) of patients were identified as having a PIM. In addition, PIMs according to STOPP contributed to 11.5% of hospital admissions, compared with only 6% according to Beers criteria.[16] In a study by Hamilton and colleagues[38] comparing Beers with STOPP criteria, Beers criteria PIMs did not significantly increase ADE risk ($P = .11$). Conversely, STOPP PIMs were significantly associated with ADE risk ($P<.001$). This study evaluated 600 patients older than 65 (median age 77) years at the point of hospital admission.

Screening tool to alert doctors to right treatment

The START criteria are the first tool to specifically evaluate errors of omission. Similar to STOPP, START is also organized according to physiologic system and each criterion is accompanied by an explanation.[17] Unlike the tools for errors of commission, this tool requires frequent updates to accurately correlate the criteria to evidence-based guidelines and recommendations. Barry and colleagues[17] found that 57.9% of hospitalized elderly patients had one or more prescribing omission. In this study, the 5 most prevalent prescribing omissions were statin use in atherosclerosis (26%), warfarin in chronic atrial fibrillation (9.5%), ACE inhibitor in heart failure (8%), antiplatelet therapy in arterial disease (7.3%), and calcium/vitamin D supplementation in patients with symptomatic osteoporosis (6%).

The STOPP and START criteria are relatively new and have yet to be validated in the outpatient setting. Although not yet validated in this setting at the time of writing, the primary care clinician could use these as reference tools in patients transitioning care between inpatient and outpatient settings. For example, the START criteria could be used to ensure proper management of disease state after hospital discharge (ie, statin use after an acute coronary syndrome or ACE-inhibitor use after a heart failure exacerbation). In addition, the STOPP criteria could be used periodically in patients followed by multiple providers to ensure that errors of commission are minimized.

MEDICATION ADHERENCE AND PERSISTENCE

Reliable medication-taking behavior includes both medication adherence and persistence, and is a major concern in the management of chronic disease. Medication adherence refers to the appropriate use of drug therapy as per the recommendations of a health care provider, whereas medication persistence describes the continued use of prescribed drug therapy.[39] It can be time consuming to evaluate medication adherence with each patient, particularly because many factors determine and effect medication adherence. Fischer and colleagues[40] found that 22% of all electronically prescribed prescriptions and 28% of all new electronically prescribed prescriptions were not filled by patients. Medications for chronic diseases were among the highest classes of medications not filled (31.4% for diabetes, 28.4% for hypertension, and 28.2% for hyperlipidemia).

In another study by Krousel-Wood and colleagues,[41] researchers found that 14.1% of patients 65 years and older with hypertension had low adherence and 27% were considered nonpersistent. Low adherence was defined as a Morisky Medication Adherence Scale (MMAS) score of less than 6 using the updated MMAS scale **(Table 1)**, whereas low persistence was defined as a medication possession ratio (MPR) of less than 0.8. In addition, patients with low MMAS scores were 2.71 (95% CI 2.31–3.18) times more likely than patients with high MMAS scores to be nonpersistent. The MMAS tool is discussed in more detail in a subsequent section.

Risk Factors for Medication Nonadherence

The World Health Organization (WHO) has categorized the reasons for nonadherence into 5 categories: (1) health system, (2) condition, (3) patient, (4) therapy, and (5) socioeconomic-related factors.[42,43] Health system–related factors include lack of communication between patients and providers and poor patient-provider relationship.[43] Medication reconciliation and discharge counseling are examples of ways to address system-related factors to improve the discrepancies that often occur during transitions in care. Condition-related factors include mental health disorders or asymptomatic chronic diseases such as hypertension. Patient-related factors include

Table 1
Comparison of the Morisky Medication Adherence Scales (MMAS)

Morisky Four-Item (1986)[62]	Morisky Eight-Item (2008)[64]
Do you ever forget to take your medications?	Do you sometimes forget to take your high blood pressure pills?
Are you careless at times about taking your medicine?	Over the past 2 weeks, were there any days when you did not take your high blood pressure medicine?
When you feel better do you sometimes stop taking your medicine?	Have you ever cut back or stopped taking your medication without telling your doctor because you felt worse when you took it?
Sometimes if you feel worse when you take the medicine, do you stop taking it?	When you travel or leave home, do you sometimes forget to bring along your medications?
	Did you take your high blood pressure medicine yesterday?
	When you feel like your blood pressure is under control, do you sometimes stop taking your medicine?
	Taking medication every day is a real inconvenience for some people. Do you ever feel hassled about sticking to your blood pressure treatment plan?
	How often do you have difficulty remembering to take all your blood pressure medication?

younger age, physical impairments, and nonwhite race.[43,44] A study by Yang and colleagues[45] found that in patients with diabetes, female gender, age younger than 65 years, and black or Hispanic race were significantly associated with nonadherence. Therapy-related factors include lack of tolerability to medications and high pill burden, and socioeconomic-related factors include cost or copayments.[43]

Cost and copayments
Socioeconomic-related factors such as higher copayments and out-of-pocket costs have been associated with nonadherence and nonpersistence in multiple disease states. For example, copayments greater than $20 for inhalers used in chronic obstructive pulmonary disease (COPD) and β-blockers in cardiovascular disease have been associated with nonadherence when compared with lower copayments.[46,47] Furthermore, Gibson and colleagues[48] found that higher copayments for statin therapy was associated with nonadherence, and Neugut and colleagues[49] found that higher copayments in patients with early-stage breast cancer were associated with nonadherence as well as nonpersistence. In a study of 77 patients with diabetes, the most common reason for nonadherence was cited as "cost of medications" (34%).[50]

Pill burden and tolerability
High pill burden, complicated dosing regimens, and medications with greater ADEs are well-known risk factors for medication nonadherence.[51,52] A meta-analysis performed by Bangalore and colleagues[51] found that fixed-dose combination therapies

significantly reduced nonadherence by 26% compared with matched free-drug medication regimens. This review evaluated a variety of disease states such as tuberculosis, hypertension, and human immunodeficiency virus. In addition, nonadherence to respiratory therapies in patients with COPD has been linked to both the quantity of medications and the number of daily doses.[53]

Beliefs

Patients' beliefs regarding their health and the potential benefit and/or harm of medication therapies can affect medication adherence. For example, in a telephone survey by Allen LaPointe and colleagues,[54] 2 factors were independently associated with adherence: greater perceived necessity for heart medications and concern about heart medication causing adverse consequences. Perceived necessity was associated with higher adherence while concern for adverse consequences was associated with lower adherence rates. Another study showed that medication beliefs affected both intentional (choosing not to take medications as prescribed) and unintentional (forgetting to take medications) medication nonadherence. Medication necessity beliefs were shown to predict intentional adherence, whereas perceptions of overuse of medication were shown to predict unintentional nonadherence.[55]

Consequences of Medication Nonadherence

Medication nonadherence and nonpersistence can be risky to a patient's health over time, as it can lead to uncontrolled or worsening of chronic conditions as well as unwanted morbidity and mortality.[56–59] In a study by DiMatteo and colleagues,[58] patients adherent to medications reduced their risk of a clinical outcome by 26%. Patients who reported missing blood-pressure pills in the last week have been shown to be 6.6 times more likely to have uncontrolled blood pressure.[60] This situation may lead to unnecessary addition of medications to a pharmacotherapy regimen to treat a chronic disease that appears uncontrolled, when in fact the patient may not be taking the medications as prescribed. In addition, nonadherence to antihypertensive and statin therapy has been shown to approximately double the patient's risk of myocardial infarction, stroke, and angina.[61] Medications are often prescribed to prevent long-term consequences associated with certain chronic diseases; poor medication-taking behavior may hinder these potential benefits.

Tools and Interventions to Reduce Medication Nonadherence

Medication-taking behavior is patient specific and is determined by a variety of different factors. Addressing an individual's contributing factors to either taking or not taking one's medications is important in improving adherence and persistence to pharmacotherapy over time. Tools such as the MMAS and the ASK-12 can be used to assess adherence. Interventions to improve adherence include a comprehensive medication history, using adherence aids, educating patients, and incorporating an interdisciplinary approach to care.

Morisky Medication Adherence Scale

The MMAS was first developed in 1986 in patients with hypertension. The tool consists of a 4-item questionnaire.[62] This questionnaire is short in length, and addresses only medication adherence and not medication efficacy. However, it has been validated in multiple disease states.[63] Recently, the MMAS was updated and validated in hypertension patients. The new version of MMAS consists of 8 items, 4 of which are derived from the original 4-item MMAS and 4 new items that address adherence behavior (see **Table 1**).[62,64] Patients are considered to have low adherence if they receive a score less than 6.[64] Muntner and colleagues[65] found that a change of 2 or more points over time in the 8-item questionnaire represented a change in adherence to antihypertensive medications. This tool is quick and easy to administer in the outpatient setting, and can be used to evaluate adherence in patients in whom "medication resistance" appears to be present (ie, patients taking 3 or more antihypertensive medications).

ASK-20 and ASK-12

The ASK-20 questionnaire is a 20-item questionnaire that was recently developed to help identify behaviors and barriers associated with medication adherence. This self-administered survey has been validated in patients with diabetes, asthma, depression, and heart failure.[66,67] Higher total scores on the ASK-20 indicate more barriers to adherence.[66,68] In a study by Matza and colleagues,[67] the questionnaire was shown to significantly correlate with the 4-item MMAS. Since then, a shortened version (ASK-12) has been evaluated in patients with asthma, diabetes, and heart failure. This version was also found to correlate with the 4-item MMAS.[68] The ASK-20 and ASK-12 surveys have only been evaluated in small studies, and further research with additional disease states and patient populations is warranted.

Adherence aids

Managing multiple medications often requires adherence aids to help patients with their complicated medication regimens. Incorporating medications into a daily routine and using pillboxes have been reported as helpful reminders by patients with diabetes.[69] A variety of adherence aids and techniques are available to patients. The following list provides some examples:

1. Using a pillbox
2. Using a calendar or log book
3. Taking medications at the same time each day
4. Incorporating medications into a daily routine and associating them with another daily activity such as brushing teeth or eating breakfast
5. Keeping medications where they are visible (away from children and pets)
6. Setting an alarm on a clock, watch, cell phone, or other device
7. Involving a family member or friend to serve as a reminder.

Education

Providing education on patient medication is a critical step toward ensuring adherence, and has been reported to enhance adherence to many types of medications including antiglycemic agents.[69] Educating patients on the long-term consequences of chronic diseases, the importance of medication adherence in potentially preventing certain sequelae, and what to expect from the medications (benefits, adverse effects, and so forth) may have a potential role in improving adherence and persistence to chronic disease medications. It is important to not only provide information, but to also confirm that the patient can understand the information that is being provided. Requesting patient feedback is of the utmost importance to judge his or her level of understanding.

Interdisciplinary approach

Multiple studies have shown that collaboration between health care providers and pharmacists have improved both medication adherence and persistence. Carter and Foppe van Mil[70] found that collaboration between physicians and pharmacists was shown to not only improve medication adherence to antihypertensive medications but also improve blood pressure control. These investigators reviewed collaboration between providers and community pharmacists as well as pharmacists incorporated in the medical home model. A recent meta-analysis also showed that pharmacist intervention involving combination strategies significantly improved both adherence to antihypertensive medications and control of blood pressure.[71]

Lee and colleagues evaluated the impact of a pharmacy care program on both medication adherence and persistence in patients who were 65 years or older and taking 4 or more chronic medications. In this study, patients were first enrolled into a pharmacy care program for 6 months (Phase 1), then randomly assigned to either continue or were returned to usual care for an additional 6 months (Phase 2). On completion of Phase 1, medication adherence increased from 61.2% at baseline to 96.9%. In addition, medication persistence was also seen after Phase 2 in the intervention group (95.5% were adherent). By contrast, adherence declined to 69.1% in the usual-care group after Phase 2.[72]

ADVERSE DRUG REACTIONS AND EVENTS

Pharmacologic management of chronic disease states is not without risk, as adverse reactions to medications can lead to serious events and consequences for patients. The FDA considers an adverse event serious if it results in one of the following outcomes: death, a life-threatening event, initial or prolonged hospitalization, disability or permanent damage, congenital anomaly or birth defect, or a serious event that jeopardizes the patient's health.[20]

In 2010 the FDA entered 673,259 ADEs into the Adverse Events Reporting System.[73] Of the adverse events reported in 2010, the FDA reported that 82,724 resulted in death and 471,291 were considered to be serious adverse events.[74] Compared with the number of deaths in the United States preliminarily reported for 2010, deaths from ADEs would rank as the seventh leading cause of death.[4,74]

A secondary analysis of 2005-2007 adult data from the National Ambulatory Medical Care Survey and the National Hospital and Ambulatory Medical Care Survey estimated that 13.5 million ADE-related visits occurred during this time period (~4.5 million/year). ADE-related visits comprised 0.5% of all ambulatory visits. Population-based ADE-related visit rates were found to increase with patient age, and those 65 years and older had the highest rate (3.8 ADE visits per 10,000 persons per year). However, the highest number of absolute ADE visits occurred in the 45- to 64-year-old age group.[75]

A cohort study of 30,397 patients 65 years and older in the ambulatory setting was conducted to identify the incidence of ADEs in a 1-year period. These events were identified via adverse event reporting by health care providers, review of hospital discharge summaries, review of emergency department notes, computer-generated signals, free text searching of electronic clinic notes, and review of incident reports of medication errors. Investigators identified 1523 adverse events. Of these events, 421 (27.6%) were characterized as preventable.[76] A prospective cohort study of 808 frail elderly veterans found 33% of patients to have at least one adverse drug reaction during a 1-year follow-up period after hospital discharge (rate of 1.92 per 1000 person days of follow-up).[77]

Risk Factors for Adverse Drug Reactions and ADEs

An expert panel identified several risk factors for adverse drug reactions in patients aged 65 years and older. Patients' characteristics identified as potential risk factors included polypharmacy, dementia, multiple chronic medical conditions, creatinine clearance less than 50 mL/min, recent hospitalization, age 85 years and older, alcohol use of more than 1 fluid ounce per day, and prior adverse drug reaction.[78] A case-control study of older adults in the ambulatory care setting also identified several factors associated with having a higher risk for an ADE. Female gender and age 80 and older were found to be independent risk factors. Increasing number of medications and higher scores on the Charlson Comorbidity Index were also associated with increased risk for having an ADE. These factors were also correlated with preventable ADEs.[79]

Several classes of medications stand out as most commonly implicated in ADEs. In the aforementioned case-control study, medication classes significantly associated with ADEs included anticoagulants, antidepressants, antibiotics, cardiovascular drugs, diuretics, hormones, and corticosteroids. Use of nonopioid analgesics, anticoagulants, diuretics, and antiseizure medications were found to be independently associated with having a preventable ADE.[79] The expert panel discussed in the previous paragraph identified anticholinergics, benzodiazepines, antipsychotics, sedative/hypnotics, nonaspirin, nonsteroidal anti-inflammatories, tricyclic antidepressants, opioids, corticosteroids, warfarin, and lithium as medication classes and medications that may put those age 65 and older at risk for ADEs.[78] In addition, in Gurwitz and colleagues'[76] cohort study conducted in elderly, ambulatory patients, the most frequent drug classes involved in the 1523 ADEs identified were cardiovascular (26%), antibiotics (14.7%), diuretics (13.3%), nonopioid analgesics (11.8%), anticoagulants (7.9%), hypoglycemics (6.8%), and steroids (5.3%). The most frequent drug classes involved in the 412 preventable ADEs were cardiovascular (24.5%), diuretics (22.1%), nonopioid analgesics (15.4%), hypoglycemics (10.9%), anticoagulants (10.2%), and opioids (6.7%). The majority of errors leading to the preventable ADEs occurred during the monitoring stage (ie, inadequate laboratory monitoring or failing to respond to signs and symptoms of drug toxicity) (60.8%) and the prescribing stage (58.4%). Patient adherence errors were identified in 21.1% of the events. Dispensing errors were identified in fewer than 2% of the events.[76]

To support the connection between polypharmacy and ADEs, an analysis of ADE rates in adult ambulatory patients found the number of daily medications taken to significantly increase the risk of an ADE. Specifically, taking 6 to 8 medications increased the odds of an ADE compared with no medications (OR 3.83 [95% CI 2.20–6.65]). There was also increased reporting of ADEs during primary care visits versus specialty visits (OR 1.82 [95% CI 1.40–2.36]).[75]

Consequences of Adverse Drug Reactions and ADEs

ADEs can lead to several serious events, as outlined earlier. According to the AHRQ's Healthcare Cost and use Project's most recent statistics in 2008, adverse effects were recorded in 1,735,000 inpatient hospital stays and 623,600 treat-and-release emergency department visits. Three percent of inpatient cases with a drug-related adverse outcome resulted in death.[80] Of the 412 preventable ADEs identified in the cohort of ambulatory elderly, electrolyte and renal events were the most prevalent (26.6%), followed by gastrointestinal tract events (21.1%), hemorrhagic (15.9%), metabolic and endocrine (13.8%), and neuropsychiatric (8.6%).[76]

Tools and Interventions to Reduce Adverse Drug Reactions and ADEs

It is thought that taking the steps to avoid polypharmacy and IP as discussed previously will in turn help to reduce ADEs. Additional ways to help avoid these events may also include being aware of risk factors for ADEs and knowing the medications most commonly implicated.[77,81] Bressler and Bahl[82] propose that health care providers must ensure that patients have a definitive diagnosis (ie, avoiding treating a side effect of another drug) and determine whether the benefits outweigh the risks before initiating drug therapy. Computerized physician order entry (CPOE) with clinical decision support (CDS), drug-drug interaction and drug-disease interaction alerts, and laboratory monitoring may also help to decrease ADEs. Increased patient education and collaborations between prescribers and pharmacists may help to reduce ADEs as well.[76]

Wolfstadt and colleagues[83] completed a systematic review of research from 1966 to March 2007 that evaluated the effect of using CPOE with CDS on the incidence of ADEs. Investigators identified 10 studies that met their inclusion criteria. Nine of these studies were conducted in the hospital setting and one in the ambulatory care setting. Five of the 10 studies found the use of CPOE with CDS to significantly reduce the number of ADEs, 4 saw a trend toward reduction but did not yield statistically significant results, and 1 found no effect. This study highlights the need for continued research on the effect of CPOE with CDS on the reduction of ADEs.

OVERALL APPROACH TO MINIMIZE MEDICATION-RELATED PROBLEMS IN OFFICE PATIENTS

To avoid or minimize the 4 pharmacologic issues discussed in this article, primary care providers should conduct a thorough review of a patient's medication list at each visit and encourage patients to bring in medication bottles at all visits. A complete medication assessment involves gathering a detailed medication history including all of a patient's current prescription medications, over-the-counter medications, vitamins, minerals, herbal products, and dietary supplements, and keeping medication lists as up to date as possible. Once completed, each medication should be matched back to a patient's disease state to identify PIMs or omitted medications. If a medication does not have an obvious indication, providers should investigate why this medication is prescribed or why the patient has elected to take this medication. Providers should also minimize the use of any medication prescribed to treat the side effect of a previously prescribed medication. Each medication should be reviewed and monitored for appropriateness at each office visit. Use of one of the tools previously discussed, such as the MAI, may also help primary care providers in assessing medication appropriateness.

Nonadherence and nonpersistence to medications is multifactorial and assessing adherence at the time of medication review may also be helpful. Health care providers can identify patients at high risk for nonadherence and patients with adherence barriers through an assessment tool, as previously described. Medication education, use of adherence aids, prescribing medications that are well tolerated and less costly (such as generic medications), and incorporating the expertise of other disciplines such as clinical pharmacists should be encouraged to overcome patients' beliefs and barriers to adherence.

The overall goal of avoiding pharmacologic-related issues is to improve patient safety. The US Department of Health and Human Services has included several objectives related to these issues in Healthy People 2020. The Medical Product Safety objectives focus on the appropriate use of drugs. Relevant objectives to the pharmacologic issues discussed include (1) increase the proportion of health care organizations that are monitoring and analyzing adverse events associated with medical therapies and their systems, (2) increase the safe and effective treatment of pain, (3) reduce the number of adverse events from medical products, and (4) reduce emergency department visits for common, preventable adverse events from medications (including anticoagulants, injectable antidiabetic agents, and narrow therapeutic index medications).[84] In addition, reducing inappropriate medication use in the elderly is included in the 2011 and 2012 HEDIS. Relevant measures include potentially harmful drug-disease interactions in the elderly and use of high-risk medications in the elderly.[33]

SUMMARY

A significant portion of the adult population uses one or more medications on a regular basis. Use of medications is not without complications. These complications may include polypharmacy, IP, medication nonadherence and nonpersistence, and ADEs. Numerous methods exist to help prevent and minimize these pharmacologic issues. By attempting to reduce polypharmacy, IP, medication nonadherence and nonpersistence, and ADEs, health care professionals will improve patient safety and well-being and optimize the medical management of chronic disease.

REFERENCES

1. Patterns of medication use in the United States 2006: a report from the Slone Survey. Slone Epidemiology Center at Boston University Web site; 2011. Available at: http://www.bu.edu/slone/SloneSurvey/AnnualRpt/SloneSurveyWebReport2006.pdf. Accessed August 15, 2011.
2. Qato DM, Alexander GC, Conti RM, et al. Use of prescription and over-the-counter medications and dietary supplements among older adults in the United States. JAMA 2008;300(24):2867–78.
3. Nahin RL, Pecha M, Welmerink DB, et al. Concomitant use of prescription drugs and dietary supplements in ambulatory elderly people. J Am Geriatr Soc 2009; 57(7):1197–205.
4. Murphy SL, Xu J, Kochanek KD. Deaths: preliminary data for 2010. National vital statistics reports, vol. 60(4). Hyattsville (MD): National Center for Health Statistics; 2012. Available at: http://www.cdc.gov/nchs/data/nvsr/nvsr60/nvsr60_04.pdf. Accessed January 15, 2012.
5. Hajjar ER, Cafiero AC, Hanlon JT. Polypharmacy in elderly patients. Am J Geriatr Pharmacother 2007;5(4):345–51.
6. Frazier SC. Health outcomes and polypharmacy in elderly individuals. J Gerontol Nurs 2005;31(9):4–11.
7. Jyrkka J, Enlund H, Korhonen MJ, et al. Patterns of drug use and factors associated with polypharmacy and excessive polypharmacy in elderly persons. Drugs Aging 2009;26(6):493–503.
8. Rollason V, Vogt N. Reduction of polypharmacy in the elderly: a systematic review of the role of the pharmacist. Drugs Aging 2003;20(11):817–32.
9. Milton JC, Jackson SH. Inappropriate polypharmacy: reducing the burden of multiple medication. Clin Med 2007;7(5):514–7.
10. Fillenbaum GG, Horner RD, Hanlon JT, et al. Factors predicting change in prescription and nonprescription drug use in a community-residing black and white elderly population. J Clin Epidemiol 1996;49:587–93.
11. Garfinkel D, Mangin D. Feasibility study of a systematic approach for discontinuation of multiple medications in older adults. Arch Intern Med 2010;170(18): 1648–54.
12. Fillit HM, Futterman R, Orland BI, et al. Polypharmacy management in Medicare managed care: changes in prescribing by primary care physicians resulting from a program promoting medication reviews. Am J Manag Care 1999;5(5):587–94.
13. Zarowitz BJ, Stebelsky LA, Muma BK, et al. Reduction of high-risk polypharmacy drug combinations in patients in a managed care setting. Pharmacotherapy 2005;25(11):1636–45.

14. Liu GG, Christensen DB. The continuing challenge of inappropriate prescribing in the elderly: an update of the evidence. J Am Pharm Assoc (Wash) 2002;42(6):847–57.

15. Gallagher PF, Barry PJ, Ryan C, et al. Inappropriate prescribing in an acutely ill population of elderly patients as determined by Beers' Criteria. Age Ageing 2008;37(1):96–101.

16. Gallagher P, O'Mahony D. STOPP (Screening Tool of Older Persons' potentially inappropriate Prescriptions): application to acutely ill elderly patients and comparison with Beers' criteria. Age Ageing 2008;37(6):673–9.

17. Barry PJ, Gallagher P, Ryan C, et al. START (screening tool to alert doctors to the right treatment)—an evidence-based screening tool to detect prescribing omissions in elderly patients. Age Ageing 2007;36(6):632–8.

18. Budnitz DS, Shehab N, Kegler SR, et al. Medication use leading to emergency department visits for adverse drug events in older adults. Ann Intern Med 2007;147(11):755–65.

19. Spinewine A, Schmader KE, Barber N, et al. Appropriate prescribing in elderly people: how well can it be measured and optimised? Lancet 2007;370(9582): 173–84.

20. What is a serious adverse event? U.S. Food and Drug Administration; 2011. Available at: http://www.fda.gov/Safety/MedWatch/HowToReport/ucm053087.htm. Accessed August 15, 2011.

21. Clinical safety data management: definitions and standards for expedited reporting. European Agency for the Evaluation of Medicinal Products, Human Medicines Evaluation Unit; 1995. Available at: http://eudravigilance.ema.europa.eu/human/docs/e2a.pdf. Accessed January 13, 2012.

22. Nixdorff N, Hustey FM, Brady AK, et al. Potentially inappropriate medications and adverse drug effects in elders in the ED. Am J Emerg Med 2008;26(6):697–700.

23. Bates DW, Spell N, Cullen DJ. The costs of adverse drug events in hospitalized patients. Adverse Drug Events Prevention Study Group. JAMA 1997;277(4):307–11.

24. Samsa GP, Hanlon JT, Schmader KE. A summated score for the Medication Appropriateness Index: development and assessment of clinimetric properties including content validity. J Clin Epidemiol 1994;47(8):891–6.

25. Beers MH, Ouslander JG, Rollingher I, et al. UCLA Division of Geriatric Medicine. Explicit criteria for determining inappropriate medication use in nursing home residents. Arch Intern Med 1991;151(9):1825–32.

26. Beers MH. Explicit criteria for determining potentially inappropriate medication use by the elderly: an update. Arch Intern Med 1997;157(14):1531–6.

27. Fick DM, Cooper JW, Wade WE, et al. Updating the Beers criteria for potentially inappropriate medication use in older adults: results of a US consensus panel of experts. Arch Intern Med 2003;163(22):2716–24.

28. Zhan C, Sangl J, Bierman AS, et al. Potentially inappropriate medication use in the community-dwelling elderly: findings from the 1996 Medical Expenditure Panel Survey. JAMA 2001;286(22):2823–9.

29. Chang CM, Liu PY, Yang YH, et al. Use of the beers criteria to predict adverse drug reactions among first-visit elderly outpatients. Pharmacotherapy 2005; 25(6):831–8.

30. Passarelli MC, Jacob-Filho W, Figueras A. Adverse drug reactions in an elderly hospitalised population: inappropriate prescription is a leading cause. Drugs Aging 2005;22(9):767–77.

31. Chrischilles EA, VanGilder R, Wright K, et al. Inappropriate medication use as a risk factor for self-reported adverse drug effects in older adults. J Am Geriatr Soc 2009;57(6):1000–6.

32. National Committee for Quality Assurance. NCQA Releases HEDIS 2006; New measures address overuse, follow-up. Available at: http://www.ncqa.org/tabid/277/Default.aspx. Accessed August 15, 2011.
33. National Committee for Quality Assurance. HEDIS, & quality measurement. Available at: http://www.ncqa.org/tabid/59/Default.aspx. Accessed August 15, 2011.
34. Lund BC, Carnahan RM, Egge JA, et al. Inappropriate prescribing predicts adverse drug events in older adults. Ann Pharmacother 2010;44(6):957–63.
35. Fitzgerald LS, Hanlon JT, Shelton PS, et al. Reliability of a modified medication appropriateness index in ambulatory older persons. Ann Pharmacother 1997; 31(5):543–8.
36. Gallagher P, Ryan C, Byrne S, et al. STOPP (Screening Toll of Older Persons' Prescriptions) and START (screening tool to alert doctors to right treatment): consensus validation. Int J Clin Pharmacol Ther 2008;46:72–83.
37. Gallagher PF, O'Connor MN, O'Mahony D. Prevention of potentially inappropriate prescribing for elderly patients: a randomized controlled trial using STOPP/START criteria. Clin Pharmacol Ther 2011;89(6):845–54.
38. Hamilton H, Gallagher P, Ryan C, et al. Potentially inappropriate medications defined by STOPP criteria and the risk of adverse drug events in older hospitalized patients. Arch Intern Med 2011;171(11):1013–9.
39. Burnier M. Medication adherence and persistence as the cornerstone of effective antihypertensive therapy. Am J Hypertens 2006;19(11):1190–6.
40. Fischer MA, Stedman MR, Lii J, et al. Primary medication non-adherence: analysis of 195,930 electronic prescriptions. J Gen Intern Med 2010;25(4):284–90.
41. Krousel-Wood MA, Muntner P, Islam T, et al. Barriers to and determinants of medication adherence in hypertension management: perspective of the cohort study of medication adherence among older adults. Med Clin North Am 2009;93(3): 753–69.
42. Adherence to long-term therapy: evidence for action. World Health Organization; 2003. Available at: http://www.who.int/chp/knowledge/publications/adherence_introduction.pdf. Accessed August 15, 2011.
43. Ho PM, Bryson CL, Rumsfeld JS. Medication adherence: its importance in cardiovascular outcomes. Circulation 2009;119(23):3028–35.
44. Friedman DS, Okeke CO, Jampel HD, et al. Risk factors for poor adherence to eyedrops in electronically monitored patients with glaucoma. Ophthalmology 2009;116(6):1097–105.
45. Yang Y, Thumula V, Pace PF, et al. Predictors of medication nonadherence among patients with diabetes in Medicare Part D programs: a retrospective cohort study. Clin Ther 2009;31(10):2178–88 [discussion: 2150–51].
46. Castaldi PJ, Rogers WH, Safran DG, et al. Inhaler costs and medication nonadherence among seniors with chronic pulmonary disease. Chest 2010;138(3): 614–20.
47. Patterson ME, Blalock SJ, Smith AJ, et al. Associations between prescription co-payment levels and β-blocker medication adherence in commercially insured heart failure patients 50 years and older. Clin Ther 2011;33(5):608–16.
48. Gibson TB, Mark TL, McGuigan KA, et al. The effects of prescription drug copayments on statin adherence. Am J Manag Care 2006;12(9):509–17.
49. Neugut AI, Subar M, Wilde ET, et al. Association between prescription co-payment amount and compliance with adjuvant hormonal therapy in women with early-stage breast cancer. J Clin Oncol 2011;29(18):2534–42.
50. Odegard PS, Gray SL. Barriers to medication adherence in poorly controlled diabetes mellitus. Educ 2008;34(4):692–7.

51. Bangalore S, Kamalakkannan G, Parkar S, et al. Fixed-dose combinations improve medication compliance: a meta-analysis. Am J Med 2007;120(8):713–9.

52. Elliott WJ. Improving outcomes in hypertensive patients: focus on adherence and persistence with antihypertensive therapy. J Clin Hypertens (Greenwich) 2009; 11(7):376–82.

53. Agh T, Inotai A, Meszaros A. Factors associated with medication adherence in patients with chronic obstructive pulmonary disease. Respiration 2011;82(4): 328–34.

54. Allen LaPointe NM, Ou FS, Calvert SB, et al. Association between patient beliefs and medication adherence following hospitalization for acute coronary syndrome. Am Heart J 2011;161(5):855–63.

55. Schüz B, Marx C, Wurm S, et al. Medication beliefs predict medication adherence in older adults with multiple illnesses. J Psychosom Res 2011;70(2):179–87.

56. Asche C, LaFleur J, Conner C. A review of diabetes treatment adherence and the association with clinical and economic outcomes. Clin Ther 2011;33(1):74–109.

57. Bae JW, Guyer W, Grimm K, et al. Medication persistence in the treatment of HIV infection: a review of the literature and implications for future clinical care and research. AIDS 2011;25(3):279–90.

58. DiMatteo MR, Giordani PJ, Lepper HS, et al. Patient adherence and medical treatment outcomes: a meta-analysis. Med Care 2002;40(9):794–811.

59. Hill MN, Miller NH, DeGeest S. American Society of Hypertension Writing Group. ASH position paper: adherence and persistence with taking medication to control high blood pressure. J Clin Hypertens (Greenwich) 2010;12(10):757–64.

60. Aggarwal B, Mosca L. Lifestyle and psychosocial risk factors predict non-adherence to medication. Ann Behav Med 2010;40(2):228–33.

61. Cherry SB, Benner JS, Hussein MA, et al. The clinical and economic burden of nonadherence with antihypertensive and lipid-lowering therapy in hypertensive patients. Value Health 2009;12(4):489–97.

62. Morisky DE, Green LW, Levine DM. Concurrent and predictive validity of a self-reported measure of medication adherence. Med Care 1986;24(1):67–74.

63. Lavsa SM, Holzworth A, Ansani NT. Selection of a validated scale for measuring medication adherence. J Am Pharm Assoc (2003) 2011;51(1):90–4.

64. Morisky DE, Ang A, Krousel-Wood M, et al. Predictive validity of a medication adherence measure for hypertension control. J Clin Hypertens 2008;10(5): 348–54.

65. Muntner P, Joyce C, Holt E, et al. Defining the minimal detectable change in scores on the eight-item Morisky Medication Adherence Scale. Ann Pharmacother 2011;45(5):569–75.

66. Hahn SR, Park J, Skinner EP, et al. Development of the ASK-20 adherence barrier survey. Curr Med Res Opin 2008;24(7):2127–38.

67. Matza LS, Yu-Isenberg KS, Coyne KS. Further testing of the reliability and validity of the ASK-20 adherence barrier questionnaire in a medical center outpatient population. Curr Med Res Opin 2008;24(11):3197–206.

68. Matza LS, Park J, Coyne KS, et al. Derivation and validation of the ASK-12 adherence barrier survey. Ann Pharmacother 2009;43(10):1621–30.

69. Morello CM, Chynoweth M, Kim H, et al. Strategies to improve medication adherence reported by diabetes patients and caregivers: results of a taking control of your diabetes survey. Ann Pharmacother 2011;45:145–53.

70. Carter BL, Foppe van Mil JW. Comparative effectiveness research: evaluating pharmacist interventions and strategies to improve medication adherence. Am J Hypertens 2010;23(9):949–55.

71. Morgado MP, Morgado SR, Mendes LC, et al. Pharmacist interventions to enhance blood pressure control and adherence to antihypertensive therapy: review and meta-analysis. Am J Health Syst Pharm 2011;68(3):241–53.
72. Lee JK, Grace KA, Taylor AJ. Effect of a pharmacy care program on medication adherence and persistence, blood pressure, and low-density lipoprotein cholesterol: a randomized controlled trial. JAMA 2006;296(21):2563–71.
73. Reports received and reports entered into AERS by year. U.S. Food and Drug Administration; 2011. Available at: http://www.fda.gov/Drugs/GuidanceComplianceRegulatoryInformation/Surveillance/AdverseDrugEffects/ucm070434.htm. Accessed August 15, 2011.
74. AERS patient outcomes by year. U.S. Food and Drug Administration; 2011. Available at: http://www.fda.gov/Drugs/GuidanceComplianceRegulatoryInformation/Surveillance/AdverseDrugEffects/ucm070461.htm. Accessed August 15, 2011.
75. Sarkkar U, Lopez A, Maselli JH, et al. Adverse drug events in U.S. adult ambulatory medical care. Health Serv Res 2011;46(5):1517–33.
76. Gurwitz JH, Field TS, Harrold LR, et al. Incidence and preventability of adverse drug events among older persons in the ambulatory setting. JAMA 2003; 289(9):1107–16.
77. Hanlon JT, Pieper CF, Hajjar ER, et al. Incidence and predictors of all and preventable adverse drug reactions in frail elderly persons after hospital stay. J Gerontol A Biol Sci Med Sci 2006;61(5):511–5.
78. Hajjar ER, Hanlon JT, Artz MB, et al. Adverse drug reaction risk factors in older outpatients. Am J Geriatr Pharmacother 2003;1(2):82–9.
79. Field TS, Gurwitz JH, Harrold LR, et al. Risk factors for adverse drug events among older adults in the ambulatory setting. J Am Geriatr Soc 2004;52(8): 1349–54.
80. Lucado J, Paez K, Elixhauser A. Medication-related adverse outcomes in U.S. hospitals and emergency departments. Agency for Healthcare Research and Quality; 2008. Available at: http://www.hcup-us.ahrq.gov/reports/statbriefs/sb109.pdf. Accessed August 15, 2011.
81. Simonson W, Feinberg JL. Medication-related problems in the elderly. Drugs Aging 2005;22(7):559–69.
82. Bressler R, Bahl JJ. Principles of drug therapy for the elderly patient. Mayo Clin Proc 2003;78(12):1564–77.
83. Wolfstadt JI, Gurwitz JH, Field TS. The effect of computerized physician order entry with clinical decision support on the rates of adverse drug events: a systematic review. J Gen Intern Med 2008;23(4):451–8.
84. Medical product safety. Healthpeople.gov; 2011. Available at: http://www.healthypeople.gov/2020/topicsobjectives2020/overview.aspx?topicid=27. Accessed August 15, 2011.

Effective Strategies to Improve the Management of Diabetes:
Case Illustration from the Diabetes Health and Wellness Institute

Donna Rice, MBA, RN, CDE[a],*, Tyson M. Bain, MS[a,b],
Ashley Collinsworth, MPH, ELS[c], Karen Boyer, MSN, RN[a],
Neil S. Fleming, PhD, CQE[d], Esteria Miller, MBA[a]

KEYWORDS

- Effective strategies • Diabetes management • Primary care
- Racial/ethnic minorities

KEY POINTS

- Using a collaborative team approach in diabetes care creates a health care environment in which the patient has access to key resources needed to improve and sustain positive health outcomes.
- The Juanita J. Craft Diabetes Health and Wellness Institute (DHWI) is a unique partnership between a large, urban integrated health care system, the City of Dallas, and a South Dallas community, aiming to improve the management of diabetes and related health outcomes in a vulnerable population.
- The Juanita J. Craft Diabetes Health and Wellness Institute provides a comprehensive approach to disease management and prevention by providing access to clinical services, a recreation facility, diabetes and health education, cooking classes, and counseling.

Diabetes is one of the most prevalent chronic diseases in the United States, affecting an estimated 25.8 million people or 8.3% of the total population, and 27% of the population aged 65 years and older.[1] Diabetes-related complications are numerous and include cardiovascular disease, nephropathy, neuropathy, and retinopathy.[1] Diabetes

This work was not supported by a specific grant.
The authors have nothing to disclose.
[a] Diabetes Health and Wellness Institute, 4500 Spring Avenue, Dallas, TX 75210, USA; [b] Department of Quantitative Sciences, Baylor Health Care System, Institute for Health Care Research and Improvement, Dallas, TX, USA; [c] Center for Health Care Research, Baylor Health Care System, Institute for Health Care Research and Improvement, 8080 North Central Expressway, Suite 500, Dallas, TX 75206, USA; [d] Baylor Health Care System, The STEEP Global Institute, 8080 North Central Expressway, Dallas, TX 75206, USA
* Corresponding author.
E-mail address: Donna.Rice@BaylorHealth.edu

is the leading cause of blindness and amputations in the United States.[1] The total esti-mated costs related to diagnosed diabetes in 2007 were $174 billion including the direct costs of medical care related to diabetes treatment and indirect costs related to disability, work loss, and premature mortality.[1]

Proper management of diabetes including glucose, blood pressure, and lipid control, and preventive care practices for eyes, feet, and kidneys, can greatly reduce a patient's risk of developing complications related to this disease.[1] Many Americans have good access to health care that enables them to benefit fully from health care in the United States. Others face barriers that make the acquisition of basic health care services difficult. Racial and ethnic minorities and people of low socioeconomic status (SES) are disproportionately represented among those with access problems.[2]

While medications play a major role in diabetes management, other elements of self-care such as diet, exercise, and glucose monitoring can substantially affect health outcomes as well as diabetes-related complications.[3] Thus, clinical care for diabetes must involve patient engagement in self-care practices. Despite the known importance of diabetes self-management, traditional care, involving professionals solving prob-lems for patients, often does not provide diabetic patients with the sufficient education, tools, resources, and empowerment to make the lifestyle changes that are necessary for improved diabetes control.[4]

The Juanita J. Craft Diabetes Health and Wellness Institute (DHWI) is a unique partner-ship between a large, urban integrated health care system, the City of Dallas, and a South Dallas community to improve the management of diabetes and related health outcomes in a vulnerable population. This article reviews key strategies including, but not limited to, reducing health disparities, establishing community-based partnerships, emphasizing interprofessional teamwork and care coordination, and improving the health care expe-rience for patients, to improve the management of diabetes in the primary care setting. The authors illustrate these strategies by describing their experiences at DHWI.

CONFRONTING AND ELIMINATING HEALTH DISPARITIES

The state of Texas faces many challenges related to the prevention and control of dia-betes. There is a high prevalence of diabetes throughout the state, higher than that of the nation. Projected increases in populations that have been identified as being at higher risk for the development of diabetes, such as Hispanics, the elderly, and persons who are overweight, highlight the need for improved diabetes management and prevention strategies. An estimated 1.7 million (9.3%) persons 18 years of age or older living in Texas have been diagnosed with diabetes,[5] which is slightly higher than the diabetes prevalence for the nation (8.0%). An additional 440,000 adult Texans are believed to be undiagnosed. Prevalence of diabetes in Texas is higher among African Americans (16.6%) and Hispanics (11.0%) than among white non-Hispanics (8%).[6] In Texas, diabetes was the seventh leading cause of death overall in 2007, and the fourth and fifth leading causes of death among African Americans and Hispanics, respectively.[7] Diabetes mortality rates for African Americans and Hispanics are twice as high as mortality rates for non-Hispanic whites.[7] Texas has more unin-sured residents than any other state.[7] Texans with diabetes are more likely to report that they cannot see a doctor because of cost than those who do not have diabetes across gender and racial groups.[8] Approximately 28% of African Americans and 39% of Hispanics with diabetes reported that they were unable to see a doctor in the 12 preceding months because of the cost.[8]

Dallas County is the second largest county in Texas and is the ninth largest county in the United States, with a population of 2.4 million. Significant health, social, and economic disparities exist within the county. Poverty rates are 30% or more in many urban areas, compared with the county's average poverty rate of 16.5%. Hispanics make up 35.6% of the population of Dallas County and are disproportionately affected by poverty.[9] A high percentage of residents in depressed socioeconomic areas lack access to basic health care and are at high risk for developing diabetes and other chronic conditions. The prevalence of diabetes in Dallas County was 11.4% in 2007, compared with the state level of 10.3%.[10] The greatest economic and health disparities exist within the southern sector of Dallas County, where DHWI resides. At present, 66% of residents in South Dallas are African American and 32% are Hispanic. More than 60% of adults in the area are unemployed. Thirty-three percent of families live below the poverty line. The median household income is less than half of the Dallas County average. Home ownership rates are 13% lower than the city as a whole.[11] The prevalence of diabetes is expanding everywhere, as shown above. Poverty and health care disparities are adversely affecting diabetes prevalence and management.

Driven by its mission as a not-for-profit, faith-based health care entity with community service and health care quality at its core, the Baylor Health Care System (BHCS) continually seeks opportunities to improve health care delivery, access, and outcomes in the communities it serves. In 2006, BHCS began to focus its efforts on eliminating health disparities. Several studies and reports have illuminated the need to reduce health disparities in order to improve overall health outcomes.[12–14] A BHCS task forced identified the Frazier Community in South Dallas as the community having the greatest need for health-equity improvement within Dallas County, and determined that the implementation of a new model of care focused on diabetes management would have the greatest impact on improving the overall health and wellness of the community. Approximately 13% of adults in the area have diabetes compared with the Dallas County average of 9.2%.[11]

COMMUNITY PARTNERSHIPS

There are many barriers to the diagnosis and effective control of diabetes in this community. Access to high-quality health care is limited. The only health clinic in the area does not actively refer patients to diabetes educators, nutritionists, or diabetes specialists such as endocrinologists or diabetologists. There is just one full-service grocery store in the area and it offers only a small selection of fresh foods, which limits the ability of residents to maintain healthy diets. Many residents do not have access to recreation facilities or a safe environment for exercise. Residents of the community commonly lack knowledge about preventing and managing diabetes (DHWI, unpublished data, 2010). A community needs assessment revealed that roughly 57% of people surveyed believe their family history of diabetes makes developing the disease "inevitable" (DHWI, unpublished data, 2010). Many people in South Dallas manage their diabetes by waiting until a crisis occurs and then entering local hospitals such as Baylor University Medical Center through the emergency department. Thirty percent of hospital admissions and emergency department visits are due to diabetes or a diabetes-related condition (BHCS, personal communication, 2009). These barriers have contributed to a significantly higher incidence rate of diabetes and diabetes-related complications in South Dallas compared with other areas of the city.

Recognizing that the disparities in health care access and outcomes faced by residents of the Frazier Community were due to an array of underlying social and economic determinants, BHCS decided to implement a comprehensive health-equity model that would not only meet immediate clinical needs related to diabetes but would also provide targeted interventions to promote wellness and behavior modification. Through community partnerships and addressing community-determined issues of health and well-being, health care organizations learn how to more effectively contribute to the overall health of the communities they serve.[15,16] At the center of this model is the Juanita J. Craft DHWI, a community center that has been repurposed through collaboration between BHCS and the City of Dallas. The center is staffed by an interprofessional team of practitioners consisting of a family medicine physician, a nurse practitioner, a clinical nurse specialist in diabetes care and education, medical assistants, a licensed social worker, certified diabetes educators, an exercise physiologist, community health educators/workers, and pastoral care. The center provides a comprehensive approach to disease management and prevention by providing access to clinical health care services, a recreation facility, diabetes and health education, cooking classes, and counseling.

OUTREACH INTO THE COMMUNITY TO IDENTIFY AND ENGAGE MAJOR STAKEHOLDERS

The DHWI model is built on 3 core concepts: (1) acting as a diabetes center of excellence, (2) promoting collaboration among community stakeholders, and (3) improving individual, family, and community health outcomes. **Fig. 1** details the collaboration among the DHWI and community partners to promote and implement clinical health care, economic development, and faith-based initiatives that support health and wellness. DHWI is a partnership between a private, nonprofit health care system and the City of Dallas, operationally funded by the health care system. A variety of services and educational opportunities are offered to encourage individual and family lifestyle changes through health screening, health education/training, programs to promote

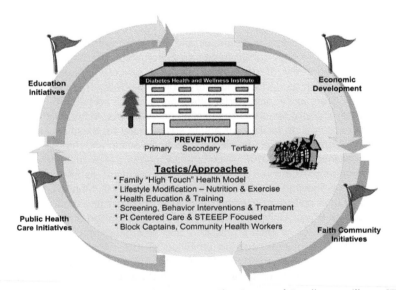

Fig. 1. Collaboration with community partners. The Center of Excellence will use STEEEP (Safety; Timeliness; Effectiveness; Efficiency; Equity; and Patient-centeredness) as a strategic imperative to ensure a high level of quality and patient satisfaction. (Copyright © 2011 Baylor Health Care System. All rights reserved; with permission.)

physical activity, behavioral interventions, and medical treatment both inside and outside DHWI's walls. This effort is similar to what has been accomplished with the REACH (Racial and Ethnic Approaches to Community Health) project in Detroit. In studying the REACH intervention, researchers found that appropriately designing a community-based program can have positive health effects such as improved knowledge, positive health behaviors, and improved glycemic control among racial and ethnic minorities with diabetes in an urban environment.[17]

The DHWI seeks to provide high-quality care as defined by the Institute of Medicine principles; care is safe, timely, effective, efficient, equitable, and patient-centered.[18] The DHWI engages in partnerships with the BHCS, the City of Dallas, and the local community. By educating schools, churches, community leaders, and local businesses on community health risks, the DHWI promotes awareness and fosters community engagement in achieving positive health outcomes. Other partnerships include the use of a ministerial advisory board representing influential community members from 40 churches and the partnership with local government, the City of Dallas, which allows for DHWI to link its preventive care and education to recreation programs. The goal of the church partnership was to set up multiple health ministries in the local community to help identify those at risk for diabetes and those in need of services. This initiative represents several innovative approaches to diabetes prevention and management that have the potential to reduce the burden of diabetes in South Dallas and abroad.

DIFFERENT APPROACHES FOR DIFFERENT AT-RISK POPULATIONS

The first part of the DHWI model (**Fig. 2**) represents the "center of excellence" concept. The DHWI strives to be a center of excellence for the treatment and prevention of diabetes.

Primary Prevention

Primary prevention initiatives focus on the prevention of diabetes, and include health promotion activities and the identification and removal of barriers to health and

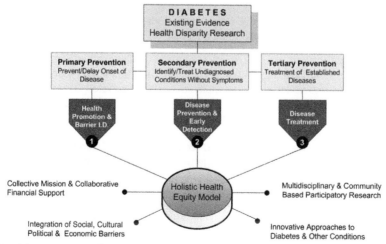

Fig. 2. Diabetes center of excellence. (Copyright © 2011 Baylor Health Care System. All rights reserved; with permission.)

wellness. The DHWI promotes primary prevention by providing low-cost access to a fitness center, exercise programs, cooking classes, health assessments, and health education in both individual and group formats throughout the day and late afternoon, and on weekends if needed. Patients can be referred to the center from the inpatient setting if they do not have a primary care provider (PCP) for their follow-up care, or they can choose to receive their primary care in the center regardless of where their care originates.

Early Identification and Secondary Prevention

Secondary prevention activities focus on individuals diagnosed with diabetes and the prevention of diabetes-related complications as well as other chronic diseases. These interventions include lifestyle programs, behavior-change strategies, psychosocial counseling, and diabetes management programs within the DHWI and community health worker–led programs at local churches. DHWI's diabetes-specific classes educate members about signs and symptoms of diabetes and related comorbidities. Members receive clinical assessments as a part of their initial enrollment to help them obtain timely and accurate diagnoses, and on an ongoing basis to monitor their response to treatment and lifestyle changes.

Tertiary Management

Tertiary prevention interventions are provided in the DHWI Family Health Clinic (the medical home for many DHWI clients), and are designed to provide treatment for persons with established diabetes and related comorbidities. DHWI works with physician groups and other health systems that provide donated services to the uninsured.

In addition to being a diabetes Center of Excellence, the DHWI strives to be a Holistic Health Equity Model by operating under 4 key areas: (1) collective mission and collaborative financial support; (2) integration of social, cultural, political, and economic barriers to health; (3) multidisciplinary and community-based participatory research; and (4) innovative approaches to diabetes and other conditions. It is a main goal of the center to achieve these key foci to ensure the provision of equitable health services to an underserved at-risk community in South Dallas.

Furthermore, establishment of the DHWI as a Center of Excellence in diabetes primary care and prevention, the following key elements and characteristics were identified by stakeholders as vital to its success:

- The establishment of an interprofessional, collaborative team of medical providers, including diabetologists and general practitioners with various levels of diabetes expertise as well as multiple levels of diabetes educators
- The provision of a personalized, individualized care plan for each patient that is outcomes-driven, based on the National Committee for Quality Assurance (NCQA) guidelines
- Care that is patient-centered and collaborative, including an individualized patient plan of care and self-management education component
- Provision of specialty care at the same site including podiatry, ophthalmology, and behavior-change counseling
- A Personalized Assistance Program that provides eligibility screening for food stamps, Medicaid, disability, cash grants, and all other forms of government assistance
- Care that is integrated across professions, community partnerships, and acute care settings

- Provision of professional development/education to continue building leaders in diabetes management

INTERPROFESSIONAL TEAMWORK

The DHWI provides personalized, individualized care involving an interprofessional health care team focusing on maintaining a center of excellence for the provision of prevention and treatment services for individuals with diabetes. At the core of this model of care is the delineation of roles among the team of diverse health care professionals. Involving a team of health care providers in care coordination requires the integration of information systems. An integrated information system ensures that the care patients receive from any member of the care team is consistent with the patient's overall care plan, is evidence based, and helps the patient to achieve improved health outcomes.[19,20] An important aspect of the model involved leveraging the expertise and practice scope of each member of the care team to prevent duplication and fragmentation of services.

The roles and skills of each member of the care team (collectively referred to as the diabetes care team), which comprises PCPs, diabetes educators, and other health care practitioners including community health workers, health educators, pastors, and social workers, must be understood and embraced to ensure that care is appropriately coordinated and that necessary collaboration occurs. Optimal care plans are developed with the input from every member of the team, including the patient. The care team's ability to enhance the patient's capacity for self-management of chronic conditions (ie, diabetes) is amplified by the variety of approaches and skills used by different team members in a coordinated manner.

Experienced diabetes education and prevention staff work with clients in between and/or in conjunction with visits with their primary provider to achieve positive health effects. Engaging a team of health care providers is an effective and efficient approach to disease management, often resulting in downstream cost savings.[21,22] This team approach promotes delineation of roles and requires that all professionals in the care team use their expertise based on their scope of practice, licensure, and related national guidelines. Although a well-functioning team with a clear division of labor might relieve physicians of some of their workload, finding the time to participate in team development is difficult for physicians.[23] One solution to this challenge as proposed by the authors is training for the functions that each team member routinely performs and cross-training to substitute for other roles in cases of absences, vacations, or periodic heavy demands on one part of the team. To facilitate the implementation of an efficient, integrated team, it is essential that all team members understand each other's roles and scope of practice and that "cross-training" be provided (as is feasible to the extent possible per role).

CARE COORDINATION

According to the American Diabetes Association Standards of Medical Care in Diabetes, glycemic control for adults with diabetes is defined as achieving a hemoglobin A_{1c} level of less than 7.0%, while a blood pressure of less than 130/80 mm Hg and a low-density lipoprotein (LDL) level of less than 100 mm/dL are additional standards of care for patients with hypertension and lipid comorbidities.[3] Standards for obesity are defined by body mass index.[24] Patients who have not achieved these standards of care, or who have a family history of diabetes, are older, and/or have barriers associated with the American Association of Diabetes Educators (AADE) 7 Key Health Behaviors (self-monitoring of blood glucose, eating a healthy diet, exercising to levels sufficient for health benefits, medications management, reducing risks, problem solving, and effective coping strategies for diabetes self-management), are triaged to one of the diabetes care team professionals to establish a diabetes prevention or management plan. This plan, based on an objective assessment of diabetes status, may include medication regimen adjustment, diabetes education, behavioral counseling, fitness assessment with exercise prescription, and dietary education. Patients with diabetes are provided with glucose self-monitoring devices as needed to promote effective self-management. Patients identified as being at high risk are assigned to a certified diabetes educator to improve their ability to self-manage their condition.

Data collected during DHWI's first year of operation indicate that patients who have participated in this new model of care have experienced improvements in diabetes-related health outcomes (DHWI, unpublished data, 2010). **Table 1** displays the outcome measures that are collected by the DHWI related to diabetes care, education, and support. More than 63% of clients have achieved a hemoglobin A_{1c} level of less than 7.0%, an increase of 16% over baseline (**Table 2**). The percentage of patients with hypertension who achieved blood-pressure control (defined as <130/80 mm/Hg) increased by 6.8% from baseline, and the percentage of patients who met the guideline for total cholesterol level less than 200 mg/dL increased by 8.1%. In addition, a major purpose of BHCS in establishing the DHWI as a center of care in South Dallas was to reduce the number of emergency department (ED) visits among South Dallas community members with diabetes to Baylor University Medical Center (BUMC). **Fig. 3** shows the BUMC ED visits by DHWI participants before and after enrollment/membership in DHWI in 2010. A total of 177 DHWI participants visited the BUMC ED at least once in the past year. Participants had 228 BUMC ED visits before enrollment in DHWI. The frequency of visits decreased to 137 after enrollment.

Table 1
DHWI diabetes-related outcomes and measures

Outcome	Measure
Glycemic control	Hemoglobin A_{1c}
Health indicators	Blood pressure Body mass index Urine albumin levels Lipid levels Flu/pneumonia vaccines
Achievement of ADA/Medicare Standards of care AADE 7 Self-Care Behaviors	Clinical, process measures, eye and foot examination Behavior change: interventions/barriers
Quality of life Satisfaction	Diabetes quality-of-life survey Patient-centeredness survey
Patient participation rates	Enrolled, % participation, dropouts/no-show rates
Health care cost	BHCS/BUMC inpatient/ED direct cost analysis/health outcomes

Abbreviations: AADE, American Association of Diabetes Educators; ADA, American Diabetes Association; BHCS, Baylor Health Care System; BUMC, Baylor University Medical Center; ED, emergency department.

Table 2
DHWI participants[a] achieving guidelines for diabetes care through May 2011

Hemoglobin A_{1c} Guidelines for Diabetes Care (<7.0%), n = 199			Blood Pressure Guidelines for Diabetes Care (<130/80 mm Hg), n = 307		
	Meets	Does Not Meet		Meets	Does Not Meet
Baseline	47.2%	52.8%	Baseline	32.6%	67.4%
Follow-up	63.3%	36.7%	Follow-up	39.4%	60.6%

Total Cholesterol Guidelines for Diabetes Care (<200 mg/dL), n = 99		
	Meets	Does Not Meet
Baseline	51.5%	48.5%
Follow-up	59.6%	40.4%

[a] Only participants with follow-up measure were used for this analysis.

The mean difference in BUMC ED visits before and after enrollment is 0.514 (95% confidence interval 0.25; 0.78) (P = .0002) (DHWI, unpublished data, 2010).

TEAM COORDINATION

The DHWI has adopted the Donabedian Model of Patient Safety[25] into the processes and procedures governing its delivery of primary care for patients with diabetes and diabetes-related complications. This model encourages the examination of how risks and hazards embedded within the structure of care have the potential to cause injury or harm to patients. In this model and its subsequent iterations, the primary goal is to improve patient outcomes. The Donabedian Model examines the role care processes have when performed within a given practice structure on health outcomes for the populations under care.

The diabetes care team works in concert to develop and support the care plan of individual patients by providing treatment, education, support, and skill building to promote self-management and lifestyle changes. If someone does not want to use the DHWI Family Health Center as their PCP, DHWI works with the patient's PCP to provide additional billable services based on referrals, such as diabetes self-management education, endocrinology, or other self-pay education classes. According to the AADE guidelines[26] for diabetes educators, a level-1 diabetes educator is a non–health care professional who has little expertise in diabetes education but provides support services to individuals with diabetes. This level includes health educators and community health workers. A level-2 diabetes educator includes health professionals who are nondiabetes educators, such as medical assistants. The third level is a noncredentialed diabetes educator or a professional who meets the AADE definition of a diabetes educator but does not have the distinction of a certified diabetes educator (CDE).[27] This level-3 role is performed by the exercise physiologist, licensed social worker, and the Family Health Center medical providers within the DHWI model. A level-4 diabetes educator is a CDE and includes the group of CDEs on the care team. The highest level, 5, includes the advanced-level diabetes educator clinical manager. The clinical nurse specialist at the DHWI fills this role by being board certified in advanced diabetes management (BC-ADM). It is this individual who

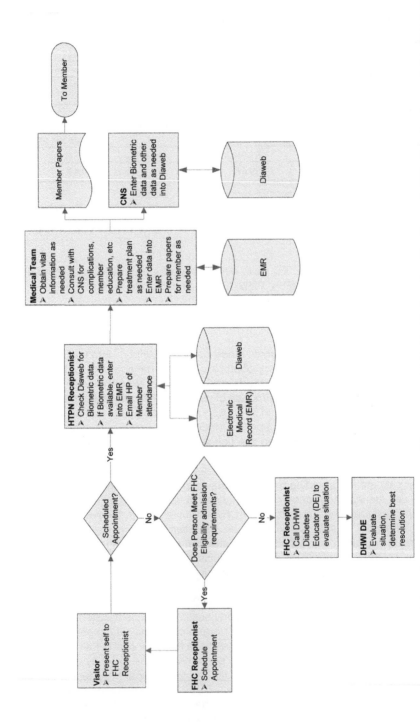

Fig. 3. DHWI Family Health Clinic (FHC) visit: integration of data systems. HTPN, Health Texas Provider Network. CNS, clinical nurse specialist; HP, health partner. (Copyright © 2011 Baylor Health Care System. All rights reserved. DHWI is a trademark of the Baylor Health Care System; with permission.)

informs the care team about best practices in diabetes education and management. DHWI currently uses all 5 levels of diabetes educators.

ELECTRONIC HEALTH RECORD

The use of patient data management systems is key to providing a coordinated, team approach to diabetes care and management and demonstrating the effectiveness of the care model. In 2008, a national survey of physicians found that only 13% reported having a basic electronic health record (EHR), and physicians in large practice groups were more likely to have an EHR in use.[19] The DHWI currently uses an EHR for its patient management. This system is used to collect and track information about clients' health risk, health behaviors, clinical outcomes, and quality of life. This EHR also provides the ability to set and manage behavior-change goals around diabetes self-management as defined by the AADE 7 Key Self-Care Behaviors.[28]

A health partner, who is one of the diabetes educators, is assigned to each patient to help coordinate diabetes care and uses the EHR to enhance coordination and management while creating and managing a patient registry. The focus is on measuring the achievement of behavior-change goals around these 7 behaviors (**Fig. 4**). The system tracks client participation in DHWI classes, and services and identifies additional programs that may be beneficial in the care plan. Educators are required to keep complete records of client encounters, including phone, e-mail, and in-person correspondence. Participants do not always have to be present at the center to receive education, counseling, and support from the diabetes care team, as staff often uses telecommunication methods. The EHR used at DHWI contains clinical decision tools, allowing for the coordination of point-of-care plans with real-time access to information that can be communicated between care team providers and patients. This immediate feedback provides staff and patients with the necessary information to treat and manage chronic conditions such as diabetes amid the fluid nature of external factors affecting one's health (see **Fig. 3**). Communication is pivotal in a collaborative care model. DHWI uses care conferences where members of staff discuss complex patients and supplement this with information from the EHR to enhance support for clinical decisions.

In selecting an EHR, physician practices should carefully consider the inclusion of clinical-decision support to facilitate quality care for individuals as well as the availability of tools, such as quality reporting and registry functions, to facilitate quality care for

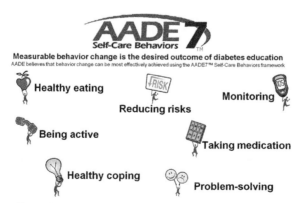

Fig. 4. AADE 7 self-care behaviors (AADE7). (Copyright © 2011 Baylor Health Care System. All rights reserved; with permission.)

populations.[20] A recent study conducted among 26 BHCS-affiliated primary care practices found that for an average 5-physician practice, implementation cost an estimated $162,000 and required 611 hours, on average, to prepare for and implement the system when considering both financial and nonfinancial (time and effort) costs.[29] Use of an integrated data system makes the coordination of care, monitoring of individual and population health outcomes, and continuous efforts to improve quality of care possible if the physician practices can afford a robust system. Although implementation of an EHR may be more feasible for larger practices or those that are part of a larger health care system from the standpoint of distributing the costs over a larger base, the potential long-term impact of better clinical outcomes resulting in lower costs may well be worth the initial investment.

IMPROVING THE CARE EXPERIENCE OF THE PATIENT

The DHWI incorporates several methodologies aimed at enhancing the care experience of patients. While addressing the AADE 7 Key Self-Care Behaviors, diabetes educators assess patients' readiness to change by using a brief questionnaire based on the Transtheoretical Model.[30] By assessing where people are in their readiness to change a diabetes-related health behavior, clinicians can more effectively design tailored plans of care rather than provide a standard prescription for all patients. Using patient feedback to improve service and program offerings is a real-time method of continuous quality improvement (CQI) to achieve positive health outcomes in the population served by PCPs. This CQI is accomplished through the use of the Client Satisfaction Questionnaire (CSQ-8),[31,32] which is collected to assess aggregate satisfaction of groups of respondents.

Additional methods to ensure individualization of care include assessments of health literacy and cultural beliefs. Educators administer the Rapids Estimate of Adult Literacy in Medicine—Short Form (REALM-SF) for English-speaking patients and the Short Assessment of Health Literacy for Spanish Adults (SAHLSA-50) to each patient to determine the degree to which individuals can comprehend information in a medical context.[33] Based on a community needs assessment that identified DHWI's target audience as having a low to very low literacy level, educational materials appropriate to that level were developed. These materials were also tailored to be culturally relevant for both the African American and Latino populations primarily served. Specific questions to elicit information about culturally relevant beliefs are also an integral part of the assessment process at DHWI.

Another goal of the DHWI is the improvement of health outcomes at the individual, family, and community level. These outcomes include improved quality of life, increased social capital, reduced costs of health care delivery, and community empowerment. An important element with which to measure efficacy of wellness services is quality of life. A baseline score for quality of life, using the EuroQol EQ-5D,[34] is obtained from each patient at initial membership and then annually to identify expected improvements in perceived health status. Evaluating and disseminating results regarding improved health outcomes with this model may inform other developing models of care in other settings and/or for other chronic conditions. Through ongoing data collection and program evaluation, the DHWI will be able to determine the impact of its interventions on improving outcomes for its members and the community of South Dallas. The DHWI provides numerous opportunities for research pertaining to health equity and best practices for diabetes management and prevention, as well as patterns of disease.

Health Partners

The DHWI coordinates care across the diabetes care team through a multistep approach (**Fig. 5**). All DHWI patients are assigned to a health partner. The health

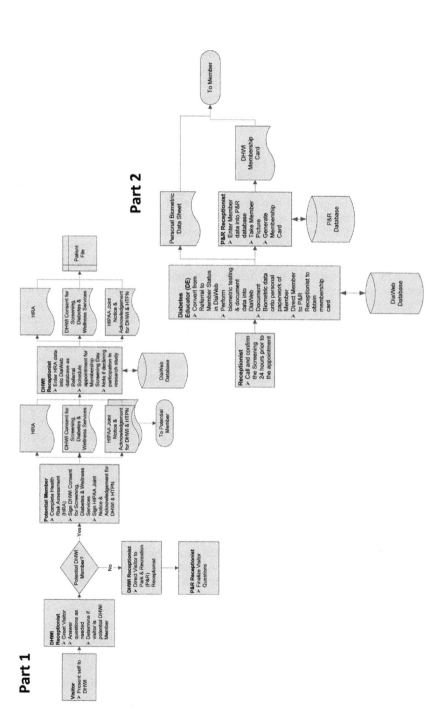

Fig. 5. Initial DHWI Member Flow (2-part). HTPN, Health Texas Provider Network (physician practice in the Family Health Clinic). (Copyright © 2011 Baylor Health Care System. All Rights Reserved. DHWI is a trademark of the Baylor Health Care System; with permission.)

partner helps the patient select and enroll in DHWI education, counseling, and exercise programs designed to improve overall health and wellness based on information collected through ongoing assessment. Patients complete a health risk assessment and receive point-of-care testing to assess level of glycemic control, hypertension, lipids, and obesity. The health risk assessment provides a triage mechanism to assign individuals to the appropriate care providers based on their level of diabetes risk. Clients with abnormal values are referred to their PCP for follow-up or to the DHWI primary care physician if they do not have a PCP.

PEERS Educator

By addressing multiple determinants of health through the team, individuals are better equipped to manage their own health. In addition, the care team reduces the burden traditionally placed on a single provider unit to improve the health of those they serve.[35,36] Through the goals of this model, the DHWI implemented a grass-roots health care initiative that trained and employed 38 community members as Diabetes PEERS (Prevention, Education, Empowerment, Resources, & Support). The PEERS educators are linked to the community via local churches. Their primary role is to advocate for diabetes awareness and prevention services on behalf of DHWI and link people to health care services. These community members received state-approved training as community health workers. A community health worker is defined as a person who, with or without compensation, provides a liaison between health care providers and patients through activities that may include assisting in case conferences, providing education, making referrals to health and social services, conducting needs assessments, distributing surveys to identify barriers to health care delivery, making home visits, and providing bilingual services.[37] The goal of this community service is to promote awareness in the community by having the diabetes PEERS educate their peers about the severity of undiagnosed and uncontrolled diabetes. The PEERS refer members of their congregation who are seeking to improve their health and their ability to self-manage their diabetes to the DHWI. Two similar projects have shown that community health workers are a familiar and cost-effective approach to producing positive health effects among community members engaged in faith-based health programs or the like.[38,39] The multidisciplinary team can then work together with the patient to meet immediate clinical needs and implement lifestyle changes that will result in sustainable improvements in health.

SUMMARY

Using a collaborative team approach in diabetes care creates a health care environment in which the patient has access to key resources needed to improve and sustain positive health outcomes. The DHWI has promoted a center without walls in an effort to engage underserved populations and increase public awareness about diabetes while promoting individual empowerment as an active constituent in their health care. The concept of the center without walls used by the DHWI provides programs and information to patients via faith-based and Web-based capabilities for community and distance learning to accommodate the personal and professional situations of the patient base.

In addition, it is recommended that health care practices and organizations in diabetes management strive to engage clinical staff specialized in diabetes self-management education across the 5 levels of diabetes educators to meet the needs of their patient population. Members of the diabetes care team provide care and support appropriate to their level of expertise and credentialing, which allows for efficient, cost-effective, high-quality care. By implementing this model, the medical provider is able to focus on his or her medical management role while other members of the care team provide education, counseling, and self-management support to optimize glucose control. Care becomes more efficient in that the medical providers can see more patients daily and can carry higher patient care loads, because other specialized clinical staff manages individual care plans in between physician visits. Developing open communication channels between members of the diabetes care team is paramount for individual patient success in achieving positive health outcomes, improving capacity for effective diabetes self-management, and coordinating services across the continuum of care.

Primary care providers can use the methods and practices in the DHWI model as a tool to enhance the prevention, early identification, and management of diabetes. It takes a coordinated team of health care providers to effectively treat and manage individuals with diabetes. Primary care practices may benefit by introducing or improving one or more components of high-performing teams: clear goals with measurable outcomes, defined tasks and roles, clinical and administrative systems with a clear division of labor, and effective communication.[23] There is no perfect way to improve diabetes health outcomes other than the plan that works best for each primary care practice and individual patient. By employing a diverse team, the burden of diabetes care can shift from the PCP to a group of providers who are trained to foster and support effective diabetes self-management skills in individuals.

REFERENCES

1. Centers for Disease Control and Prevention. National diabetes fact sheet, 2011. Atlanta (GA): Department of Health and Human Services, Centers for Disease Control and Prevention; 2011.
2. Agency for Healthcare Research and Quality. National health care disparities report. Available at: http://www.ahrq.gov/qual/nhdr08/Chap3.htm. Accessed November 2011.
3. American Diabetes Association. Standards of medical care in diabetes. Diabetes Care 2010;33(Suppl 1):S11–61.
4. Bodenheimer T, Lorig K, Holman H, et al. Patient self-management of chronic disease in primary care. JAMA 2002;288(19):2469–75.
5. Texas Diabetes Council. Texas diabetes fact sheet. 2011. Austin (TX): Texas Diabetes Council; 2011.
6. Centers for Disease Control and Prevention (CDC), editor. Behavioral risk factor surveillance system survey data. Atlanta (GA): C. f. U.S. Department of Health and Human Services; 2010.
7. Texas Department of State Health Services. Austin (TX): Texas Vital Statistics; Annual Report 2008.
8. Texas Diabetes Council, Texas Department of State Health Services. Austin (TX): Diabetes: a comprehensive approach 2010–2011. p. E45–10524.
9. U.S. Census Bureau. The Hispanic population. Washington, DC: census 2000 Brief.
10. Texas Department of State Health Services. 2007 Texas behavioral risk factor surveillance system. Texas Department of State Health Services; 2007.
11. Frazier Revitalization Initiative. Frazier Neighborhood Initiative Weed & Seed Proposal: FY 2010 Weed and Seed Communities Competitive Application. Dallas (TX): Frazier Revitalization Inc; 2010.
12. Adler NE. U.S. disparities in health: descriptions, causes, and mechanisms. Annu Rev Public Health 2008;29:235–52.

13. Michaud CM, Murray CJ, Bloom BR. Burden of disease—implications for future research. JAMA 2001;285(5):535–9.
14. Nelson AR. Unequal treatment: report of the Institute of Medicine on racial and ethnic disparities in healthcare. Ann Thorac Surg 2003;76(4):S1377–81.
15. Meyer D, Armstrong-Coben A, Batista M. How a community-based organization and an academic health center are creating an effective partnership for training and service. Acad Med 2005;80(4):327–33.
16. Roussos ST, Fawcett SB. A review of collaborative partnerships as a strategy for improving community health. Annu Rev Public Health 2000;21:369–402.
17. Two Feathers J, Kieffer EC, Palmisano G, et al. Racial and Ethnic Approaches to Community Health (REACH) Detroit partnership: improving diabetes-related outcomes among African American and Latino adults. Am J Public Health 2005;95(9):1552–60.
18. Institute of Medicine. Clinical practice guidelines we can trust. Available at: http://www.iom.edu/~/media/Files/Report%20Files/2011/Clinical-Practice-Guidelines-We-Can-Trust/Clinical%20Practice%20Guidelines%202011%20Insert.pdf. Accessed April 12, 2011.
19. DesRoches CM, Campbell EG, Rao SR, et al. Electronic health records in ambulatory care—a national survey of physicians. N Engl J Med 2008;359(1):50–60.
20. Linder JA, Ma J, Bates DW, et al. Electronic health record use and the quality of ambulatory care in the United States. Arch Intern Med 2007;167(13):1400–5.
21. Funnell MM, Anderson RM. Changing office practice and health care systems to facilitate diabetes self-management. Curr Diab Rep 2003;3(2):127–33.
22. Jackson GL, Lee SY, Edelman D, et al. Employment of mid-level providers in primary care and control of diabetes. Prim Care Diabetes 2011;5(1):25–31.
23. Grumbach K, Bodenheimer T. Can health care teams improve primary care practice? JAMA 2004;291(10):1246–51.
24. National Heart Lung and Blood Institute. Calculate your body mass index. Available at: http://www.nhlbisupport.com/bmi/. Accessed July 14, 2011.
25. Baker DP, Gustafson S, Beaubien J, et al. Medical teamwork and patient safety: the evidence-based relation. Literature review. AHRQ Publication No. 05-0053. Available at: http://www.ahrq.gov/qual/medteam/. Accessed June 29, 2011.
26. American Association of Diabetes Educators (AADE). Competencies for Diabetes Educators: a companion document to the Guidelines for the Practice of Diabetes Education. Chicago (IL); 2011.
27. American Association of Diabetes Educators (AADE). Diabetes education definition. Available at: http://www.diabeteseducator.org/DiabetesEducation/Definitiona.html. Accessed April 12, 2011.
28. AADE. AADE7 Self-Care Behaviors. Diabetes Educ 2008;34(3):445–9.
29. Fleming NS, Culler SD, McCorkle R, et al. The financial and nonfinancial costs of implementing electronic health records in primary care practices. Health Aff (Millwood) 2011;30(3):481–9.
30. Prochaska JO, DiClemente CC. Stages and processes of self-change of smoking: toward an integrative model of change. J Consult Clin Psychol 1983; 51(3):390–5.
31. Attkisson CC, Greenfield TK. The UCSF client satisfaction scales; the client satisfaction questionnaire-8. In: ME M, editor. Psychological testing: treatment planning and outcome assessment. 3rd edition. Hillsdale (NJ): Erlbaum; 2004. p. 799–812.
32. Larsen DL, Attkisson CC, Hargreaves WA, et al. Assessment of client/patient satisfaction: development of a general scale. Eval Program Plann 1979;2(3): 197–207.

33. Health literacy measurement tools. Agency for Healthcare Research and Quality; 2009. Available at: http://www.ahrq.gov/populations/sahlsatool.htm. Accessed January 5, 2012.

34. EuroQol Group. EQ-5D. Available at: http://www.euroqol.org/eq-5d/what-is-eq-5d. html. Accessed January 5, 2012.

35. Donohoe ME, Fletton JA, Hook A, et al. Improving foot care for people with diabetes mellitus–a randomized controlled trial of an integrated care approach. Diabet Med 2000;17(8):581–7.

36. Stroebel RJ, Broers JK, Houle SK, et al. Improving hypertension control: a team approach in a primary care setting. Jt Comm J Qual Improv 2000;26(11):623–32.

37. State of Texas. Texas constitution and statutes; 2011. Available at: http://www. statutes.legis.state.tx.us/Docs/HS/htm/HS.48.htm#48.001. Accessed April 12, 2011.

38. DeHaven MJ, Hunter IB, Wilder L, et al. Health programs in faith-based organizations: are they effective? Am J Public Health 2004;94(6):1030–6.

39. Fedder DO, Chang RJ, Curry S, et al. The effectiveness of a community health worker outreach program on healthcare utilization of west Baltimore City Medicaid patients with diabetes, with or without hypertension. Ethn Dis 2003; 13(1):22–7.

Childhood Asthma

Considerations for Primary Care Practice and Chronic Disease Management in the Village of Care

Michael P. Rosenthal, MD

KEYWORDS

- Asthma • Chronic disease • Care coordination • Patient-centered medical home
- Community intervention

KEY POINTS

- The example of childhood asthma can help us to understand the importance of the awareness of the many social, economic, environmental, behavioral, and cultural aspects of care that contribute to better health outcomes.
- Our ability to be more successful as primary care providers can be greatly enhanced by building connections to, integrating with, and incorporating community-based supports and approaches to care for our patients.
- Successful "community-included" approaches to childhood asthma may also serve as examples for other chronic disease care.

INTRODUCTION

Primary care practice development and related considerations for approaches to chronic disease management are significant topics in this era of rapid change in health care. The burden of chronic disease in the United States has been increasing, and there has been an increased recognition of the need for primary care to address this problem.[1] Interacting issues (the chronic disease model of care, the patient-centered medical home [PCMH], the Patient Centered Affordable Care Act) have developed during the past decade have led to an increased recognition of the need for an advanced model of primary care to improve the health of patients in the context of their families, homes, and communities.[2,3]

This article presents a practical question-oriented approach to considerations for chronic disease care, using childhood asthma as an example, to help primary care providers (PCPs) appreciate the wide-ranging concept of advanced primary care.

The author has nothing to disclose.
Department of Family and Community Medicine, Christiana Care Health System, 1400 North Washington Street, Suite 420, Wilmington, DE 19801, USA
E-mail address: mrosenthal@christianacare.org

Prim Care Clin Office Pract 39 (2012) 381–391
doi:10.1016/j.pop.2012.04.001   primarycare.theclinics.com
0095-4543/12/$ – see front matter © 2012 Elsevier Inc. All rights reserved.

How do primary care practices develop efforts within the context of a PCMH that can be linked to community-based efforts for addressing chronic disease care? Also, specifically, how does a PCP envision the role of an individual practice in the practice neighborhood (community)?[4] There is a stated need and new emphasis for PCPs to not only consider a transformed model of care in a PCMH but also shift the paradigm from an individual practice and one-on-one care to population-based approaches, with coordination and integration of care in the medical neighborhood.[4] The neighborhood of the medical system includes specialists, health care institutions, and health care teams, and PCPs need to help patients navigate the system to ensure that plans of all entities are coordinated and work together as a whole for patients' health care needs.[4] Importantly, the neighborhood can and likely should be extended to include developing better relationships and supports through community services.[4] PCPs need to consider a new paradigm of care that includes population-based approaches, positioning their practice efforts within a broader context of health care at a community level and developing a community-included system integration model of care for chronic diseases.

However, as much as there is a developing emphasis on providing a supportive primary care environment and PCMH, it is important to recognize that the real medical home is the patient's home. In other words, using the example of childhood asthma, children and their families must be seen as central to addressing their issues in care and to making health care most effective. We need to find new and innovative ways to reach children and their families, via a potential array of community-based services and supports, and work with them to improve care.

This article highlights the value of community-based contributions to childhood asthma care and discusses how that value might be linked to evolving practice and health system needs. It underscores the concept of enhancing practice connections to local community services to build a local "village of care."

QUESTION 1: WHY DOES THIS RELATE TO MY PRACTICE AND THE CARE I PROVIDE

Traditional medical training, in both medical school and primary care residencies, has emphasized care of the individual patient. Even when the context of patient care has been expanded to the understanding of inclusion of the family within the home and the home environment, there has been a disconnection, much more often than not, from the consideration of the people living in their community, the village of care. The community has its own culture, attitudes, and beliefs about health and health care. Those attributes provide the community with an enormous potential to influence the attitudes, education, medical literacy, behaviors, and health actions of the individuals who live within it. Many community-based efforts can influence health care via community-based organizations and institutions (eg, schools, health care institutions, advocacy agencies). Furthermore, the community establishes the environment for living and health care through policies (eg, outdoor air quality, smoking in public venues, housing standards) that affect those who live within it.

QUESTION 2: WHY SHOULD WE USE CHILDHOOD ASTHMA TO CONSIDER A MODEL OF ADVANCED PRIMARY CARE

Despite a redefinition of the approach to and care for childhood asthma more than 2 decades ago (eg, routine use of anti-inflammatory medications, such as inhaled corticosteroids for persistent asthma) under the National Asthma Education and Prevention Program (NAEPP), the incidence of childhood asthma has increased to historically high levels and disparities in care remain high.[5–7] Furthermore, high rates of emergency department (ED) visits and hospitalizations indicate a lack of control of this disease from a population perspective.[5–8]

Childhood asthma presents an excellent opportunity to understand control and management of a chronic disease from a broad-based advanced primary care perspective. It has a multifactorial nature related to indoor and external environments; it produces intermittent challenges through unpredictable exacerbations; and, as a health system, we are falling short in consistently reaching and caring for those who are most at risk.

It is apparent that the burden of childhood asthma remains extraordinarily high, even in the face of a better understanding of the disease process, improved medications, and more expenditures on care in the medical system. Primary care efforts are underutilized and have not been well coordinated with EDs and hospital care.[8] Community-based services and supports may be available, but they are not routinely coordinated with practice-based efforts. Fragmentation of care in the medical system is high, and care coordination is, on the whole, lacking.[9,10] There is significant room and an imperative for improvement. An advanced model of primary care, which leads to a higher degree of patient- and family-centered support, partnerships in care, integration of health services, care coordination, and improved understanding and self-management abilities, has the potential to make an enormous difference.[2]

QUESTION 3: WHY IS IT IMPORTANT TO CONTROL CHILDHOOD ASTHMA

Childhood asthma is frequently underappreciated in terms of its effect on children, families, and the costs of health care. It is the most prevalent chronic disease in children and causes absenteeism from school (a marker for poor school performance), missed workdays for parents, and lost productivity for employers.[5–7,11–13] Costs of medical care related to unnecessary or excessive ED visits are high, as well as hospitalizations for children with uncontrolled asthma. In the United States by 2007, for all types of asthma, an estimated $56 billion was spent on medical costs, lost school days and workdays, and early deaths.[13,14]

The prevalence of asthma continues to increase.[14] Childhood asthma has also been found to be significantly higher in poor children and in those from minority populations. Among all children younger than 18 years, the prevalence in 2009 was 9.6% nationally but was highest among poor children (13.5%) and non-Hispanic black children (17%). In addition, disparities in care are apparent; mortality rates in black children are 6 times higher than that in white children.[13,15]

QUESTION 4: WHY HAS IT BEEN DIFFICULT TO CONTROL CHILDHOOD ASTHMA

Asthma is a multifactorial illness with a variety of causes and triggers. Identification and removal of triggers can be problematic. Common triggers and/or environmental irritants may include outdoor air quality (pollution, fumes), indoor air quality, environmental tobacco smoke, mold, pets, rodents, dust, and many others.[5,6,9]

Furthermore, the transient intermittent nature of childhood asthma often results in decreased understanding and underestimation of the disease or its importance.[7,11,12] Children, parents, and providers alike may be caught in the trap of lines of thought such as "this is only a mild case of asthma," "it's normal to have a little shortness of breath," or "this is just reactive airway disease, it's nothing severe." Many patients and families accept short of breath or wheezing as a normal part of having asthma. This relative lack of appreciation for the seriousness of the disease and need for control may result in lack of visits for primary care (because the asthma is perceived to be "stable") and/or decreased adherence by children/families. Costs of medications and insurance coverage for needed medications are also responsible for decreased control. In a fragmented health system with incomplete insurance coverage, many children do not have primary providers, or do not routinely see them, and their parents are often unsure of when to get assistance or where to turn during an exacerbation or attack.[5–9]

In addition, providers may be unaware that they play a role in the underappreciation and undertreatment of childhood asthma. Despite years of national recommendations and specific guidelines under the NAEPP to prescribe anti-inflammatory medications for childhood asthma beyond mild status, many providers do not do so on a routine basis.[5–7,16] Moreover, some providers are reluctant to provide a diagnosis of asthma because they do not want to label a patient, but this may actually do patients a disservice; referring to childhood asthma as multiple episodes of reactive airway disease or bronchitis may delay appropriate treatment because it builds into the belief that the patients/families are not dealing with a significant disease. In fact, it is important to improve partnerships between patients, families, and providers.[5–7,16,17] Structured provider education on caring for children with asthma has been shown to be beneficial in improving outcomes without needing to increase provider office time.[16,17] Directly communicating the diagnosis of asthma with children and families to help them appreciate the nature of the disease and accept the need for care and support, as well as providing specific clear recommendations, have been show to decrease asthma symptoms, acute office visits, ED use, and hospitalizations.[16,17]

It would be beneficial for children with asthma and their families if providers establish Asthma Action Plans (AAPs). There are several forms of AAPs that can be easily included in office practice to provide medications and document approaches at times of asthma exacerbations (**Fig. 1**).[18,19] AAPs also provide a mechanism for building patient-provider communication and partnerships; help in documentation; and, because they can "travel" with the patient, serve as a "vehicle" to build consistency among multiple providers and sites of care.[18] Importantly, AAPs are not routinely prescribed by many providers, and, even if they are, they may not be used.[14] AAPs, as part of an overall approach to education about asthma care and services, may be beneficial to improving asthma outcomes.[10,20]

QUESTION 5: HOW DOES THE AFFORDABLE CARE ACT APPLY TO THESE CONSIDERATIONS FOR CHILDHOOD ASTHMA AND CHRONIC DISEASE CARE

The Patient Protection and Affordable Care Act (ACA), signed into law in March, 2010, will have far-reaching effects for fostering change in primary care practice. Emphasis is placed on "reaching" the practice population at risk, electronic health records with "meaningful use," developing patient registries (eg, all children in a practice with asthma), coordination of care, and incentives for improved patient outcomes, and there is an expanded emphasis on community-based care. These emphases of the ACA fit into the developing concept of the PCMH.[2,3]

In many locales, care for childhood asthma, the most prevalent chronic disease in children, serves as a quality indicator for tracking and outcomes under meaningful use. Capitated rates or bundled payments from health insurers to control costs will need to include broad-based strategies for reaching children and families to keep their asthma under control and prevent unnecessary or excessive ED visits and hospitalizations. Developing effective practice strategies that are well integrated with community efforts fosters increased communication among patients and providers, more effective care coordination via integration of care and support services, improved access to care, more support at times of need, better asthma control, and decreased ED and hospital use.

Asthma Action Plan

(To be completed by Doctor/Nurse)

ALLIES AGAINST ASTHMA

Name	Birth Date	Effective Date
School	Parent/Guardian	Parent's Phone
Doctor/Nurse's Name	Doctor/Nurse's Office Phone	
Emergency Contact After Parent		Contact Phone

Asthma Severity: ☐ Mild Intermittent ☐ Mild Persistent ☐ Moderate Persistent ☐ Severe Persistent

Asthma Triggers: ☐ Colds ☐ Exercise ☐ Animals ☐ Dust ☐ Smoke ☐ Food ☐ Weather ☐ Other: _____

TAKE THESE MEDICINES EVERYDAY

Child feels good:
- Breathing is good
- No cough or wheeze
- Can work/play
- Sleeps all night

Peak flow in this area:
_____ to _____

MEDICINE:	HOW MUCH:	WHEN TO TAKE IT:

20 MINUTES BEFORE EXERCISE USE THIS MEDICINE:

(Green)

IF NOT FEELING WELL — TAKE EVERYDAY MEDICINES AND (ADD) THESE RESCUE MEDICINES

Child has any of these:
- Cough
- Wheeze
- Tight Chest

Peak flow in this area:
_____ to _____

MEDICINE:	HOW MUCH:	WHEN TO TAKE IT:

Call your doctor/nurse's office if the symptoms don't improve in 2 days OR if the flare lasts for longer than ___ days. After _____ days go back to GREEN ZONE and take everyday medications as instructed.

(Yellow)

IF FEELING VERY SICK CALL THE DOCTOR OR NURSE NOW! TAKE THESE MEDICINES

Child has any of these:
- Medicine not helping
- Breathing is hard and fast
- Lips and fingernails are blue
- Can't walk or talk well

Peak flow below:
_____

MEDICINE:	HOW MUCH:	WHEN TO TAKE IT:

IF UNABLE TO CONTACT YOUR DOCTOR OR NURSE:
Call 911 or go to the nearest emergency room and bring this form with you!

(Red)

I give permission to the doctor, nurse, health plan, and other health care providers to share information about my child's asthma to help improve the health of my child.

_____ Parent/Guardian Signature _____ Date

_____ Health Care Provider Signature

Adapted from the NYC Childhood Asthma Initiative
Adapted from the NHLBI
Printed 2004
To download additional forms go to: www.hpcpa.org

Fig. 1. Asthma Action Plan (AAP). This was developed by the Health Promotion Council (HPC) of Southeastern Pennsylvania with collaborating partners of the Philadelphia Allies Against Asthma Coalition. (*Courtesy of* Health Promotion Council, Philadelphia, PA; with permission.)

QUESTIONS 6 AND 7: WHAT IS THE IMPORTANCE OF CHILDHOOD ASTHMA IN THE CONTEXT OF THE CHRONIC CARE MODEL AND HOW DO WE REACH THOSE WHO CANNOT BE REACHED

Plumb and colleagues in an article elsewhere in this issue discuss the importance of community-based partnerships for improving chronic disease management. The investigators emphasize the importance of expanding the Chronic Care Model developed by Wagner and colleagues to include community-based approaches to enable patients and families to become better, informed partners in care.[21–23] Furthermore, Plumb and colleagues develop the concept that the Social Ecology Model can provide the framework for integrating community partnerships and chronic disease management. Examples are provided regarding improved education and awareness and the opportunity for approaches to multiple chronic disease states.

From a PCPs' viewpoint, the considerations of working with community-based efforts may be seen as "not part of my practice" and "unrelated to my patients' care." However, if viewed in the context of the ACA, the importance of reaching an entire practice's population of patients or those with a certain disease state takes on new significance.[2,3] The provider's accountability for all patients in a practice with childhood asthma, a population-based consideration, is different from the individual accountability for the individual patient "seen in my office." Having a disease registry to identify and track patients who may not routinely visit the office implies the need to reach all patients and provide them needed care and services, but any practice may be limited by its resources and ability to bring patients to its "PCMH."

Furthermore, PCPs are often disappointed in their ability to influence their patients' care. PCPs' impact on the daily lives of patients may be limited, and they often wrestle with the difficulty of helping patients become informed partners in care. This is not surprising when considering that most patients spend a maximum of only a few hours, total, each year within a practice seeing their provider and/or staff, even in a well-developed PCMH.

Including community efforts to help patients become informed partners in care, enhanced by community-based programs and education, developed and administered in the context of people's lives, where they live and what they do, may be a great help. In addition, educators, health workers, and other health care personnel, working in the home or community, may be in an advantageous position to develop influential relationships with children and their families to improve understanding, build positive attitudes, promote healthy behaviors, and enhance self-care.

More traditional views of medical education and care may raise questions about the evidence regarding community-based approaches and how they might be helpful in achieving outcomes in care. There is a growing evidence base, however, that such community-based approaches have been beneficial in addressing the burden of childhood asthma and are important to consider in building a more comprehensive and successful approach.[5,6]

QUESTION 8: WHAT HAVE WE LEARNED FROM COMMUNITY COALITION EXAMPLES TO ADDRESS THE BURDEN OF CHILDHOOD ASTHMA

Two national multisite projects (Allies Against Asthma, Robert Wood Johnson Foundation; Merck Childhood Asthma Network [MCAN], Merck Foundation),[13,24] developed via foundation support, provide examples and considerable insight into the ability of communities to form coalitions and collaborative approaches to address the burden of childhood asthma. The key tenet for both efforts relies on the capacity of a coalition or collaborative partnership to bring many local stakeholders together to form a unique entity with infrastructure support to focus on a common health care issue. Coalitions bring many experiences and perspectives together to identify discrepancies in health care, develop innovative approaches that cross traditional boundary lines, implement creative programs that reach many difficult-to-reach individuals, address health literacy, enhance coordination of care, integrate systems, influence policy, promote education and behavior change, and lead to improved health outcomes. Even though they were part of national efforts, the community site-specific efforts (discussed later) included local coalition/partnership formation and project development specific to the local community. Each national project had a coordinating center for approach, evaluation, periodic sharing of experiences among sites via telephone conferences and annual meetings, and a national expert advisory panel.[10,11,13,24]

The Robert Wood Johnson Foundation supported the Allies Against Asthma project from 2000 to 2004. This project required 2 key goals: to form a local coalition and to address the burden of childhood asthma in the community. Through a competitive grant application process, 7 communities (Long Beach, California; Kings County/Seattle, Washington; Philadelphia, Pennsylvania; Hampton Roads, Virginia; Washington, DC; Milwaukee, Wisconsin; and, San Juan, Puerto Rico) were chosen to undergo a planning year and subsequent 3-year intervention.[11] Lead institutions were identified, and plans for coalition infrastructure and development were proposed as part of each proposal. Every coalition progressed through stages of formation to the action of addressing the burden of childhood asthma in each community.[9,25] Allies Against Asthma was coordinated via a national program office at the University of Michigan in Ann Arbor.[11,24]

Multisite evaluation showed that the Allies Against Asthma project was successful in developing system and policy changes in all sites and contributing to broad-based childhood asthma care in its communities.[26] Local change and influences included a variety of approaches, developed by each community in response to its assessment and needs. Examples of interventions ranged from legislative outdoor air policy change (Long Beach) to redesigned and integrated health care delivery (Milwaukee) to incorporation of wide-scale community health worker education and care coordinator programs (Kings County), home care assessment and education (Philadelphia), physician and nurse education (Virginia), electronic data sharing and case coordination (Washington, DC), and community health worker coordination with nurses and provider teams (Puerto Rico).[9] In total, there were 89 policy or system changes in the 7 sites during the 3-year implementation phase of the project. Asthma symptoms were reduced in children who were involved in the coalition programs of Allies Against Asthma in comparison with a group of children who were not involved.[26] In addition, the Philadelphia Allies Against Asthma program established the Child Asthma Link Line (Link Line), an interactive telephonic care coordination system with asthma educators who provided basic asthma education and administrative links to care and support services for children who were primarily seen at ED visits.[9] The Link Line intervention was designed to get appropriate and timely support services and care from children and their families. This program decreased asthma morbidity as measured by decreased ED visits and hospitalizations for those who received the Link Line intervention in comparison with a matched group who did not; it demonstrated the ability of a coalition to implement a community-wide program to affect changes in end point outcomes of care.[27]

The Merck Foundation supports the MCAN. Five sites (New York, New York; Philadelphia, Pennsylvania; Chicago, Illinois; Los Angeles, California; and, San Juan, Puerto Rico) were chosen for the initial MCAN project, which ran from 2005 through 2009.[13] The MCAN national office in Washington, DC, coordinated the project that emphasized the need for coalitions or partnerships to identify children with asthma in their communities and provide them evidence-based interventions and care.[10,13,28,29] All sites were involved in aspects of system delivery change, implementation of care coordination at a community level, and inclusion of components from evidence-based interventions such as Yes We Can (a medical-social model of asthma care for children and families), the Inner-City Asthma Study Environmental Intervention, and the National Cooperative Inner-City Asthma Study.[28] The comprehensive cross-site evaluation of the programs demonstrated that the community-based care coordination achieved via MCAN efforts improved patient/family education, enhanced the processes of care, and significantly reduced morbidity as measured by ED visits and hospitalizations.[10,29]

QUESTION 9: HOW DO THESE EXPERIENCES WITH LARGE COMMUNITY COALITIONS RELATE TO DEVELOPING INTEGRATED PRACTICE AND COMMUNITY-BASED APPROACHES IN A LOCAL COMMUNITY ON A SMALLER SCALE

The community coalition experiences described earlier indicate the ability to assess community needs and bring stakeholders together to plan effective programs for childhood asthma care and services in a variety of communities. Every primary care practice exists within the context of its own community. The people or families that any practice serves are community members who are affected by the community's circumstances, economics, institutions, structure, supports, and services. Each practice has the opportunity to consider ways to build supports for its patients' care by working with community members, organizations, or institutions.

The coalitions mentioned had funding and infrastructure support for developing interventions. An individual practice might consider it difficult to become involved in integrating practice-based care with community efforts. On the other hand, the imperative of the PCMH movement and the ACA, based on a greater focus on health care for the US population, emphasizes the need for broader practice and population-based approaches to care in local practice.[2–4]

QUESTION 10: HOW DO WE LINK COMMUNITY-BASED APPROACHES WITH PRACTICE-BASED APPROACHES TO CARE

For the provider in primary care practice, it may seem beyond the scope of care to include community-based care and services in a practice-based approach. This article is intended to encourage thought about how to consider expanding the reach of care to create a more coordinated, comprehensive, and inclusive arrangement of practice and community-based services to support children with asthma, and their families, to improve outcomes in care. As the health system moves toward a higher degree of expectation regarding each practice's responsibility for its population of patients, population-based approaches to care, including involvement of community-based organizations, institutions, and services, become increasingly important.

Community providers and practices do not have the same infrastructure and support provided by the community coalitions described earlier. On the other hand, they do not need to have that level of support to begin building the bridges necessary to overcome the gap between practice and community efforts that is commonly seen.

Each practice has to assess its own needs as well as the opportunities for increasing community-based supports in its local environment. A thoughtful, steady, and practical effort, which builds relationships and collaborations, one step at a time, is more likely to succeed than overwhelmingly complex endeavors. Straightforward considerations that intend to building partnerships among patients, their families, community supports, and primary care practices are needed. Setting common goals with partners and working together to align strategies to achieve them are also more likely to predict success.

There are many ways to consider building a bridge. The following are a few among them: discuss a need for a comprehensive approach to childhood asthma in your community with health care agencies, institutions, and hospitals; coordinate efforts with other medical providers in your community; identify and contact community-based organizations that have programs and services for childhood asthma (eg, American Lung Association, grassroots advocacy groups); connect with schools (where children spend a majority of their time), as schools have a vested interest in lower absenteeism to improve scholastic performance; coordinate care with school nurses and provide education for children with asthma and their parents; work with housing professionals, local officials, public health, and/or other health-oriented community-based organizations; obtain materials and information about creating better home and school environment for children with asthma from the US Environmental Protection Agency and the Department of Health and Human Services; provide support for patients and families with education, information, and plans for care; and enhance access and availability in community practices, so children and their families can get to the site of care when needed.

The understanding that any one model will not work in every community is essential to achieving success. The best approach includes an assessment of local community needs and opportunities that can lead to thoughtful and creative plans to improve childhood asthma care and support. Care providers should define a specific intervention and implement it. This intervention could start with something that is reasonable and achievable. PCPs should learn from it, modify it as needed, and then build from there.

Most importantly, being actively involved in the development and inclusion of new approaches to primary care, in an enhanced and advanced model, supported and integrated with community efforts, can be extremely rewarding. Creating opportunities to promote an improved local system of patient- and family-centered health care can augment providers' accomplishments and sense of satisfaction, while improving health outcomes for patients that help them achieve a better quality of life.

SUMMARY

The example of childhood asthma can help us to understand the importance of the awareness of the many social, economic, environmental, behavioral, and cultural aspects of care that contribute to better health outcomes. The care for children with asthma depends on the many factors and influences of life beyond the office time spent with the children and their families or caregivers. Our ability to be more successful as PCPs will be greatly enhanced by building connections to, integrating with, and incorporating community-based supports and approaches to care for our patients.

Some PCPs may choose to be champions and look to directly become involved in building community-based contributions to care or influencing relevant policy change. Some may not. However, every provider can be proactive in developing a PCMH that better connects to and works with the many system supports available in our communities to foster better care, health outcomes, and quality of life for those who live in our village.

ACKNOWLEDGMENTS

The author acknowledges the many colleagues and partners who participated in the Robert Wood Johnson Foundation Allies Against Asthma Coalitions and the Merck Childhood Asthma Network of the Merck Foundation. Also appreciated are the efforts of the staff of the Health Promotion Council of Southeastern Pennsylvania, which served as the infrastructure organization supporting the Philadelphia Allies Against Asthma Coalition and the Philadelphia Merck Childhood Asthma Network Project.

REFERENCES

1. Starfield B, Shi L, Macinko J. Contribution of primary care to health systems and health. Milbank Q 2005;83(3):457–502.
2. Patient-Centered Primary Care Collaborative. Available at: http://www.pcpcc.net/. Accessed March 25, 2012.
3. The Patient Protection and Affordable Care Act. Available at: http://www. healthcare.gov/law/index.html. Accessed March 25, 2012.
4. Taylor EF, Lake T, Nysenbaum J, et al. Coordinating care in the medical neighbor-hood. AHRQ Publication No. 11–0064, 2011. Available at: www.ahrq.gov. Accessed March 25, 2012.
5. National Asthma Education and Prevention Program. Expert Panel Report 3 (EPR-3): Guidelines for the Diagnosis and Management of Asthma—Summary Report 2007. Report of the National Asthma Education and Prevention Program of the National Heart, Lung, and Blood Institute (NHLBI) of the National Institutes of Health, US Department of Health and Human Services. Bethesda, MD, August, 2007.
6. National Asthma Education and Prevention Program. Guidelines implementation panel report for Expert Panel Report 3—Guidelines for the Diagnosis and Management of Asthma. Partners Putting Guidelines into Action. Report of the National Asthma Education and Prevention Program of the National Heart, Lung, and Blood Institute (NHLBI) of the National Institutes of Health, US Department of Health and Human Services. Bethesda, MD, December, 2008.
7. Wechsler ME. Managing asthma in primary care: putting new guideline recom-mendations into context. Mayo Clin Proc 2009;84(8):707–17.
8. Baren JM, Boudreaux ED, Brenner BE, et al. Randomized controlled trial of emer-gency department interventions to improve primary care follow-up for patients with acute asthma. Chest 2006;129:257–65.
9. Rosenthal MP, Butterfoss FD, Doctor LJ, et al. The coalition process at work: building care coordination models to control chronic disease. Health Promot Pract 2006;7(Suppl 2):117S–26S.
10. Findley S, Rosenthal M, Bryant-Stephens T, et al. Community-based care coordi-nation: practical applications for childhood asthma. Health Promot Pract 2011;12: 52S.
11. Clark NM, Doctor L, Friedman AR, et al. Community coalitions to control chronic disease: Allies Against Asthma as a model and case study. Health Promot Pract 2006;7(Suppl 2):14S–22S.
12. Gupta RS, Weiss KB. The 2007 National Asthma Education and Prevention Program Asthma Guidelines: accelerating their implementation and facilitating their impact on children with asthma. Pediatrics 2009;123(Suppl 3):S193–8.
13. Merck Childhood Asthma Network. Available at: http://www.mcanonline.org/. Accessed March 25, 2012.
14. Centers for Disease Control and Prevention (CDC). Vital signs: asthma preva-lence, disease, and self-management education: United States, 2001–2009. MMWR Morb Mortal Wkly Rep 2011;60(17):547–52.
15. Akinbami LJ, Moorman JE, Garbe PL, et al. Status of childhood asthma in the United States, 1980–2007. Pediatrics 2009;123(Suppl 3):S131–45.
16. Clark NM, Cabana M, Kaciroti N, et al. Long-term outcomes of physician peer teaching. Clin Pediatr (Phila) 2008;47(9):883–90.
17. Cabana MD, Slish KK, Evans D, et al. Impact of physician care education on patient outcomes. Pediatrics 2006;117(6):2149–57.

18. Pennsylvania Asthma Partnership. Available at: http://www.paasthma.org/. Accessed March 25, 2012.
19. National Heart Lung and Blood Institute, Asthma Action Plan. Available at: http://www. nhlbi.nih.gov/health/public/lung/asthma/asthma_actplan.htm. Accessed March 25, 2012.
20. Brouwer AF, Brand PL. Asthma education and monitoring: what has been shown to work. Paediatr Respir Rev 2008;9:193–200.
21. Wagner EH, Austin BT, Davis C, et al. Improving chronic illness care: translating evidence into action. Health Aff 2001;20:64–78.
22. Bodenheimer TM, Wagner EH, Grumbach KM. Improving primary care for patients with chronic illness. JAMA 2002;288:1775–9.
23. Bodenheimer TM, Wagner EH, Grumbach KM. Improving primary care for patients with chronic illness: the Chronic Care Model, part 2. JAMA 2002;288: 1909–14.
24. Allies Against Asthma: The Center for Chronic Disease Management, University of Michigan. Available at: http://cmcd.sph.umich.edu/Allies-Against-Asthma.html. Accessed March 25, 2012.
25. Butterfoss FD, Gilmore LA, Krieger JW, et al. From formation to action: how allies against asthma coalitions are getting the job done. Health Promot Pract 2006; 6(Suppl 2):34S–43S.
26. Clark NM, Lachance L, Doctor LJ, et al. Policy and system change and community coalitions: outcomes from allies against asthma. Am J Public Health 2010; 5(100):904–12.
27. Coughey K, Klein G, West C, et al. The child asthma link line: a coalition-initiated, telephone-based, care coordination intervention for childhood asthma. J Asthma 2010;47(3):303–9.
28. Lara M, Bryant-Stephens T, Damitz M, et al. Balancing "Fidelity" and community context in the adaptation of asthma evidence-based interventions in the "Real World". Health Promot Pract 2011;12(Suppl 1):63S–72S.
29. Mansfield C, Viswanathan M, Woodell C, et al. Outcomes from a cross-site evaluation of a comprehensive pediatric asthma initiative incorporating translation of evidence-based interventions. Health Promot Pract 2011;12:34S.

Effective Strategies to Improve the Management of Heart Failure

Geoffrey D. Mills, MD, PhD[a,b,]*, Christopher V. Chambers, MD[c]

KEYWORDS

- Heart failure • Primary care physicians • Acute decompensated heart failure
- Self-care behavior

KEY POINTS

- Primary care physicians play multiple roles in the care of acute decompensated heart failure (ADHF), including prevention of heart failure (HF), in-office diagnosis of ADHF, transitions of care to and from the hospital, and postdischarge care and routine outpatient disease management.
- The early identification of HF shows promise in improving the natural course of the disease, and primary care physicians may play a future role in broader screening for asymptomatic left ventricular dysfunction. Primary care providers should promote adherence to treatment plans through patient education, fostering behavior change, and action planning.
- Early intervention, team-based disease management, and consistent follow-up are keys to improving outcomes. Patients with end-stage HF should be considered for focused goals-of-care discussions to improve quality of life and limit hospitalizations for recurrent HF exacerbations.

Heart failure (HF) is a common, progressive syndrome defined as the inability of the heart to deliver sufficient blood to meet the changing demands of tissues and organs. HF affects approximately 6 million people in the United States, with 670,000 people newly diagnosed each year.[1,2] The progressive nature of this syndrome, lack of clear diagnostic criteria or screening tools, and the heterogeneous nature of its root causes make HF a challenging management problem for cardiologists and generalists alike. Primary care physicians play an important role in the care of patients with HF from primary prevention to end-of-life care. Despite the availability of clinical guidelines

Funding Sources: Dr Mills, NHLBI. Dr Chambers, Merck, GlaxoSmithKline, NHLBI-research support.
Conflict of Interest: The authors have no conflict of interest.
[a] Department of Family and Community Medicine, Jefferson Medical College, 833 Chestnut Street, Suite 301, Philadelphia, PA 19107, USA; [b] Department of Physiology, Jefferson Medical College, Jefferson Alumni Hall, 4th Floor, 1020 Locust Street, Philadelphia, PA 19107, USA; [c] Department of Family and Community Medicine, 1015 Walnut Street, Suite 401, Philadelphia, PA 19107, USA
* Department of Family and Community Medicine, Jefferson Medical College, 833 Chestnut Street Suite 301, Philadelphia, PA 19107.
E-mail address: Geoffrey.Mills@jefferson.edu

Prim Care Clin Office Pract 39 (2012) 393–413
doi:10.1016/j.pop.2012.03.009

for the management of acute and chronic HF, there is wide variability in clinical practice, particularly between primary care providers and cardiologists.[3]

The purpose of this article is to provide primary care providers with an evidence-based resource for management of HF and to describe effective strategies to facilitate transitions in care, self-care education, and action planning. The pharmacologic management of patients with HF is described in detail elsewhere and should be familiar to the primary care physician.[4–6] Adherence to published guidelines has been shown to be lower for generalist physicians relative to cardiology specialists and may account for poorer outcomes in patients with HF cared for by primary care physicians.[7]

Knowledge of appropriate medical therapies is crucial, but evidence suggests that improved systems of care for patients with HF that involve collaborative care with specialists, multidisciplinary teams (including primary care), with a focus on transitions of care and chronic disease management, improve adherence to published guidelines and, as a result, clinical outcomes.[8] Primary care plays a central role in the early identification of HF, transitions to and from acute care settings, self-care promotion, managing comorbid conditions, and end-of-life care in HF.

EARLY IDENTIFICATION OF HF AND TRANSITION TO HIGHER LEVELS OF CARE

The 2 most common causes of HF are chronic hypertension and coronary artery disease (CAD) leading to ischemic cardiomyopathy. Primary prevention of hypertension and management of risk factors for CAD through early identification and treatment may prevent the development and progression of HF. Prevention of HF requires recognition of early symptoms in appropriate patients and optimal medical management of CAD once present. Hypertension accounts for approximately one-third of new cases of HF in men and up to 60% of new cases in women.[9] Chronic hypertension is the most common cause of HF in African American patients.[10] Pressure overload causes ventricular hypertrophy, which causes increased myocardial oxygen demand and eventually diastolic and/or systolic dysfunction. Treatment of hypertension can significantly reduce the risk of hypertrophy and the development of chronic HF.[11,12]

CAD is present in approximately two-thirds of patients with HF and is a common cause of left ventricular (LV) dysfunction. Acute myocardial infarction can result in sudden changes in LV systolic function and symptomatic acute decompensated HF (ADHF), but LV dysfunction may be present for months or years before symptoms develop.[13] Primary prevention of CAD through risk factor reduction (treatment of dyslipidemia, smoking cessation, hypertension management) is the standard of care, and treatment guidelines should be followed.[12,14,15] Patients who have had prior ischemia or myocardial infarction benefit from the use of β-blockers and angiotensin-converting enzyme (ACE) inhibitors to prevent reinfarction. Moreover, the use of ACE inhibitors in patients with asymptomatic LV systolic dysfunction after myocardial infarction improves survival and decreases the risk of developing HF by 20% to 30%.[16,17]

Primary care physicians should address cardiac risk factors at every visit and should implement strategies aimed at maximizing the quality of chronic disease management for patients with hypertension, diabetes, and CAD. These management strategies may include disease-specific group visits, goal-directed therapy, the formation of multidisciplinary care teams, and partnering with the patient to improve self-care behaviors.

SCREENING FOR HF IN ASYMPTOMATIC PATIENTS

Prevention of HF requires the management of predisposing conditions and risk factors. In patients with chronic hypertension or CAD, early detection of asymptomatic

LV systolic dysfunction before HF has the potential to modify the course of the HF syndrome. The rationale for this argument comes from studies showing that appropriate medical therapy can prevent progression of asymptomatic HF (as measured by LV systolic function).[17,18] Early identification (before symptoms) depends on the availability of an effective screening strategy for asymptomatic pre-HF. However, limited data are available on appropriate screening strategies.[19] Any screening strategy for HF must show that identification in the preclinical state and early intervention lead to improved clinical outcomes. In addition, it must be safe, cost effective, and widely available.[20]

Studies have shown that appropriate pharmacologic therapy with ACE inhibitors can reduce the risk of progression of HF in patients with asymptomatic LV systolic dysfunction, suggesting that early detection is a promising intervention.[17,18,21]

The SOLVD ([Studies of Left Ventricular Dysfunction] enalapril), SAVE ([Survival and Ventricular Enlargement] captopril), and TRACE ([Trandolapril Cardiac Evaluation] trandolapril) trials studied asymptomatic patients with an LV ejection fraction (LVEF) by echocardiography of 35% to 40% or less. The exact prevalence of asymptomatic systolic dysfunction with an LVEF less than 40% is unclear, but population studies have shown that it is present in 0.9% to 2.1% of adults aged 45 to 74 years.[22,23] Whether pharmacologic intervention with ACE inhibitors improves outcomes in patients with modestly reduced LVEF (>40%) has not been established.

The promise of echocardiography as a noninvasive test for LVEF assessment is based on both its wide availability in the community and its high sensitivity.[21] Choosing echocardiography as a screening test for asymptomatic LV dysfunction is challenging because of 2 key factors: assessment of LV function with formal transthoracic echocardiography might need to be repeated if the initial test results were negative and the cost of formal transthoracic echocardiography is too high for widespread screening, even in patients with preexisting chronic hypertension and CAD, given the prevalence of these conditions.[19]

Two strategies proposed to reduce the cost of screening and improve sensitivity of echocardiography are prescreening and risk stratification. Prescreening with plasma brain natriuretic peptide (BNP) levels or using hand-held ultrasound in community clinics may be able to determine when formal echocardiography is warranted.[19] However, the test value cutoffs for these preliminary measurements have not been established.[24,25] Another strategy to improve the efficiency of screening for preclinical HF is using risk stratification to determine who is likely to have abnormal LVEF by formal echocardiography. The use of a clinical multivariate risk assessment can identify high-risk candidates for HF who may have positive findings by echocardiography. In an investigation of Framingham Study data,[21] the investigators created a multivariate risk calculation to identify high-risk candidates for HF who would be likely to have abnormal echocardiography. Risk factors included age, the presence of LV hypertrophy by electrocardiography, cardiomegaly on chest radiography, heart rate, blood pressure, vital capacity, and the presence of hypertension, diabetes, and a history of myocardial infarction or valvular disease. This approach, if combined with biomarkers such as BNP, may hold future promise as a screening strategy, but its real-world application has not been tested.[26] Although the benefits of screening for asymptomatic LV dysfunction have been demonstrated for patients with LVEF of 35% to 40%, routine screening for asymptomatic LV dysfunction is not currently recommended by the 2009 update of the American College of Cardiology/American Heart Association (ACC/AHA) Guidelines for the Diagnosis and Management of Heart Failure in Adults.[5]

More studies are needed to determine the appropriateness of screening in asymptomatic patients. Primary care physicians likely play an important role in recognizing at-risk individuals and may be tasked with screening for asymptomatic LV dysfunction. Screening strategies likely involve in-office LVEF assessment and HF risk stratification.

MANAGEMENT OF HF AS A CHRONIC DISEASE

Strategies for the management of chronic systolic and diastolic HF are divided into pharmacologic and nonpharmacologic approaches. There have been major advances in the outpatient treatment of chronic HF, especially in patients with systolic dysfunction and LVEF less than 40%. Patients are classified based on symptom severity by the commonly used New York Heart Association (NYHA) scale: class I, patients with no symptoms and no limitation in ordinary physical activity; class II, patients with mild symptoms such as mild shortness or breath or angina with slight limitations in activity; class III, patients with limitations in activity because of symptoms even with walking short distances; and class IV, patients with severe limitations, even with rest.[27] The use of ACE inhibitors, angiotensin receptor blockers (ARBs), β-blockers, spironolactone, diuretics, and other pharmacologic agents is reviewed in depth elsewhere.[5,28] Primary care physicians should be aware of these therapeutic modalities and should approach each patient with the goal of ensuring that he/she is taking optimal doses of medications that will improve clinical outcomes. In general, pharmacologic therapies are aimed at normalizing blood pressure and volume status and preventing worsening myocardial dysfunction. Pharmacologic therapy should also be focused on controlling risk factors by treating diabetes and CAD.

Pharmacologic Management of Patients with Chronic HF

All patients with systolic dysfunction should be taking the maximally tolerated dose of an ACE inhibitor, regardless of HF severity, unless contraindicated. These medications reduce mortality and morbidity in patients with HF with significant benefit in hospitalization rate.[29] There is no evidence that one ACE inhibitor is better than the other in HF, and they are equally well-tolerated.[30] For patients who cannot tolerate ACE inhibitors, ARBs are an effective but more costly substitute. ARBs also reduce all-cause mortality and hospitalizations in NYHA class II and III HF.[31,32] The addition of an ARB to ACE inhibitors is safe and should be considered in patients who are symptomatic despite therapy with diuretics, ACE inhibitors, and β-blockers.[33]

For all symptomatic patients (NYHA class II–IV) and for most asymptomatic patients, β-blockers should be added unless they are acutely decompensated. Most β-blockers (carvedilol, metoprolol, bisoprolol) have been shown to reduce mortality in systolic HF.[30] The ACC/AHA guidelines recommend the use of these β-blockers in stable patients with current or prior symptoms of HF and who have a reduced LVEF.[5]

Aldosterone antagonists (spironolactone or eplerenone, which is more costly) prolong survival in patients with severe HF (class III–IV) and an LVEF of 35% or less.[34,35] Their use should be considered in these patients as long as serum potassium levels can be monitored and who have no underlying renal dysfunction (glomerular filtration rate <50 mL/min).[5]

Diuretics are often needed in patients with severe HF (class III–IV) to manage volume overload. There have been no large trials of diuretics in HF to examine the effect of these agents on morbidity and mortality, but most trials of other medications (described earlier) included diuretics as baseline therapy. The loop diuretics are the most potent diuretics, but serum potassium and creatinine levels should be monitored periodically, especially when used in combination with ACE inhibitors or ARBs.[36]

Details about the use of digoxin, calcium channel blockers, and nitrates are available elsewhere and are beyond the scope of this article.[5,30] For patients with chronic diastolic dysfunction, calcium channel blockers or β-blockers should be used to promote LV filling by controlling heart rate, diuretics to control volume overload, and ACE inhibitors to promote myocardial remodeling. Each patient with chronic HF should be approached with an at-goal or not-at-goal approach with respect to medication management, and primary care physicians should strive to adhere to the guidelines cited earlier.

Nonpharmacologic Management of Patients with Chronic HF

Medication compliance

Data from large randomized clinical trials have shown that β-blockers and ACE inhibitors (or ARBs) reduce hospitalization and mortality for patients with HF.[5] Nonadherence to prescribed medications is a common cause for ADHF but may only account for a small percentage of acute exacerbations relative to dietary noncompliance.[37] Reports of adherence rates vary widely,[38] but patients who have better adherence have improved survival.[39,40]

Medication management at home requires the filling of prescriptions provided by a provider or at hospital discharge, reconciling changes and updating new medication regimens, recognizing and understanding the benefits and potential side effects of medications, and changing medication routines as needed. Adherence to recommended daily medications greater than 88% is the critical rate predicting improved clinical outcomes.[39] This point should be emphasized by primary care providers at each visit. Medication adherence rates are higher in older patients, in those with higher NYHA class, in those with less comorbidity, and for those who are married.[41]

After hospitalization for ADHF, early postdischarge follow-up should focus on performing a thorough medication assessment, reinforcing proper medication use, counseling regarding potential benefits and side effects, and teaching effective strategies for self-management of medications. Outpatient physicians should recognize and clarify any new or changed medications during a transition of care with the patient and caregiver to ensure that they have accurately rectified the medication at home.

NUTRITION

Dietary education is recommended at each visit for patients with HF.[4,40] Nutritional interventions include dietary sodium restriction of less than 2 grams per day and, in some patients with serum sodium abnormalities, free water restriction. Sodium restriction is known to reduce mean arterial blood pressure and may also prevent urinary potassium loss in patients taking diuretics for hypertension or HF.[42,43] Although almost 20% of patients with ADHF have excessive salt intake identified as the primary cause for exacerbation, no clinical trials have evaluated the effect of a low-sodium diet on important clinical outcomes.[37] In one study of patients being discharged with ADHF and preserved systolic function, those with documented discharge instructions for a low-sodium diet were found to have significantly reduced odds (0.43) of 30-day death or readmission for ADHF.[44] Adherence to a low-sodium diet is improved by face-to-face education from a registered dietician when compared with written instructions alone at 3 months postdischarge from a hospitalization for ADHF.[40] Providers should consider outpatient consultation with nutritionists or registered dieticians and at every visit should assess patient adherence and understanding of this key self-care behavior.

Activity Level and Exercise Recommendations

Severity of HF is defined by limitations in activity and exercise capacity based on symptoms of dyspnea and fatigue.[45] The 2010 Heart Failure Society of America (HFSA) guidelines and 2009 ACC/AHA guidelines suggest that patients with HF should be provided with details regarding their recommended activity level and that exercise training is effective at improving clinical status in ambulatory patients (a Class I recommendation).[4,5] The physiologic rationale for aerobic exercise in HF includes demonstrable improvements in peak oxygen consumption, peripheral blood flow and symptoms of dyspnea and fatigue.[46]

Exercise training may reduce readmission for HF and may improve survival in patients with NHYA class II or III HF.[47] However, a large trial (HF-ACTION) showed only modest benefits in all-cause mortality or hospitalization in patients with NYHA class II to IV HF receiving supervised exercise training.[48] During this trial, patients were guided to exercise at an intensity of 70% of heart rate reserve (as determined by an exercise test done before the trial) for 2 months. Adherence to physical activity is low even in supervised exercise studies.[49]

Although adherence is low and costs are high, exercise programs may be appropriate for some patients. Primary care physicians should consider specific exercise recommendations for patients with stable class II or III HF without other limitations to exercise.[50] Specialized cardiac rehabilitation programs should be recommended if available, and, with supervision, higher intensity activity can be recommended. Recommendations for home exercise on a stationary bicycle or treadmill (if appropriate) should include the intensity of exercise (moderate, 40%–50% of maximum capacity), duration (titrate from 2 minutes to 15–30 minute sessions), and frequency (3–5 times per week), and patients should be instructed to avoid isometric exercise (such as weight lifting).[51] A prolonged warm-up period may be necessary. Because higher exercise intensity is likely necessary to achieve meaningful results, cardiac rehabilitation should be considered for patients with stable class II or III HF, where available.[5]

SELF-CARE BEHAVIORS

In addition to dietary and medication adherence, nonpharmacologic management of HF also includes self-care behaviors such as early symptom recognition. Patients and their families or caregivers are responsible for at-home self-care behaviors. Self-care is a "decision-making process that patients use in choosing behaviors that maintain physiologic stability and the response to symptoms when they occur."[52] Daily monitoring for signs and symptoms of HF improves early identification of worsening clinical status potentially to avoid hospitalization. However, the impact of positive self-care behaviors is unclear.[53] Recommended self-care instructions are shown in **Table 1**.[4]

Daily weighing can be an important tool for the detection of worsening HF; however, measurement of daily weights ranges from 12% to 75%, even for patients with access to a bathroom scale at home.[41,54] Furthermore, measured changes in weight do not reliably result in medication adjustments perhaps because one-half of patients rate sudden weight gain as not important and fail to inform their doctor of the weight gain.[55,56] Reinforcing these self-care behaviors at each visit is critical to improving adherence and to preventing readmissions.

A validated self-care instrument is available for measuring self-care in HF (Self-Care of Heart Failure Index) and is adapted in **Fig. 1**.[52,57] The main purpose of this tool is to study self-care behaviors in research settings where it may be scored and individual

Table 1
Recommended self-care behaviors for patients with HF

Behavior	Frequency	Notes
Daily weight	Daily at the same time: after urination but before eating in the morning	Notify provider if >2 lb gained in 1 d or >5 lb gained in 1 wk
Check for edema	Daily	Examine legs for swelling (new or increase in existing swelling) and describe if swelling reaches ankle, shin, or knee
Check exercise tolerance	Daily	Follow NYHA class definitions for shortness of breath at rest, mild exertion, moderate exertion, or none at all
Check for orthostatic dyspnea	Daily	Follow number of pillows used at night or increase in waking at night with dyspnea
Salt/sodium restriction	Daily	Calculate total sodium intake in a day from nutrition labels and food charts. Understand hidden sources of salt intake (goal of <2 g/d)

Data from 2005 Writing Committee Members, Hunt SA, Abraham WT, et al. 2009 focused update incorporated into the ACC/AHA 2005 guidelines for the diagnosis and management of heart failure in adults. Circulation 2009;119(14):e391–479.

behaviors can be studied. Although this tool is not widely used in current clinical practice, it may be useful to use to reinforce positive self-care behaviors and stress the importance of physician communication when symptoms are worsening and may identify educational opportunities.

Adherence to positive self-care behaviors has the potential to influence outcomes in HF and reduces ADHF admissions.[58] However, overall adherence to treatments and lifestyle modification is low for patients with HF. Lack of understanding of medication instructions (57%) and lack of true medication reconciliation at home are common causes of poor adherence rates.[59] Patients often delay seeking care for symptoms of HF.[60] In the first week after discharge for ADHF, only 14% patients check their weight daily.[61] In addition, most patients with HF have difficulty following a low-sodium diet.[37] Comorbid psychosocial issues and other medical conditions may make HF self-care challenging for patients. Despite significant barriers to HF self-care, there are limited data available for interventions that improve self-care compliance in the HF.

Successful Interventions Promoting HF Self-Care and Improving HF Outcomes

Educational and behavioral interventions

Patient understanding of medication usage and symptom monitoring may be increased using validated techniques for adult education, such as the teach-back technique, where a provider addresses a few key teaching points per educational session, as well as repetition and reinforcement at regular intervals or follow-up session.[62] In this case, patients are regularly scheduled until self-care goals are met. Some patients require multiple educational interventions, and knowledge skills may improve over time and with practice.

Listed below are common recommendations for persons with heart failure. How often do you do the following?

	Never or rarely	Sometimes	Frequently	Always
Weigh yourself daily?	1	2	3	4
Eat a low-salt diet?	1	2	3	4
Take part in regular physical activity?	1	2	3	4
Keep your weight down?	1	2	3	4
Get a flu shot every year?	1	2	3	4

Many patients have symptoms due to their heart failure. *Trouble breathing and ankle swelling are symptoms of heart failure.*

In the past three months, have you had trouble breathing or ankle swelling? CIRCLE ONE

1) NO
2) YES

The last time you had trouble breathing or ankle swelling:
How quickly did you recognize it as a symptom of heart failure?

I did not recognize it	Not quickly	Somewhat quickly	Quickly	Very quickly
0	1	2	3	4

Listed below are remedies that people with heart failure use. When you have trouble breathing or ankle swelling, how likely are you to try one of these remedies?

	Not likely	Somewhat likely	Likely	Very Likely
Reduce your salt intake ?	1	2	3	4
Reduce your fluid intake?	1	2	3	4
Take an extra water pill?	1	2	3	4
Call your doctor for guidance?	1	2	3	4

If you tried any of these remedies the last time you had trouble breathing or ankle swelling, how sure were you that the remedy helped or not?

I did not try anything N/A	Not sure	Somewhat sure	Sure	Very sure
	1	2	3	4

	Not confident	Somewhat confident	Very confident	Extremely confident
How confident are you that you can evaluate the importance of your symptoms?	1	2	3	4
Generally, how confident are you that you can recognize changes in your health if they occur?	1	2	3	4
Generally, how confident are you that you can do something that will relieve your symptoms?	1	2	3	4
How confident are you that you can evaluate the effectiveness of whatever you do to relieve your symptoms?	1	2	3	4

Fig. 1. Self-Care of Heart Failure Index. (*From* Riegel B, Carlson B, Moser DK, et al. Psychometric testing of the self-care of heart failure index. J Card Fail 2004;10(4):353; with permission.)

Although education that increases HF knowledge is important, knowledge alone is not sufficient.[63] Interventions causing behavioral change and those focused on changing patient perceptions of self-care have shown the most promise. For example, brief motivational interviewing in patients with HF improves short-term physical activity adherence in older patients with HF.[64]

This study[64] involved phone calls, using which patients were encouraged to articulate their own ambivalence toward self-care behaviors, and education was offered only if the participant requested information. The investigators' approach was to identify a behavior (in this case exercise) and facilitate patient problem solving to address barriers to performing this behavior. More research is needed to determine what educational and behavioral interventions are most effective at improving HF care and reducing admission rates, but primary care providers (and their care team) can use this approach to improve self-care behavior.

Systems-based interventions

Many studies have looked at multifaceted, system-based interventions to reduce hospital readmissions. These interventions often include multiple educational components, assessments by registered dieticians and pharmacists, home-care plans, phone follow-up, and outpatient appointments after discharge. They are designed to facilitate transitions across care settings and may begin in the hospital and extend into the postdischarge period at home, in outpatient primary care, or in cardiology practices. In a meta-analysis of published studies, HF self-care programs reduce HF-specific and all-cause hospitalization but have little effect on overall mortality.[65] Unfortunately, most studies were nonrandomized, and it is unclear which elements of these multidisciplinary and multifaceted interventions are most effective. However, it is clear that strategies incorporating follow-up monitoring by specially trained staff (home nursing, physicians, or pharmacists) and access to specialty HF clinics can reduce mortality and hospitalizations.[65]

Outpatient disease management programs involving team-based approaches improve self-care knowledge and daily weighing behavior. More importantly, recommended medication use is improved and the frequency of hospitalization is decreased while quality of life improves over time.[66] In one study, 2 internists and clinic nurses conducted a primary care HF clinic one half-day per week for patients with symptomatic HF. In this study, inadequate resources for patient education and for phone visits by the multidisciplinary team were cited as barriers that might be encountered by other practices.[66] The implementation of a protocol-driven HF disease management program in a specialty-run cardiology practice increased adherence to medication guidelines, reduced cardiac-related hospitalizations, and was cost saving.[67,68] This protocol included a patient education manual that was given to patients, scheduled telephone calls by trained nurses, and scheduled clinic visits with a physician, nurse, or nurse practitioner.

Incorporating an HF disease management team into a primary care practice is feasible and may make HF management less opportunistic and more proactive; staff dedicated to make follow-up phone calls can reinforce self-care behaviors and medication adherence and identify patients who need to be evaluated in person.

HF action planning
A useful tool for incorporating self-care behaviors into the management of patients with HF is the HF action plan. The 2010 HFSA guidelines recommend that patients with HF have a plan for how and when to notify a provider of changes in symptoms or medications, but no studies have looked at the effect of this intervention alone on HF outcomes such as readmission and mortality.[4] An HF action plan includes information that reinforces daily self-care behaviors (weighing, symptom checking, and changes in ability to do everyday things) as well as a color-coded severity-based action plan for seeking medical care. A sample HF action plan is shown in **Fig. 2**.

A central element in managing HF is recognizing it as a chronic disease and promoting self-care with frequent patient engagement. A team-based approach that bridges inpatient and outpatient care is effective at improving HF outcomes, including hospitalizations and quality of life. The details of this approach may be tailored to fit individual institution and practice needs but should include the following: early identification of HF to facilitate HF education focused on behavior change from a multidisciplinary team, care coordination that may include home nursing, pharmacy, and case management. Patients should be specifically instructed in the following self-care activities: medication use and management, daily monitoring of signs and symptoms, and adherence to a low-sodium diet. Outpatient disease management programs are cost effective and improve important outcomes. The use of HF action planning should be considered for most patients.

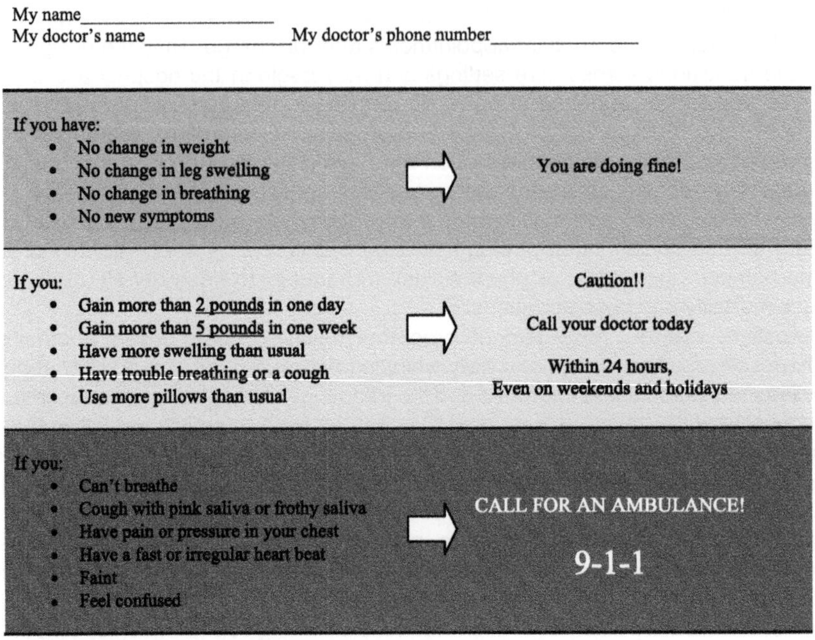

My name_____
My doctor's name_____My doctor's phone number_____

If you have:
- No change in weight
- No change in leg swelling
- No change in breathing
- No new symptoms

You are doing fine!

If you:
- Gain more than 2 pounds in one day
- Gain more than 5 pounds in one week
- Have more swelling than usual
- Have trouble breathing or a cough
- Use more pillows than usual

Caution!!

Call your doctor today

Within 24 hours,
Even on weekends and holidays

If you:
- Can't breathe
- Cough with pink saliva or frothy saliva
- Have pain or pressure in your chest
- Have a fast or irregular heart beat
- Faint
- Feel confused

CALL FOR AN AMBULANCE!

9-1-1

Fig. 2. Heart Failure Action Plan.

RECOGNITION AND MANAGEMENT OF ADHF

The classic signs and symptoms of ADHF include fatigue, volume overload, and adrenergic stimulation (tachycardia, peripheral vasoconstriction). However, these are not unique to HF, and their presence and severity vary from patient to patient. Moreover, these signs and symptoms do not correlate with the degree of LV dysfunction or with NHYA functional class.[69] False-positive diagnosis of ADHF is common (up to 34%) in primary care, and accurate diagnosis is more difficult in women and obese patients.[69] Therefore, a systematic approach to the patient with suspected ADHF that includes appropriate point-of-care testing and referral to higher levels of care is necessary.

ADHF occurs most commonly from LV systolic or diastolic dysfunction secondary to ischemic CAD or chronic pressure-overload hypertrophy. However, it may occur in the absence of cardiac pathologic conditions with iatrogenic fluid overload, severe hypertension, or renal failure. ADHF is a syndrome characterized by the development of dyspnea and accumulation of fluid in the lung interstitium and alveolar space.[1]

Data gathering by history taking and examination in the office should be focused on determining the cause, onset, duration, chronicity, and severity of decompensation. The presenting clinical features of cardiogenic ADHF and noncardiogenic dyspnea and volume overload are similar. The history taking should be focused on uncovering symptoms of ischemia, arrhythmia, dyspnea, syncope, and failures in adhering to medical therapies and diet. Paroxysmal nocturnal dyspnea or orthopnea suggests cardiogenic pulmonary edema, whereas signs of infection, vomiting, or trauma may suggest noncardiogenic causes of edema. Easy fatigue and dyspnea on exertion are common features of ADHF, and the level of activity (or duration) causing dyspnea should be defined. Pulmonary examination may reveal tachypnea with increased work of breathing, whereas chest auscultation usually reveals crackles or wheezing (so-called cardiac asthma present in up to one-third of patients with HF).[70] Patients with ADHF may have an audible S3 sound, but the sensitivity of this finding is low (9%–51%).[71] The presence of peripheral edema is not a specific finding for ADHF and may have noncardiogenic causes. Cardiogenic edema is often associated with distended neck veins, an enlarged and tender liver, and respiratory findings in addition to symmetric edema. Examination should be focused on uncovering potential causes for ADHF. For example, an irregular pulse may suggest new-onset atrial fibrillation, or a new murmur may suggest unrecognized valvular disease.

Patients who do not meet hospital admission criteria with adequate follow-up potential, good self-care behaviors, and family support may only need additional short-term diuretic therapy and outpatient assessment of renal function or electrocardiography, for instance, and may not require additional imaging or urgent testing.[5] In addition, some patients who are homebound or in hospice may not be appropriate for inpatient management.

Recognition of ADHF in the office is the first step in managing ADHF. In-office electrocardiography may identify precipitating factors such as LV hypertrophy, left atrial enlargement, ischemia, or atrial fibrillation. Common findings in ADHF include tachycardia, T-wave inversion, and QT prolongation. Repolarization abnormalities may occur due to subendocardial ischemia from increased demand (increased wall stress) and/or decreased supply (decreased coronary blood flow from tachycardia and increased end-diastolic pressure).[72]

In most patients with suspected ADHF seen in the outpatient setting, additional testing is necessary and the decision to transfer the care of the patient to the emergency department for additional laboratory and imaging tests is made.

Transitions in Care

In the emergency department, plasma BNP levels are used in the initial evaluation of ADHF. BNP is a natriuretic hormone that is released from ventricular myocardium in response to high filling pressures. It is cleaved from a prohormone pro-BNP into its biologically active component and causes diuresis, natriuresis, and vasodilation.[73] In patients with HF, plasma BNP correlates with LV end-diastolic pressure,[74] and cutoffs have been established for circulating BNP and pro-BNP levels that are associated with high, moderate, and low likelihood of ADHF.[75,76] Both measurements are helpful at determining ADHF from other causes of dyspnea or edema. These cutoff values are listed in **Table 2** but may vary in different laboratories. Plasma BNP and pro-BNP levels can be elevated in critically ill patients without ADHF and patients with a glomerular filtration rate less than 60 mL/min. For this reason, the main value would

Table 2
Evidence-based cutoff values of BNP and pro-BNP for diagnosing ADHF

| | BNP (pg/mL) | | Pro-BNP (pg/mL) | |
Criterion	CHF unlikely	CHF likely	CHF unlikely	CHF likely
All ages	<100	>500	<300	-
21–50 y	-	-	-	>450
50–75 y	-	-	-	>900
>75 y	-	-	-	>1800
Estimated GFR <60 mL/min	<200	>500	-	-

Abbreviations: GFR, glomerular filtration rate; -, not defined.
   Data from Refs.[74,97,98]

be a low plasma BNP or pro-BNP level, which would exclude ventricular dysfunction. Other causes of elevated plasma BNP include acute pulmonary embolism and pulmonary hypertension from cor pulmonale or chronic hypoxia.[77] The use of these assays should supplement clinical judgment when the cause of dyspnea is uncertain, particularly in patients with intermediate probability of ADHF.

Other useful tests available in the emergency department are chest radiography, arterial blood gas analysis, and serum cardiac enzymes. The ACC/AHA and HFSA guidelines recommend echocardiography to aid in the diagnosis and classification of symptomatic HF. The use of routine invasive hemodynamic monitoring with flow-directed pulmonary artery catheters is not recommended.[5]

Hospital Admission

Primary care physicians are often involved in the decision to admit a patient to hospital and may be the primary caregiver in the acute care setting. Another consideration in managing the transition to hospitalization is the option of observation units in managing ADHF treatment if available.

Hospital admission criteria are listed in **Table 3**. HF guidelines recommend hospitalization for patients with abnormal vital signs, arrhythmia, and suspected acute coronary syndromes and consideration for hospitalization in patients with associated comorbid conditions, new HF, implantable cardioverter-defibrillator firing, or progressive fluid overload.

The initial management of ADHF is focused on hemodynamic stabilization, oxygenation, and ventilation followed by symptom relief. Although the details of medical therapy for ADHF are beyond the scope of this review, the general goals of treatment include restoration of oxygenation and normalization of volume status. It is important to document the etiology and nature (systolic vs diastolic) of HF as well as precipitating factors. Patients with acute coronary syndrome may need revascularization, and those with very low ejection fractions may need anticoagulation to prevent mural thrombus formation. Patients with ischemic or nonischemic cardiomyopathy may be candidates for implantable defibrillator devices.[4]

Table 3	
Recommendations for hospitalizing patients presenting with ADHF	
Recommendation	**Clinical Scenario**
Hospitalization recommended	ADHF with hypotension, worsening renal function, altered mental status
	Dyspnea at rest: resting tachypnea or oxygen saturation <90%
	Hemodynamically significant arrhythmia including new-onset atrial fibrillation
	Acute coronary syndromes
Hospitalization should be considered	Worsened systemic or pulmonary congestion without dyspnea or weight gain
	Major electrolyte disturbance
	Comorbid pneumonia, suspected pulmonary embolism, diabetic ketoacidosis, stroke
	Implantable cardioverter-defibrillator firing
	Previously undiagnosed HF with signs of systemic or pulmonary congestion

Data from Heart Failure Society of America. HFSA 2010 comprehensive heart failure practice guideline. J Card Fail 2010;16(6):e1–2.

DISCHARGE PLANNING FOR ADHF

In-hospital mortality related to ADHF admissions has decreased 40% in the last 10 years, and mean length of stay has decreased 30% over the same period.[2] However, 30-day readmission rates for ADHF remain in the range of 20% to 30%.[78] Primary care physicians not directly involved in inpatient care of their patients should be involved in the discharge planning early in the hospitalization. Discharge planning should happen early and should involve a multidisciplinary team focusing on self-care education (and caregiver education), healthy behavior promotion, and early hospital follow-up.

A critical role for the primary care physician in the care of the patient with HF is in the transition from hospital to home and postdischarge office follow-up. Multidisciplinary discharge planning should begin as soon as possible during admission and may include efforts from nursing, nutrition, social work, physical therapy, and pharmacy. The criteria for hospital discharge are listed in **Table 4**. The use of plasma BNP as a discharge marker is controversial, and further studies are needed to determine its utility in predicting when patients are safe to discharge and in identifying patients at risk for readmission.[79]

The days following discharge are critical for patients with HF because of medication changes and transition to new self-care behaviors. The duration of time to outpatient follow-up with a generalist or cardiologist after discharge varies from hospital to hospital, and different physicians may care for patients in the hospital and outpatient settings. Early physician follow-up (within 7 days) reduces readmission events significantly regardless of whether the follow-up is with a generalist or cardiologist.[80]

Collaborative Care with Specialists

Approximately 60% of ambulatory visits for HF occur in primary care offices.[81] Cardiology consultation may be necessary in both the inpatient and outpatient settings for diagnostic purposes, to troubleshoot failure of recommended therapies, and to assist

Table 4	
Discharge criteria for patients with ADHF	
Recommendation	**Criteria**
All patients with HF	Exacerbating factors addressed
	Volume status near optimal
	Oral diuretic use
	Patient and family education completed
	LVEF documented
	Smoking cessation counseling initiated
	Near optimal pharmacotherapy initiated with ACE inhibitor and β-blocker if appropriate
	Follow-up visit scheduled for within 7–10 d
Consider for patients with advanced HF or recurrent admissions	Oral medication regimen stable for 24 h
	No intravenous vasodilator or inotropic agent for 24 h
	Ambulation before discharge and functional capacity assessment
	Postdischarge plan for visiting nursing, telephone follow-up (<3 d after discharge)
	Multidisciplinary care plan if available

Data from Heart Failure Society of America. HFSA 2010 comprehensive heart failure practice guideline. J Card Fail 2010;16(6):e1–2.

in the management of patients with complex HF.[13] Patients with NYHA class IV HF have very high annual mortality (nearly 50%) and benefit from evaluation for potential transplant or advanced therapies offered by a specialist. Early collaborative care between a primary care physician and cardiologist improves survival at 30 days after discharge and is associated with higher rates of LVEF assessment, stress testing, revascularization, and device implantation.[82] Inpatient care by cardiology specialists results in better physician adherence to recommended medical therapies but is also associated with increased invasive testing and cost.[7,83] Referral and collaboration with cardiac specialists is an important factor in HF outcomes and should be considered with every patient, where appropriate.

HF AND COMORBIDITIES

Patients with HF often have multiple comorbidities. Therefore, primary care physicians play a central role in the careful management of coexisting conditions. Studies have shown that more than two-thirds of patients with HF have 2 or more noncardiac comorbidities.[84] The impact of these conditions on older adults with HF is particularly profound; patients older than 65 years with HF and 5 comorbidities have nearly twice the risk of hospitalization for any cause relative to patients with no comorbidity.[84] Renal dysfunction is common in patients with HF and may be worsened by diuretic use and ACE inhibitors and may contribute to volume overload. Anemia is a common complication of chronic renal dysfunction, and both are independently associated with an increased risk of death after discharge from community hospitals with ADHF.[85] These conditions should be assessed at each visit and treated as part of the outpatient HF management plan.

The prevalence of HF in patients with diabetes is between 9% and 22%, which is higher compared with the general population (approximately 4%). In addition, the prevalence of diabetes in patients hospitalized for ADHF is high (44%) and patients with diabetes and HF have a poorer prognosis and quality of life.[86] There is a connection between risk for CAD and diabetes, and there may be other direct pathophysiologic links between diabetes and HF. ACE inhibitors or ARBs should be used in patients with diabetes and HF. β-Blockers should also be used in patients with diabetes and HF, but evidence from subgroup analyses in HF trials show a more modest benefit in patients with diabetes and HF than in nondiabetic patients with HF.[86] Intense blood sugar control confers no additional benefit in patients with diabetes and HF as demonstrated in the ACCORD (Action to Control Cardiovascular Risk in Diabetes) trial.[87]

Metformin is generally safe and is the preferred oral agent for diabetes in patients with HF, associated with better clinical outcomes than other agents.[8] Coadministration of metformin, diuretics, and ACE inhibitors or ARBs may warrant more frequent monitoring of renal function. Insulin may be necessary for glucose control but is correlated with higher mortality and HF hospitalization. Thiazolidinediones (pioglitazone and particularly rosiglitazone) are associated with fluid retention and increase the risk of worsening HF. Pioglitazone is generally not recommended for patients with symptomatic HF and are contraindicated in patients with class III and IV HF.[88] Rosiglitazone is associated with an increased risk of cardiovascular morality and should not be used in patients with heart disease and diabetes.[89]

Another diagnosis relevant to the primary care management of patients with HF is coexisting depression. Depression is more common in patients with HF (24%–40% prevalence) than in other adults and is associated with poor outcomes, including recurrent admissions and increased mortality.[90] Patients with depression and HF are more likely to take medication inappropriately, have poor dietary compliance, and have difficulty with self-care behaviors.[56,91] However, the data are limited regarding optimal management strategies for depression in patients with HF. These patients should be identified early, with validated depression screening tools, and aggressively treated within the context of a care team that includes behavioral health providers.

ADVANCE DIRECTIVES AND END-OF-LIFE CARE IN HF

Overall, the average life expectancy for patients diagnosed with HF is less than 6 years, but the course of HF is variable, and patients with good medication response and self-care behaviors can live 10 years or more. An important role for the primary care physician is discussing prognosis and end-of-life care planning in all patients with HF. A long-standing patient-physician relationship can help facilitate these discussions, but end-of-life discussions can be time consuming, and physicians may be uncomfortable with the topic of death and dying or with prognostication.[92]

Patients who have had 3 or more hospitalizations for HF, who are 85 years or more, who have multiple comorbidities, or who have had a rapid decline in functional status should be considered for a dedicated goals-of-care discussion.[93] All patients with HF should have advanced directives, and office practices should have mechanisms to provide written resources to develop these documents as well as to provide a place to store them in patient charts and to access from the hospital.

Prognostic tools are available to predict survival and supplement clinical judgment to guide these decisions.[94] One predictive model that is useful in the inpatient setting is called the EFFECT (Enhanced Feedback for Effective Cardiac Treatment) model. An online calculator is available at www.ccort.ca/CHF riskmodel.aspx. Vital signs, laboratory values (respiratory rate, systolic blood pressure, serum urea nitrogen, serum sodium), and the presence of comorbid conditions are used in a multivariate analysis to estimate 30-day mortality.[95] This model has been validated in a large number of patients and can be used in any patient admitted for ADHF at the time of admission. Another model that is available for use in non-ADHF outpatients is the Seattle Heart Failure Model, which is derived from a broad HF population including both outpatients and patients with advanced HF. It can provide accurate estimates of 1-, 2-, and 3-year survival estimates. An online calculator for the Seattle Model is also available at www. SeattleHeartFailureModel.org. An important aspect of this model is that it can be used to determine the estimated effect of adding new therapies on the risk of mortality.[96]

Patients diagnosed with HF should have regular estimates of severity and NYHA class at every visit along with LVEF assessment when there are apparent changes in clinical status. Physicians should consider the use of prognostic models to guide patient selection for end-of-life care discussions in conjunction with clinical judgment and knowledge of individual patient values and advance directives.

SUMMARY

HF is a common progressive syndrome that, despite major advances in pharmacotherapy, is associated with significant morbidity and mortality and high rates of hospital admission for ADHF. Factors leading to ADHF include noncompliance with self-care behaviors and medications, worsening disease, hypertension, and new arrhythmias. Self-care behaviors include adherence to diet (salt, water, and alcohol intake), symptom monitoring, following an action plan for changing symptoms, and communication with the care team. Primary care physicians play multiple roles in the care of ADHF, including prevention of HF, in-office diagnosis of ADHF, transitions of care to and from the hospital, and post-discharge care and routine outpatient disease management. The early identification of HF shows promise in improving the natural course of the disease and primary care physicians may play a future role in broader screening for asymptomatic LV dysfunction. Primary care providers should promote adherence to treatment plans through patient education, fostering behavior change, and action planning. Early intervention, team-based disease management, and consistent follow-up are keys to improving outcomes. Patients with end-stage HF should be considered for focused goals-of-care discussions to improve quality of life and limit hospitalizations for recurrent HF exacerbations.

REFERENCES

1. Ware LB, Matthay MA. Acute pulmonary edema. N Engl J Med 2005;353(26): 2788–96. Available at: http://dx.doi.org/10.1056/NEJMcp052699. Accessed October 1, 2011.
2. Lloyd-Jones D, Adams R, Carnethon M, et al. Heart disease and stroke statistics—2009 update. A report from the American Heart Association Statistics Committee and Stroke Statistics Subcommittee. Circulation 2008;117(4):e25–146.
3. Hunt SA, Baker DW, Chin MH, et al. ACC/AHA guidelines for the evaluation and management of chronic heart failure in the adult: executive summary: a report of the American College of Cardiology/American Heart Association Task Force on practice guidelines (committee to revise the 1995 guidelines for the evaluation and management of heart failure) developed in collaboration with the International Society for Heart and Lung Transplantation endorsed by the Heart Failure Society of America. J Am Coll Cardiol 2001;38(7):2101–13.
4. Heart Failure Society of America. HFSA 2010 comprehensive heart failure practice guideline. J Card Fail 2010;16(6):e1–2.
5. 2005 Writing Committee Members, Hunt SA, Abraham WT, et al. 2009 focused update incorporated into the ACC/AHA 2005 guidelines for the diagnosis and management of heart failure in adults. Circulation 2009;119(14):e391–479.
6. Hunt SA, Baker DW, Chin MH, et al. ACC/AHA guidelines for the evaluation and management of chronic heart failure in the adult: executive summary. A report of the American College of Cardiology/American Heart Association Task Force on practice guidelines (committee to revise the 1995 guidelines for the evaluation and management of heart failure). J Am Coll Cardiol 2001;38(7):2101–13.
7. Edep M, Shah N, Tateo I, et al. Differences between primary care physicians and cardiologists in management of congestive heart failure: relation to practice guidelines. J Am Coll Cardiol 1997;30(2):518–26.
8. Eurich DT, McAlister FA, Blackburn DF, et al. Benefits and harms of antidiabetic agents in patients with diabetes and heart failure: systematic review. BMJ 2007;335(7618):497.
9. Levy D, Larson MG, Vasan RS, et al. The progression from hypertension to congestive heart failure. JAMA 1996;275(20):1557–62.
10. Ferdinand K, Serrano C, Ferdinand D. Contemporary treatment of heart failure: is there adequate evidence to support a unique strategy for African-Americans? Con position. Curr Hypertens Rep 2002;4(4):311–8.
11. Kostis JB, Davis BR, Cutler J, et al. Prevention of heart failure by antihypertensive drug treatment in older persons with isolated systolic hypertension. JAMA 1997; 278(3):212–6.
12. Chobanian AV, Bakris GL, Black HR, et al. Seventh report of the Joint National Committee on Prevention, Detection, Evaluation, and Treatment of High Blood Pressure. Hypertension 2003;42(6):1206–52.

13. Diller PM, Smucker DR. Management of heart failure. Prim Care Clin Office Pract 2000;27(3):651–75.
14. Pearson TA, Blair SN, Daniels SR, et al. AHA guidelines for primary prevention of cardiovascular disease and stroke: 2002 update. Circulation 2002;106(3): 388–91.
15. Expert Panel on Detection, Evaluation, and Treatment of High Blood Cholesterol in Adults. Executive summary of the third report of the National Cholesterol Education Program (NCEP) expert panel on detection, evaluation, and treatment of high blood cholesterol in adults (adult treatment panel III). JAMA 2001;285(19): 2486–97.
16. Køber L, Torp-Pedersen C, Carlsen JE, et al. A clinical trial of the angiotensin-converting–enzyme inhibitor trandolapril in patients with left ventricular dysfunction after myocardial infarction. N Engl J Med 1995;333(25):1670–6. Available at: http://dx.doi.org/10.1056/NEJM199512213332503. Accessed October 1, 2011.
17. Effect of enalapril on survival in patients with reduced left ventricular ejection fractions and congestive heart failure. N Engl J Med 1991;325(5):293–302. Available at: http://dx.doi.org/10.1056/NEJM199108013250501. Accessed October 1, 2011.
18. Pfeffer MA, Braunwald E, Moyé LA, et al. Effect of captopril on mortality and morbidity in patients with left ventricular dysfunction after myocardial infarction. N Engl J Med 1992;327(10):669–77. Available at: http://dx.doi.org/10.1056/NEJM199209033271001. Accessed October 1, 2011.
19. Galasko GI, Barnes SC, Collinson P, et al. What is the most cost-effective strategy to screen for left ventricular systolic dysfunction: natriuretic peptides, the electrocardiogram, hand-held echocardiography, traditional echocardiography, or their combination? Eur Heart J 2006;27(2):193–200.
20. Herman CR, Gill HK, Eng J, et al. Screening for preclinical disease: test and disease characteristics. AJR Am J Roentgenol 2002;179(4):825–31.
21. Kannel WB, D'Agostino RB, Silbershatz H, et al. Profile for estimating risk of heart failure. Arch Intern Med 1999;159(11):1197–204.
22. Devereux RB, Roman MJ, Paranicas M, et al. A population-based assessment of left ventricular systolic dysfunction in middle-aged and older adults: the Strong Heart Study. Am Heart J 2001;141(3):439–46.
23. Davies M, Hobbs F, Davis R, et al. Prevalence of left-ventricular systolic dysfunction and heart failure in the Echocardiographic Heart of England Screening study: a population based study. Lancet 2001;358(9280):439–44.
24. Vasan RS, Benjamin EJ, Larson MG, et al. Plasma natriuretic peptides for community screening for left ventricular hypertrophy and systolic dysfunction. JAMA 2002;288(10):1252–9.
25. Luchner A, Burnett JC, Jougasaki M, et al. Evaluation of brain natriuretic peptide as marker of left ventricular dysfunction and hypertrophy in the population. J Hypertens 2000;18(8):1121–8.
26. Velagaleti RS, Gona P, Larson MG, et al. Multimarker approach for the prediction of heart failure incidence in the community/clinical perspective. Circulation 2010; 122(17):1700–6.
27. Nomenclature and criteria for diagnosis of diseases of the heart and great vessels. Ann Intern Med 1974;80(5):678.
28. McConaghy JR, Smith SR. Outpatient treatment of systolic heart failure. Am Fam Physician 2004;70(11):2157–64.
29. Flather MD, Yusuf S, Køber L, et al. Long-term ACE-inhibitor therapy in patients with heart failure or left-ventricular dysfunction: a systematic overview of data from individual patients. Lancet 2000;355(9215):1575–81.

30. Chavey WE, Bleske BE, Van Harrison R, et al. Pharmacologic management of heart failure caused by systolic dysfunction. Am Fam Physician 2008;77(7): 957–64.

31. Pitt B, Poole-Wilson PA, Segal R, et al. Effect of losartan compared with captopril on mortality in patients with symptomatic heart failure: randomised trial—the Losartan Heart Failure Survival Study ELITE II. Lancet 2000;355(9215):1582–7.

32. Cohn JN, Tognoni G. A randomized trial of the angiotensin-receptor blocker valsartan in chronic heart failure. N Engl J Med 2001;345(23):1667–75. Available at: http://dx.doi.org/10.1056/NEJMoa010713. Accessed October 1, 2011.

33. Granger CB, McMurray JJ, Yusuf S, et al. Effects of candesartan in patients with chronic heart failure and reduced left-ventricular systolic function intolerant to angiotensin-converting-enzyme inhibitors: the CHARM-alternative trial. Lancet 2003;362(9386):772–6.

34. Pitt B, Zannad F, Remme WJ, et al. The effect of spironolactone on morbidity and mortality in patients with severe heart failure. N Engl J Med 1999;341(10): 709–17. Available at: http://dx.doi.org/10.1056/NEJM199909023411001. Accessed October 1, 2011.

35. Zannad F, McMurray JJV, Krum H, et al. Eplerenone in patients with systolic heart failure and mild symptoms. N Engl J Med 2011;364(1):11–21. Available at: http://dx.doi.org/10.1056/NEJMoa1009492. Accessed October 1, 2011.

36. Faris Rajaa F, Flather M, Purcell H, et al. Diuretics for heart failure. Chichester (United Kingdom): John Wiley & Sons, Ltd; 2006 (1).

37. Tsuyuki RT, McKelvie RS, Arnold JM, et al. Acute precipitants of congestive heart failure exacerbations. Arch Intern Med 2001;161(19):2337–42.

38. Wu JR, Moser DK, Lennie TA, et al. Medication adherence in patients who have heart failure: a review of the literature. Nurs Clin North Am 2008;43(1):133–53, vii–viii.

39. Wu J, Moser DK, De Jong MJ, et al. Defining an evidence-based cutpoint for medication adherence in heart failure. Am Heart J 2009;157(2):285–91.

40. Arcand JA, Brazel S, Joliffe C, et al. Education by a dietitian in patients with heart failure results in improved adherence with a sodium-restricted diet: a randomized trial. Am Heart J 2005;150(4):716.e1–5.

41. van der Wal MH, Jaarsma T, van Veldhuisen DJ. Non-compliance in patients with heart failure; how can we manage it? Eur J Heart Fail 2005;7(1):5–17.

42. Appel LJ, Espeland MA, Easter L, et al. Effects of reduced sodium intake on hypertension control in older individuals: results from the Trial of Nonpharmacologic Interventions in the Elderly (TONE). Arch Intern Med 2001;161(5):685–93.

43. Ram CV, Garrett BN, Kaplan NM. Moderate sodium restriction and various diuretics in the treatment of hypertension: effects of potassium wastage and blood pressure control. Arch Intern Med 1981;141(8):1015–9.

44. Hummel SL, DeFranco AC, Skorcz S, et al. Recommendation of low-salt diet and short-term outcomes in heart failure with preserved systolic function. Am J Med 2009;122(11):1029–36.

45. Dolgin M. Nomenclature and criteria for diagnosis of diseases of the heart and great vessels. 9th edition. Boston: Little, Brown; 1994.

46. McKelvie RS, Teo KK, McCartney N, et al. Effects of exercise training in patients with congestive heart failure: a critical review. J Am Coll Cardiol 1995;25(3):789–96.

47. Exercise training meta-analysis of trials in patients with chronic heart failure (ExTraMATCH). BMJ 2004;328(7433):189.

48. O'Connor CM, Whellan DJ, Lee KL, et al. Efficacy and safety of exercise training in patients with chronic heart failure. JAMA 2009;301(14):1439–50.

49. Evangelista LS, Shinnick MA. What do we know about adherence and self-care? J Cardiovasc Nurs 2008;23(3):250–7.
50. Georgiou D, Chen Y, Appadoo S, et al. Cost-effectiveness analysis of long-term moderate exercise training in chronic heart failure. Am J Cardiol 2001;87(8):984–8.
51. Experience from controlled trials of physical training in chronic heart failure. Protocol and patient factors in effectiveness in the improvement in exercise tolerance. European Heart Failure Training Group. Eur Heart J 1998;19(3):466–75.
52. Riegel B, Carlson B, Moser DK, et al. Psychometric testing of the self-care of heart failure index. J Card Fail 2004;10(4):350–60.
53. Jovicic A, Holroyd-Leduc J, Straus S. Effects of self-management intervention on health outcomes of patients with heart failure: a systematic review of randomized controlled trials. BMC Cardiovasc Disord 2006;6(1):43. Available at: http://www.biomedcentral.com/1471-2261/6/43. Accessed October 1, 2011.
54. Sulzbach-Hoke LM, Kagan SH, Craig K. Weighing behavior and symptom distress of clinic patients with CHF. Medsurg Nurs 1997;6(5):288–93, 314.
55. Jaarsma T. Self-care behaviour of patients with heart failure. Scand J Caring Sci 2000;14(2):112.
56. Carlson B, Riegel B, Moser DK. Self-care abilities of patients with heart failure. Heart Lung 2001;30(5):351–9.
57. Riegel B, Carlson B, Glaser D. Development and testing of a clinical tool measuring self-management of heart failure. Heart Lung 2000;29(1):4–15.
58. Clark AM, Savard LA, Thompson DR. What is the strength of evidence for heart failure disease-management programs? J Am Coll Cardiol 2009;54(5):397–401.
59. Riegel B, Moser DK, Anker SD, et al. State of the science. Circulation 2009;120(12):1141–63.
60. Evangelista LS, Dracup K, Doering LV. Treatment-seeking delays in heart failure patients. J Heart Lung Transplant 2000;19(10):932–8.
61. Moser DK, Doering LV, Chung ML. Vulnerabilities of patients recovering from an exacerbation of chronic heart failure. Am Heart J 2005;150(5):984.e7–13.
62. Doak CC, Doak LG, Root JH, editors. Teaching patients with low literacy skills. 2nd edition. Philadelphia: J.B. Lippincott Company; 1996.
63. Durose CL, Holdsworth M, Watson V, et al. Knowledge of dietary restrictions and the medical consequences of noncompliance by patients on hemodialysis are not predictive of dietary compliance. J Am Diet Assoc 2004;104(1):35–41.
64. Brodie DA, Inoue A. Motivational interviewing to promote physical activity for people with chronic heart failure. J Adv Nurs 2005;50(5):518–27.
65. McAlister FA, Stewart S, Ferrua S, et al. Multidisciplinary strategies for the management of heart failure patients at high risk for admission: a systematic review of randomized trials. J Am Coll Cardiol 2004;44(4):810–9.
66. Hershberger RE, Nauman DJ, Byrkit J, et al. Prospective evaluation of an outpatient heart failure disease management program designed for primary care: the Oregon model. J Card Fail 2005;11(4):293–8.
67. Whellan DJ, Gaulden L, Gattis WA, et al. The benefit of implementing a heart failure disease management program. Arch Intern Med 2001;161(18):2223–8.
68. Rich MW, Baldus Gray D, Beckham V, et al. Effect of a multidisciplinary intervention on medication compliance in elderly patients with congestive heart failure. Am J Med 1996;101(3):270–6.
69. Remes J, Miettinen H, Reunanen A, et al. Validity of clinical diagnosis of heart failure in primary health care. Eur Heart J 1991;12(3):315–21.

70. Gehlbach BK, Geppert E. The pulmonary manifestations of left heart failure. Chest 2004;125(2):669–82.

71. Marcus GM, Gerber IL, McKeown BH, et al. Association between phonocardiographic third and fourth heart sounds and objective measures of left ventricular function. JAMA 2005;293(18):2238–44.

72. Littmann L. Large T wave inversion and QT prolongation associated with pulmonary edema: a report of nine cases. J Am Coll Cardiol 1999;34(4):1106–10.

73. Kinnunen P, Vuolteenaho O, Ruskoaho H. Mechanisms of atrial and brain natriuretic peptide release from rat ventricular myocardium: effect of stretching. Endocrinology 1993;132(5):1961–70.

74. Maisel AS, Krishnaswamy P, Nowak RM, et al. Rapid measurement of B-type natriuretic peptide in the emergency diagnosis of heart failure. N Engl J Med 2002;347(3):161–7. Available at: http://dx.doi.org/10.1056/NEJMoa020233. Accessed October 1, 2011.

75. McCullough PA, Nowak RM, McCord J, et al. B-type natriuretic peptide and clinical judgment in emergency diagnosis of heart failure: analysis from Breathing Not Properly (BNP) Multinational Study. Circulation 2002;106(4):416–22.

76. Januzzi JL, van Kimmenade R, Lainchbury J, et al. NT-proBNP testing for diagnosis and short-term prognosis in acute destabilized heart failure: an international pooled analysis of 1256 patients. Eur Heart J 2006;27(3):330–7.

77. Silver M. BNP consensus panel 2004: a clinical approach for the diagnostic, prognostic, screening, treatment monitoring, and therapeutic roles of natriuretic peptides in cardiovascular diseases. Congest Heart Fail 2004;10(Suppl 5):1–30.

78. Jencks SF, Williams MV, Coleman EA. Rehospitalizations among patients in the Medicare fee-for-service program. N Engl J Med 2009;360(14):1418–28. Available at: http://dx.doi.org/10.1056/NEJMsa0803563. Accessed October 1, 2011.

79. Caldwell MA, Howie JN, Dracup K. BNP as discharge criteria for heart failure. J Card Fail 2003;9(5):416–22.

80. Hernandez AF, Greiner MA, Fonarow GC, et al. Relationship between early physician follow-up and 30-day readmission among Medicare beneficiaries hospitalized for heart failure. JAMA 2010;303(17):1716–22.

81. Schappert SM, Rechsteiner EA. Ambulatory medical care utilization estimates for 2007. Vital Health Stat 13 2011;(169):1–38.

82. Lee DS, Stukel TA, Austin PC, et al. Improved outcomes with early collaborative care of ambulatory heart failure patients discharged from the emergency department/clinical perspective. Circulation 2010;122(18):1806–14.

83. Patel JA, Fotis MA. Comparison of treatment of patients with congestive heart failure by cardiologists versus noncardiologists. Am J Health Syst Pharm 2005; 62(2):168–72.

84. Braunstein JB, Anderson GF, Gerstenblith G, et al. Noncardiac comorbidity increases preventable hospitalizations and mortality among Medicare beneficiaries with chronic heart failure. J Am Coll Cardiol 2003;42(7):1226–33.

85. McClellan WM, Flanders WD, Langston RD, et al. Anemia and renal insufficiency are independent risk factors for death among patients with congestive heart failure admitted to community hospitals: a population-based study. J Am Soc Nephrol 2002;13(7):1928–36.

86. Voors AA, van der Horst IC. Diabetes: a driver for heart failure. Heart 2011;97(9): 774–80.

87. Skyler JS, Bergenstal R, Bonow RO, et al. Intensive glycemic control and the prevention of cardiovascular events: implications of the ACCORD, ADVANCE, and VA diabetes trials. Circulation 2009;119(2):351–7.

88. Nesto RW, Bell D, Bonow RO, et al. Thiazolidinedione use, fluid retention, and congestive heart failure. Circulation 2003;108(23):2941–8.
89. Erdmann E, Charbonnel B, Wilcox RG, et al. Pioglitazone use and heart failure in patients with type 2 diabetes and preexisting cardiovascular disease. Diabetes Care 2007;30(11):2773–8.
90. Vaccarino V, Kasl SV, Abramson J, et al. Depressive symptoms and risk of functional decline and death in patients with heart failure. J Am Coll Cardiol 2001; 38(1):199–205.
91. Ziegelstein RC, Fauerbach JA, Stevens SS, et al. Patients with depression are less likely to follow recommendations to reduce cardiac risk during recovery from a myocardial infarction. Arch Intern Med 2000;160(12):1818–23.
92. Curtis JR, Patrick DL, Caldwell ES, et al. Why don't patients and physicians talk about end-of-life care? Barriers to communication for patients with acquired immunodeficiency syndrome and their primary care clinicians. Arch Intern Med 2000;160(11):1690–6.
93. Setoguchi S, Stevenson LW, Schneeweiss S. Repeated hospitalizations predict mortality in the community population with heart failure. Am Heart J 2007; 154(2):260–6.
94. Goldberg LR, Jessup M. A time to be born and a time to die. Circulation 2007; 116(4):360–2.
95. Lee DS, Austin PC, Rouleau JL, et al. Predicting mortality among patients hospitalized for heart failure. JAMA 2003;290(19):2581–7.
96. Levy WC, Mozaffarian D, Linker DT, et al. The Seattle Heart Failure Model. Circulation 2006;113(11):1424–33.
97. Maisel AS, McCord J, Nowak RM, et al. Bedside B-type natriuretic peptide in the emergency diagnosis of heart failure with reduced or preserved ejection fraction: results from the Breathing Not Properly Multinational Study. J Am Coll Cardiol 2003;41(11):2010–7.
98. Januzzi JL Jr, Camargo CA, Anwaruddin S, et al. The N-terminal pro-BNP investigation of dyspnea in the emergency department (PRIDE) study. Am J Cardiol 2005;95(8):948–54.

Strategies to Improve the Management of Depression in Primary Care

Jürgen Unützer, MD, MPH, MA*, Mijung Park, PhD, RN

KEYWORDS

- Depression • Primary care • Collaborative care

KEY POINTS

- Depression can be effectively treated in primary care settings using an evidence-based collaborative approach in which primary care providers are systematically supported by mental health providers in caring for a caseload of patients.
- Core components of effective collaborative care programs include a focus on populations of patients identified with depression, measurement-based care, treatment to target, and stepped care in which treatments are systematically adjusted and "stepped up" if patients are not improving as expected. Such an approach can dramatically improve patient satisfaction and health outcomes.
- These principles of collaborative care are highly consistent with the notion of patient-centered medical homes and accountable care and can help effectively position primary care practices for health care reform and coming changes in health care delivery and financing.

INTRODUCTION

Depression is one of the most common and disabling chronic health problems encountered in the primary care setting. In this article, opportunities and strategies to improve care for depression in primary care practice are reviewed and collaborative care, an evidence-based approach to chronic disease management for depression is introduced. In this approach, primary care providers (PCPs) and care managers look after a caseload of depressed patients with systematic support from mental health experts. Lessons from implementing evidence-based collaborative care programs in diverse primary care practice settings are summarized to convey relatively simple changes that can improve patient outcomes in primary care practices.

Financial disclosure: Authors have nothing to disclose.

Department of Psychiatry and Behavioral Sciences, University of Washington, 1959 NE Pacific Street 356560, Seattle, WA 98195-6560, USA

* Corresponding author.

E-mail address: unutzer@uw.edu

Prim Care Clin Office Pract 39 (2012) 415–431

doi:10.1016/j.pop.2012.03.010

primarycare.theclinics.com

THE CLINICAL EPIDEMIOLOGY OF DEPRESSION IN PRIMARY CARE

Behavioral health problems, such as depression, anxiety, and alcohol or substance abuse, are among the most common and disabling health conditions worldwide[1] and are common in primary care settings.[2–9] Depending on the clinical setting, between 5% and 20% of adult patients,[10,11] including adolescents[12–14] and older adults,[15] seen in primary care have clinically significant depressive symptoms. Depression is one of the most common conditions treated in primary care and nearly 10% of all primary care office visits are depression related.[16] From 1997 to 2002, the proportion of depression visits that took place in primary care increased from 51% to 64%.[17] For many patients, depression is a chronic or recurrent illness.[18] For example, up to 40% of depressed older adults meet criteria for chronic depression.[19] Depressed patients with chronic medical illnesses are at greater risk for a chronic course of depression or less complete recovery.[20]

National surveys have consistently demonstrated that more Americans receive mental health care from PCPs than from mental health specialists,[9,21] and primary care has been identified as the "de facto mental health services system"[2,9] for adults, children, and older adults with common mental disorders.[22,23] Most patients would prefer an integrated approach in which primary care and mental health providers work together to address medical and behavioral health needs.[24] In reality, however, we have a fragmented system in which medical, mental health, substance abuse, and social services are delivered in geographically and organizationally separate "silos" with little to no effective collaboration. A recent national survey[25] concluded that two-thirds of PCPs reported that they could not get effective mental health services for their patients. Barriers to mental health care access included shortage of mental health care providers and lack of insurance coverage.

INTERACTION OF DEPRESSION WITH OTHER CHRONIC ILLNESSES

Successful management of depression in primary care settings is particularly important considering complex interactions between mental and physical health.[26] Major depression is associated with high numbers of medically unexplained symptoms,[27–29] such as pain and fatigue, and poor general health outcomes.[1,30] Untreated depression is independently associated with morbidity,[30–33] delayed recovery, and negative prognosis among those with medical illness; elevated premature mortality associated with comorbid medical illness[34]; and increased health care costs.[35–37] Depression also increases functional impairment[38–43] and decreases work productivity.[44] Depression significantly decreases quality of life for patients and their family members.[45,46] In a study of 2558 elderly primary care patients, participants with depression had greater losses in quality adjusted life years (QALYs) than those with emphysema, cancer, chronic foot problems, or hypertension.[46] Depression can also be a barrier to positive and productive relationships between patients and providers.[47,48] PCPs tend to rate patients with depression as more difficult to evaluate and treat compared with those without depression,[47] and depressed patients have been shown to be less satisfied with their PCPs.[48]

Screening/Diagnosing Depression

Depression in primary care is underdetected, underdiagnosed, and undertreated. Older adults, men, patients with medical comorbidities, and patients from ethnic minority groups are at particularly high risk of not being recognized as depressed or treated effectively.[49–52] The US Preventive Services Task Force issued recommendations, encouraging primary care physicians to routinely screen their adult patients for depression in clinical settings that have systems in place to ensure effective treatment and follow-up.[53]

Brief screening tools for depression are available. A simple question "Do you often feel sad or depressed?" to which the patient is required to answer either "yes" or "no" was tested in a sample of medically ill patients in the community and had a sensitivity of 69% and a specificity of 90%.[54] The Patient Health Questionaire-2 (PHQ-2) consists of 2 questions about depressed mood: (1) "During the past weeks have you often been bothered by feeling down, depressed, or hopeless?" and (2) "During the past month have you often been bothered by little interest or pleasure in doing things?"[55] Such brief screening tools can be easily administered by office staff or physicians during a primary care visit. Positive response to these questionnaires should alert the PCP to further evaluate the patient for depression. Not all depressed patients will answer positively to these questionnaires. To address the possible "false-negatives," clinicians may wish to ask additional questions about depressive symptoms for patients who appear depressed, who have a difficulty engaging in care, or whose functional impairment seems inconsistent with objective medical illness.

TREATMENT OF DEPRESSION

More than 25 medications have been approved by the Food and Drug Administration for the treatment of major depression, and there is strong and increasing evidence about the effectiveness of psychotherapies that can be delivered in primary care or specialty mental health care settings.[56–58] A number of guidelines have been developed to guide the effective management of depression in primary care[59] and in specialty mental health settings.[60] These guidelines succinctly summarize the evidence base for pharmacologic and nonpharmacological treatment options. If nonpharmacologic treatments are available, PCPs should ask patients who are initiating depression treatment about preferences for medications or psychotherapy because the ability to address a patient's treatment preference has been shown to be related to the likelihood of entering depression treatment[61] and better treatment outcomes.[62] Patients' clinical outcomes should be tracked with structured depression rating scales, such as the 9-item Patient Health Questionnaire (PHQ-9), similar to the way PCPs follow clinical outcomes of other treatments, such as blood pressure or blood lipids. Treatments should be systematically adjusted for patients who do not improve with initial treatments using evidence-based medication treatments and/or psychotherapies. The flowchart in **Fig. 1** summarizes a comprehensive guideline for the treatment of major depression in primary care developed by the Institute of Clinical Systems Improvement (ICSI).[59]

Effective management of depression in primary care requires a number of steps: detection and diagnosis, patient education and engagement in treatment, initiation of evidence-based pharmacotherapy or psychotherapy, close follow-up focusing on treatment adherence, treatment effectiveness, and treatment side effects. Consistent follow-up is crucial, as treatment adherence is a major problem in primary care. Response to specific depression treatments varies among individuals and data from large treatment trials in primary care and specialty care settings point out that initial treatments are effective in about 30% to 50% of patients regardless of the choice of initial pharmacotherapy or psychotherapy.[61,63–65]

There is little information to guide initial selection of treatments except for treatment history in patients and family members. Clinicians should follow existing guidelines and take into account patients' treatment preferences when selecting initial treatments. Perhaps most importantly, they should be prepared to adjust and intensify

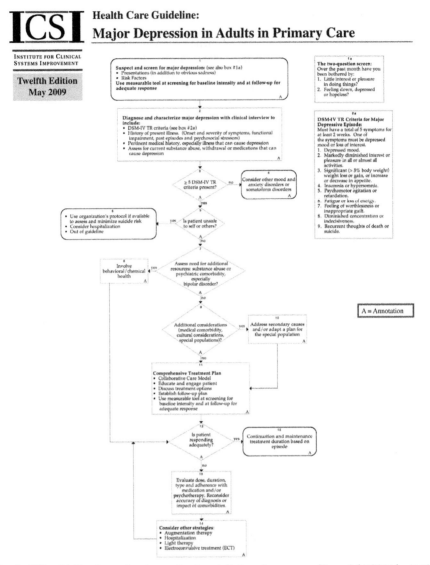

Fig. 1. ICSI guideline for major depression in adults in primary care. (Copyright 2011 by Institute for Clinical Systems Improvement. Used with permission. Available at: www.icsi.org.)

treatment for the 50% to 70% of patients who will not improve with initial treatment.[66] Data from the Sequenced Treatment Alternatives to Relieve Depression trial indicates that most patients who failed an initial trial of an antidepressant medication improved with sequential adjustments in dosage, agent, or both in treatment.[67] Patients with particularly challenging cases of depression (ie, those who do not respond to several treatment adjustments, patients with comorbid psychiatric problems, such as psychosis, or patients considered to be at high risk for self-harm) should be considered for a psychiatric consultation or referral to specialty mental health care for additional treatments, such as inpatient treatment and electroconvulsive therapy.

QUALITY OF CARE FOR DEPRESSION

There is a large gap between the efficacy of treatments for depression under research conditions and the effectiveness of treatments as they occur in "real-world" primary care settings.[68] Although a number of effective pharmacologic and nonpharmacological treatments exist for depression, studies in the United States and Canada have consistently demonstrated that few patients receive adequate dosages or courses of such treatments.[49,69–71] Almost 30 million Americans receive prescriptions for antidepressants each year, which are most often prescribed by PCPs. Unfortunately, many patients stop medication early because of side effects or other concerns and do not follow-up with their PCP to change treatments. Few patients have access to or use evidence-based psychotherapies in primary care settings. Others continue on ineffective dosages and medications because of clinical inertia[72] and a lack of appropriate treatment intensification in patients who are not improving with initial treatments. As a result, as few as 20% to 40% of patients started on depression treatment in primary care show substantial clinical improvements.[73,74] Similar problems have been identified for patients treated in specialty mental health care settings,[75] but patients treated in specialty settings often have greater severity of illness and receive treatment that is more consistent with existing guidelines. Patients referred to psychotherapy often receive inadequate trials of such treatments and treatment response rates can be as low as 20%.[76] Barriers include limited availability of evidence-psychotherapy and costs.

Time constraints and conflicting demands in "real-world" primary care settings are a major challenge for effectively treating depression in primary care settings.[77] Generalist physicians also have limited training in the diagnosis and treatment of depression and other mental illnesses. Patients may feel reluctance to discuss their emotional distress, family problems, or behavioral problems with PCPs because of the stigma associated with mental disorders and concerns that the PCP might not take their other health problems seriously.

STRATEGIES TO IMPROVE THE MANAGEMENT OF DEPRESSION IN PRIMARY CARE

Efforts to improve the management of depression and other common mental disorders in primary care have focused on screening, education of PCPs, development of treatment guidelines, and referral to mental health specialty care. Although well intended, these efforts have by and large not been effective in reducing the substantial burden of depression and other common mental disorders in primary care.[78] Another approach to improve care for patients with depression is to colocate mental health specialists into primary care clinics. Having a mental health professional, such as a psychologist, a clinical social worker, or a psychiatrist, available to see patients in primary care can improve access to mental health services but there is little evidence that such colocation of a behavioral health provider in primary care by itself is sufficient to improve patient outcomes for large populations of primary care patients.[79]

Collaborative Care and Stepped Care

Over the past 15 years, more than 40 randomized controlled trials have established a robust evidence base for an approach called "collaborative care for depression."[80–82] More recent studies have documented the effectiveness of such collaborative approaches for anxiety disorders[83] and for depression and comorbid medical disorders, such as diabetes and heart disease.[84] In such programs, PCPs are part of a collaborative care team that includes a depression care manager (usually a nurse or clinical social worker and in some cases a trained medical assistant under supervision from a mental health provider) and a designated psychiatric consultant to augment the management of depression in the primary care setting. The depression care manager supports medication management prescribed by PCPs through patient education, close and proactive follow-up, and brief, evidence-based psychosocial treatments, such as behavioral activation or problem-solving treatment in primary care. The care manager may also facilitate referrals to additional services as needed. A designated psychiatric consultant regularly (usually weekly) reviews all patients in the care manager's caseload who are not improving as expected and provides focused treatment recommendations to the patient's PCP. The psychiatric consultant is also available to the care manager and the PCP for questions about patients. **Table 1**[80,85–87] summarizes key roles and tasks of the 2 new team members: the depression care manager and the psychiatric consultant.

Effective collaborative care adhere to the principle of stepped care in which treatment is systematically changed, intensified, or "stepped up" if patients are not improving as expected (eg, 8–10 weeks after the initiation of evidence-based pharmacotherapy).[88] Stepped care approaches can enhance the cost-effectiveness of depression care by focusing the use of limited resources, such as care management and specialist consultation, on those patients who cannot be effectively managed by the PCP alone. Patients initiating care are educated on this systematic approach to treatment and provided tools, such as the PHQ-9,[89,90] that help them track symptoms of depression over time. They are also encouraged and empowered to request changes in treatment if treatments are not effective or cause significant side effects. Patients who continue to have depressive symptoms after initial treatment trials with medication or psychotherapy are systematically reviewed with a psychiatric consultant and considered for additional treatments as summarized in **Table 2**.

Because of the high risk of depression relapse,[91] patients who have responded to treatment receive relapse-prevention plans that help them maintain treatment gains made. Such relapse-prevention plans include advice on the continuation of maintenance medications as clinically indicated, personal warning signs if depression should

Table 1
Key processes and roles for collaborative care team members

Process	Role	
	Depression Care Manager	Psychiatric Consultant
1. Systematic diagnosis and tracking of patient outcomes	Patient engagement, education/self-management support Close follow-up to make sure patients don't "fall through the cracks"	Systematic caseload review Diagnostic consultation on difficult cases
2. Stepped Care a. Change treatment according to evidence-based algorithm if patient is not improving b. Relapse prevention once patient is improved	Support medication management by primary care provider (PCP) Brief counseling (eg, behavioral activation or problem-solving treatment in primary care) Facilitate treatment change/referral to mental health as needed Relapse prevention planning	Consultation focused on patients not improving as expected Recommendations to PCP for additional treatment or referral to specialty care

From Advancing Integrated Mental Health Solutions (AIMS) Center; with permission. Available at: http://uwaims.org/.

Table 2
Stepped-care activities for depression in evidence-based collaborative care programs

Stepped Care Activity	Depression	Local Considerations
Patient identification/ screening	Provider referral or screening with PHQ-2/PHQ-9.	• Who provides key treatment components: primary care provider, mental health staff in primary care, care manager, other?
Patient education and engagement	Patient education. Shared goal setting. Screening for bipolar disorder and substance use.	
Close follow-up and behavioral activation	Close telephone or in-person follow-up. Support of medical management. Behavioral activation strategies used at each contact.	• Where are treatments provided? (eg, what can happen in primary care clinic vs in referral center) • How do team members communicate & collaborate effectively? • Who is responsible for tracking patient and program outcomes?
Medication management prescribed by primary care provider with guidance from psychiatric consultant	Antidepressant medications. Anxiolytics and hypnotics as clinically indicated.	• How is psychiatric caseload consultation provided? • What kind of training and ongoing clinical support is needed for the program to succeed?
Evidence-based psychotherapy.	Problem-Solving Treatment in Primary Care (PST-PC) or other evidence-based psychotherapy (eg, cognitive behavioral therapy or interpersonal therapy).	
Community-based resources	Local community-based resources and support services	
Specialty mental health / substance abuse referral and treatment	Mental health specialty care for severe or persistent depression or comorbidities (eg, suicidal, dual diagnosis, psychotic).	

From Advancing Integrated Mental Health Solutions (AIMS) Center; with permission. Available at: http://uwaims.org/.

recur, strategies to maintain clinical gains made (eg, continued systematic scheduling of pleasant events), and advice on what to do if depression symptoms should recur. Relapse prevention may be particularly important in patients with comorbid medical conditions who are at higher risk for relapse than those with depression only.[20]

RESEARCH EVIDENCE FOR COLLABORATIVE CARE

Studies of collaborative care programs have been conducted in small and large primary care practices, in diverse health care settings under fee-for-service or capitated payment arrangements, with different patient populations, including both insured and uninsured/safety-net populations, and with different mental health conditions, including depression[80,82] and anxiety disorders.[92] The literature has consistently demonstrated that collaborative management of depression in primary care is more effective than usual primary care.[80,93]

In the largest trial of collaborative care to date, the study entitled "Improving Mood—Promoting Access to Collaborative Treatment for Late-Life Depression" (IMPACT), 1801 primary care patients with depression and an average of 3.5 chronic medical disorders from 18 primary care clinics in 5 states were randomly assigned to a collaborative stepped care program or to care as usual. IMPACT participants were more than twice as likely as those in usual care to experience a substantial improvement (a 50% or greater improvement in the depression severity score of the Hopkins Symptom Checklist over 12 months).[73] They also had less physical pain, better social and physical functioning, and better overall quality of life than patients in care as usual.[94] Patients and providers participating in collaborative care were more satisfied than those in the usual care group.[95] More recent studies have demonstrated the effectiveness of the IMPACT program in depressed adolescents,[96] depressed patients with cancer,[97,98] and patients with diabetes,[99,100] including low-income Spanish-speaking patients.[101]

Long-term cost-effectiveness analyses from the IMPACT study found that patients who received collaborative care for depression had substantially lower overall health care costs than those in usual care.[102] An initial "investment" in 12 months of collaborative care of approximately $522 resulted in savings in total health care costs of $3363. Similar cost savings have been identified in other collaborative care trials in patients with depression and diabetes[100] and other chronic medical conditions, and in patients with severe anxiety (panic disorder).[103] Large-scale implementations outside of research trials in several large health care systems, such as Kaiser Permanente[104] and Intermountain Healthcare,[105] also point to savings in overall health care costs when collaborative care is effectively implemented. Collaborative care interventions also generate important social benefits in terms of QALYs.[106] Finally, and perhaps most importantly, collaborative care has been shown to improve both patient[73] and provider[95] satisfaction with care.

Collaborative care programs, such as the approach tested in IMPACT, have been recommended as an evidence-based practice by the Substance Abuse and Mental Health Services Administration and recommended as a "best practice" by the Surgeon General's Report on Mental Health,[107] the President's New Freedom Commission on Mental Health,[108] and a number of national organizations, including the National Business Group on Health.[109] In a recent evidence-based practice report by the Agency for Healthcare Research and Quality that reviewed the existing literature on approaches to integration of mental health/substance abuse and primary care, the IMPACT program was profiled as one of the most successful models of integrated mental health care to date.[110]

LARGE-SCALE IMPLEMENTATIONS OF COLLABORATIVE CARE

Although there are some variations in the components of collaborative care programs, most effective programs build on several core clinical principles and components. These include the core components of chronic illness care as proposed by Wagner and colleagues[111]: (1) the use of explicit treatment plans and protocols; (2) the reorganization of the practice to meet the needs of patients who require more time, a broad array of resources, and closer follow-up; (3) systematic attention to the information and behavioral change needs of patients; (4) ready access to necessary expertise; and (5) supportive information systems and strategies, such as "measurement-based care,"[112] "treatment to target," and "stepped care."[88] Systematic measurement of clinical outcomes using brief, patient-rating scales, such as the PHQ-9 for depression,[89] helps clinicians keep track if patients are improving as expected or if treatment needs to be adjusted. On the PHQ-9, a drop in 5 points has been identified as a clinically meaningful reduction in symptoms, but the ultimate treatment target is remission, which is captured by a PHQ-9 score of less than 5.[89] Psychiatric consultation, a limited resource in most settings, can then be focused on patients who are not improving as expected. Such systematic "treatment to target" can overcome the "clinical inertia"[72] that is often responsible for ineffective treatments of common mental disorders in primary care.

Several health care organizations have undertaken large-scale implementations of evidence-based collaborative care programs for depression. These include national health plans, such as Kaiser Permanente, and the Depression Improvement Across Minnesota, Offering a New Direction (DIAMOND) program in Minnesota in which the ICSI has worked with 8 commercial health plans, 25 medical groups, and more than 80 primary care clinics to implement collaborative care for depression.[113,114] In Washington State, the Mental Health Integration Program, sponsored by the Community Health Plan of Washington and Seattle King County Public Health,[115] includes more than 100 community health centers and more than 30 community mental health centers that work together to provide integrated care for poor, underserved, uninsured, or underinsured clients with medical and behavioral health needs. Other large-scale implementations include the Army's Re-Engineering Systems of Primary Care Treatment in the Military (RESPECT-MIL) program,[116] implemented in Army primary care clinics in the United States and abroad; and the Department of Veterans Affairs' Veterans Health Administration,[117] which has implemented collaborative care in hundreds of primary care clinics across the United States.

IMPLEMENTING EFFECTIVE COLLABORATIVE CARE PROGRAMS

Over the past 10 years, the Advancing Integrated Mental Health Solutions (AIMS) Center at the University of Washington[94] has provided technical assistance and training to more than 5000 clinicians in more than 600 primary care practices to implement effective collaborative care. Some key lessons from the implementation of such programs in diverse practice settings are as follows.

- Fragmented financing streams are an important barrier to integrating mental health and primary care services,[118] but financial integration does not guarantee clinical integration and practices have to develop effective clinical workflows where PCPs and supporting mental health providers communicate and collaborate effectively.
- Simply colocating a mental health provider into a primary care setting may improve access to behavioral health care but it does not guarantee improved health outcomes for the large population of primary care patients with mental health needs.
- Effective treatment requires a move from episodic acute care in which we provide the equivalent of "behavioral health urgent care" to patients presenting for care to a population-based approach in which all patients with behavioral health needs are systematically tracked until the problem is resolved. A "registry" or clinical tracking system is required to identify patients who are "falling through the cracks" and to support effective stepped care. This can be accomplished using the registry functions of electronic health record systems or a freestanding registry tool.[119]
- Initial treatments (be they pharmacologic or psychosocial) are rarely sufficient to achieve desired health outcomes. Systematic outcome tracking, treatment adjustment, and consultation for patients who are not improving can help achieve the desired health outcomes. This requires systematic caseload review by the

treating providers and psychiatric consultation, focusing on patients who are not improving as expected.

- Effective collaboration in primary care requires flexibility in both mental health specialists and PCPs. Mental health providers should maintain regular and effective communication with patients' PCP be open to interruption during therapy sessions, use the telephone to reach patients who cannot make clinic appointments. Several brief, evidence-based therapies can be provided in the context of a busy primary care practices, such as motivational interviewing, behaivoral activation, problem solving, or brief cognitive behavioral therapy.
- Training mental health specialists and primary care providers in integrated care is important but not sufficient. Effective implementation of depression treatment in primary care setting requires ongoing support from clinical champions in primary care and behavioral health, financial support, operational support, and a clear set of shared and measureable goals and objectives. As with all efforts to improve chronic illness care, such support may be easier to obtain in large delivery systems and under managed care arrangements than in small fee-for-service medical practices.
- There are many ways to implement effective integrated care for behavioral health problems in primary care. Treatment manuals used in research studies have been "translated" into job descriptions and clear operational manuals that help busy practices implement the program in their unique settings.
- Attention to core principles, such as measurement-based care and careful tracking of desired outcomes at the patient and clinic levels, can help make sure that integrated care programs "live up to their promise," as they are implemented in diverse real-world settings.

Although the full-scale implementation of evidence-based collaborative care programs may be challenging for small to moderate-sized primary care practices under current fee-for-service health care financing mechanisms,[118] relatively "simple" changes can help practices improve care and gain important experience on the way to becoming a fully integrated patient-centered health care home. Such changes include the following:

- Routine use of brief, structured rating scales for common mental disorders, such as the PHQ-9 for depression, to help with screening but more importantly to determine if patients started on treatment are improving as expected.
- Incorporation of such behavioral health rating scales into paper or electronic health records, creating a "registry" function that allows PCPs and clinic managers to identify patients who are "falling through the cracks" or not improving as expected.
- Stepped care and "treatment to target," in which treatments (medications, psychosocial treatments, or referrals to mental health) are actively changed and adjusted until the desired health outcomes are achieved.
- Incorporation of evidence-based motivational interviewing strategies into patient encounters to help patients engage in and adhere to effective treatment for behavioral health problems. Both physicians and other office staff can be trained in these techniques.
- Training office-based personnel to help perform core support functions of behavioral health care managers, such as proactive outreach and tracking of treatment adherence, medication side effects, referrals (if appropriate), and treatment effectiveness.
- Development of relationships and "shared workflows" with behavioral health providers that are not simply referrals but include active dialogue and

collaboration between the PCP and the behavioral health provider to ensure patients achieve the desired clinical outcomes.

These strategies are highly compatible with approaches to improve patient care and outcomes through patient-centered medical homes.

SUMMARY

Depression can be effectively treated in primary care settings using an evidence-based collaborative approach in which PCPs are systematically supported by mental health providers in caring for a caseload of patients. Core components of effective collaborative care programs include a focus on populations of patients identified with depression, measurement-based care, treatment to target, and stepped care in which treatments are systematically adjusted and "stepped up" if patients are not improving as expected. Such an approach can dramatically improve patient satisfaction and health outcomes. These principles of collaborative care are highly consistent with the notion of patient-centered medical homes and accountable care and can help effectively position primary care practices for health care reform and coming changes in health care delivery and financing.

REFERENCES

1. Moussavi S, Chatterji S, Verdes E, et al. Depression, chronic diseases, and decrements in health: results from the World Health Surveys. Lancet 2007; 370(9590):851–8.
2. Regier DA, Goldberg ID, Taube CA. The de facto US mental health services system: a public health perspective. Arch Gen Psychiatry 1978;35(6):685–93.
3. Barrett JE, Barrett JA, Oxman TE, et al. The prevalence of psychiatric disorders in a primary care practice. Arch Gen Psychiatry 1988;45(12):1100–6.
4. Ansseau M, Dierick M, Buntinkx F, et al. High prevalence of mental disorders in primary care. J Affect Disord 2004;78(1):49–55.
5. Leon AC, Olfson M, Broadhead WE, et al. Prevalence of mental disorders in primary care: implications for screening. Arch Fam Med 1995;4(10):857–61.
6. Kroenke K, Spitzer RL, Williams JB, et al. Anxiety disorders in primary care: prevalence, impairment, comorbidity, and detection. Ann Intern Med 2007;146(5): 317–25.
7. Sherbourne CD, Jackson CA, Meredith LS, et al. Prevalence of comorbid anxiety disorders in primary care outpatients. Arch Fam Med 1996;5(1):27–34 [discussion: 35].
8. Brienza RS, Stein MD. Alcohol use disorders in primary care. J Gen Intern Med 2002;17(5):387–97.
9. Regier DA, Narrow WE, Rae DS, et al. The de Facto US mental and addictive disorders service system: epidemiologic catchment area prospective 1-year prevalence rates of disorders and services. Arch Gen Psychiatry 1993;50(2): 85–94.
10. Katon W, Schulberg H. Epidemiology of depression in primary care. Gen Hosp Psychiatry 1992;14(4):237–47.
11. Zung W, Broadhead W, Roth M. Prevalence of depressive symptoms in primary care. J Fam Pract 1993;37(4):337–44.
12. Schubiner H, Tzelepis A, Wright K, et al. The clinical utility of the safe times questionnaire. J Adolesc Health 1994;15(5):374–82.

13. Winter LB, Steer RA, Jones-Hicks L, et al. Screening for major depression disorders in adolescent medical outpatients with the Beck Depression Inventory for primary care. J Adolesc Health 1999;24(6):389–94.

14. Johnson JG, Harris ES, Spitzer RL, et al. The patient health questionnaire for adolescents: validation of an instrument for the assessment of mental disorders among adolescent primary care patients. J Adolesc Health 2002;30(3):196–204.

15. Lyness JM, Caine ED, King DA, et al. Psychiatric disorders in older primary care patients. J Gen Intern Med 1999;14(4):249–54.

16. Stafford RS, Ausiello JC, Misra B, et al. National patterns of depression treatment in primary care. Primary Care Companion J Clin Psychiatry 2000;2:211–6.

17. Harman JS, Veazie PJ, Lyness JM. Primary care physician office visits for depression by older Americans. J Gen Intern Med 2006;21(9):926–30.

18. Klein DN, Shankman SA, Rose S. Ten-year prospective follow-up study of the naturalistic course of dysthymic disorder and double depression. Am J Psychiatry 2006;163(5):872–80.

19. Alexopoulos G, Chester JG. Outcomes on geriatric depression, vol. 8. New York: Elsevier; 1992.

20. Iosifescu DV, Nierenberg AA, Alpert JE, et al. Comorbid medical illness and relapse of major depressive disorder in the continuation phase of treatment. Psychosomatics 2004;45(5):419–25.

21. Wang PS, Demler O, Olfson M, et al. Changing profiles of service sectors used for mental health care in the United States. Am J Psychiatry 2006;163(7):1187–98.

22. Burns BJ, Costello EJ, Angold A, et al. Children's mental health service use across service sectors. Health Aff 1995;14(3):147–59.

23. Kessler RC, Birnbaum H, Bromet E, et al. Age differences in major depression: results from the National Comorbidity Survey Replication (NCS-R). Psychol Med 2010;40(02):225–37.

24. Mauksch LB, Tucker SM, Katon WJ, et al. Mental illness, functional impairment, and patient preferences for collaborative care in an uninsured, primary care population. J Fam Pract 2001;50(1):41–7.

25. Cunningham PJ. Beyond parity: primary care physicians' perspectives on access to mental health care. Health Aff 2009;28(3):w490–501.

26. Katon WJ. Clinical and health services relationships between major depression, depressive symptoms, and general medical illness. Biol Psychiatry 2003;54(3):216–26.

27. Simon GE, VonKorff M. Somatization and psychiatric disorder in the NIMH epidemiologic catchment area study. Am J Psychiatry 1991;148(11):1494–500.

28. Henningsen P, Zimmermann T, Sattel H. Medically unexplained physical symptoms, anxiety, and depression: a meta-analytic review. Psychosom Med 2003;65(4):528–33.

29. Gureje O, Von Korff M, Simon GE, et al. Persistent pain and well-being. JAMA 1998;280(2):147–51.

30. Van der Kooy K, van Hout H, Marwijk H, et al. Depression and the risk for cardiovascular diseases: systematic review and meta analysis. Int J Geriatr Psychiatry 2007;22(7):613–26.

31. Knol M, Twisk J, Beekman A, et al. Depression as a risk factor for the onset of type 2 diabetes mellitus. A meta-analysis. Diabetologia 2006;49(5):837–45.

32. Mezuk B, Eaton WW, Golden SH. Depression and type 2 diabetes over the lifespan: a meta-analysis. Diabetes Care 2009;32(5):e57.

33. Bonnewyn A, Katona C, Bruffaerts R, et al. Pain and depression in older people: comorbidity and patterns of help seeking. J Affect Disord 2009;117(3):193–6.

34. Cuijpers P, Smit F. Excess mortality in depression: a meta-analysis of community studies. J Affect Disord 2002;72(3):227–36.
35. Katon WJ, Lin E, Russo J, et al. Increased medical costs of a population-based sample of depressed elderly patients. Arch Gen Psychiatry 2003;60(9):897–903.
36. Simon G, Ormel J, VonKorff M, et al. Health care costs associated with depressive and anxiety disorders in primary care. Am J Psychiatry 1995; 152(3):352–7.
37. Unützer J, Patrick DL, Simon G, et al. Depressive symptoms and the cost of health services in HMO patients aged 65 years and older. A 4-year prospective study. JAMA 1997;277(20):1618–23.
38. Wells K, Stewart A, Hayes R, et al. The functioning and well-being of depressed patients. Results from the medical outcomes study. JAMA 1989;262:914–9.
39. Alexopoulos GS, Buckwalter K, Olin J, et al. Comorbidity of late life depression: an opportunity for research on mechanisms and treatment. Biol Psychiatry 2002; 52(6):543–58.
40. Kessler RC, Ormel J, Demler O, et al. Comorbid mental disorders account for the role impairment of commonly occurring chronic physical disorders: results from the national comorbidity survey. J Occup Environ Med 2003;45(12):1257–66.
41. Barry LC, Allore HG, Bruce ML, et al. Longitudinal association between depressive symptoms and disability burden among older persons. J Gerontol A Biol Sci Med Sci 2009;64(12):1325–32.
42. Ciechanowski PS, Katon WJ, Russo JE. Depression and diabetes: impact of depressive symptoms on adherence, function, and costs. Arch Intern Med 2000;160(21):3278–85.
43. Lin EH, Katon W, Von Korff M, et al. Relationship of depression and diabetes self-care, medication adherence, and preventive care. Diabetes Care 2004; 27(9):2154–60.
44. Greenberg PE, Kessler RC, Birnbaum HG, et al. The economic burden of depression in the United States: how did it change between 1990 and 2000? J Clin Psychiatry 2003;64(12):1465–75.
45. Sewitch MJ, McCusker J, Dendukuri N, et al. Depression in frail elders: impact on family caregivers. Int J Geriatr Psychiatry 2004;19(7):655–65.
46. Unützer J, Patrick DL, Diehr P, et al. Quality adjusted life years in older adults with depressive symptoms and chronic medical disorders. Int Psychogeriatr 2000;12(01):15–33.
47. Hahn S, Kroenke K, Spitzer R, et al. The difficult patient. J Gen Intern Med 1996; 11(1):1–8.
48. Callahan E, Bertakis K, Azari R, et al. The influence of depression on physician-patient interaction in primary care. Fam Med 1996;28(5):346–51.
49. Ettner SL, Azocar F, Branstrom RB, et al. Association of general medical and psychiatric comorbidities with receipt of guideline-concordant care for depression. Psychiatr Serv 2010;61(12):1255–9.
50. Gonzalez HM, Vega WA, Williams DR, et al. Depression care in the United States: too little for too few. Arch Gen Psychiatry 2010;67(1):37–46.
51. Unützer J, Katon W, Callahan CM, et al. Depression treatment in a sample of 1,801 depressed older adults in primary care. J Am Geriatr Soc 2003;51(4):505–14.
52. Mojtabai R, Olfson M. Proportion of antidepressants prescribed without a psychiatric diagnosis is growing. Health Aff 2011;30(8):1434–42.
53. Screening for depression: recommendations and rationale. U.S. Preventive Services Task Force; 2002. Available at: http://www.uspreventiveservicestaskforce.org/3rduspstf/depression/depressrr.htm. Accessed October 30, 2011.

54. Watkins CL, Lightbody CE, Sutton CJ, et al. Evaluation of a single-item screening tool for depression after stroke: a cohort study. Clin Rehabil 2007; 21(9):846–52.

55. Kroenke K, Spitzer RL, Williams JB. The Patient Health Questionnaire-2: validity of a two-item depression screener. Med Care 2003;41(11):1284–92.

56. Mynors-Wallis L, Gath D, Day A, et al. Randomised controlled trail of problem solving treatment, antidepressant medication, and combined treatment for major depression in primary care. BMJ 2000;320:26–30.

57. Kuyken W, Byford S, Taylor RS, et al. Mindfulness-based cognitive therapy to prevent relapse in recurrent depression. J Consult Clin Psychol 2008;76(6): 966–78.

58. Cuijpers P, van Straten A, Warmerdam L. Behavioral activation treatments of depression: a meta-analysis. Clin Psychol Rev 2007;27(3):318–26.

59. Health care guideline: major depression in adults in primary care. Bloomington (MN): Institute for Clinical Systems Improvement (ICSI); 2009.

60. APA working group on major depressive disorder. Practice guideline for the treatment of patients with major depressive disorder. Arlington (VA): American Psychiatric Association; 2010.

61. Dwight-Johnson M, Unutzer J, Sherbourne C, et al. Can quality improvement programs for depression in primary care address patient preferences for treatment? Med Care 2001;39(9):934–44.

62. Lin P, Campbell D, Chaney E, et al. The influence of patient preference on depression treatment in primary care. Ann Behav Med 2005;30(2):164–73.

63. Trivedi M, Rush A, Wisniewski S, et al. Evaluation of outcomes with citalopram for depression using measurement-based care in STAR*D: implications for clinical practice. Am J Psychiatry 2006;163(1):28–48.

64. Hansen NB, Lambert MJ, Forman EM. The psychotherapy dose-response effect and its implications for treatment delivery services. Clin Psychol Sci Pract 2002; 9(3):329–43.

65. Thase M, Haight B, Richard N, et al. Remission rates following antidepressant therapy with bupropion or selective serotonin reuptake inhibitors: a meta-analysis of original data from 7 randomized controlled trials. J Clin Psychiatry 2005;66(8):974–81.

66. Simon GE, Perlis RH. Personalized medicine for depression: can we match patients with treatments? Am J Psychiatry 2010;167(12):1445–55.

67. Rush AJ, Trivedi MH, Wisniewski SR, et al. Acute and longer-term outcomes in depressed outpatients requiring one or several treatment steps: a STAR*D report. Am J Psychiatry 2006;163(11):1905–17.

68. Unutzer J, Katon W, Sullivan M, et al. Treating depressed older adults in primary care: narrowing the gap between efficacy and effectiveness. Milbank Q 1999; 77(2):225–56, 174.

69. Young AS, Klap R, Sherbourne CD, et al. The quality of care for depressive and anxiety disorders in the United States. Arch Gen Psychiatry 2001;58(1): 55–61.

70. Duhoux A, Fournier L, Nguyen CT, et al. Guideline concordance of treatment for depressive disorders in Canada. Soc Psychiatry Psychiatr Epidemiol 2009; 44(5):385–92.

71. Wells KB, Schoenbaum M, Unutzer J, et al. Quality of care for primary care patients with depression in managed care. Arch Fam Med 1999;8(6):529–36.

72. Henke RM, Zaslavsky AM, McGuire TG, et al. Clinical inertia in depression treatment. Med Care 2009;47(9):959–67, 910.

73. Unutzer J, Katon W, Callahan CM, et al. Collaborative care management of late-life depression in the primary care setting: a randomized controlled trial. JAMA 2002;288(22):2836–45.

74. Rush AJ, Trivedi M, Carmody TJ, et al. One-year clinical outcomes of depressed public sector outpatients: a benchmark for subsequent studies. Biol Psychiatry 2004;56(1):46–53.

75. Simon GE, Von Korff M, Rutter CM, et al. Treatment process and outcomes for managed care patients receiving new antidepressant prescriptions from psychiatrists and primary care physicians. Arch Gen Psychiatry 2001;58(4):395–401.

76. Hansen N. The psychotherapy dose-response effect and its implications for treatment delivery services. Clin Psychol Sci Pract 2002;9:329–43.

77. Tai-Seale M, McGuire T, Colenda C, et al. Two-minute mental health care for elderly patients: inside primary care visits. J Am Geriatr Soc 2007;55(12):1903–11.

78. Unutzer J, Schoenbaum M, Druss BG, et al. Transforming mental health care at the interface with general medicine: report for the President's Commission. Psychiatr Serv 2006;57(1):37–47.

79. Uebelacker LA, Smith M, Lewis AW, et al. Treatment of depression in a low-income primary care setting with colocated mental health care. Fam Syst Health 2009;27(2):161–71.

80. Gilbody S, Bower P, Fletcher J, et al. Collaborative care for depression: a cumulative meta-analysis and review of longer-term outcomes. Arch Intern Med 2006; 166:2314–21.

81. Simon G. Collaborative care for depression. BMJ 2006;332(7536):249–50.

82. Simon G. Collaborative care for mood disorders. Curr Opin Psychiatry 2009; 22(1):37–41.

83. Roy-Byrne P, Craske MG, Sullivan G, et al. Delivery of evidence-based treatment for multiple anxiety disorders in primary care. JAMA 2010;303(19):1921–8.

84. Katon WJ, Lin EH, Von Korff M, et al. Collaborative care for patients with depression and chronic illnesses. N Engl J Med 2010;363(27):2611–20.

85. Katon W, Unutzer J. Collaborative care models for depression: time to move from evidence to practice. Arch Intern Med 2006;166(21):2304–6.

86. Katon W, Unutzer J, Wells K, et al. Collaborative depression care: history, evolution and ways to enhance dissemination and sustainability. Gen Hosp Psychiatry 2010;32(5):456–64.

87. Katon W, Von Korff M, Lin E, et al. Rethinking practitioner roles in chronic illness: the specialist, primary care physician, and the practice nurse. Gen Hosp Psychiatry 2001;23(3):138–44.

88. Von Korff M, Tiemens B. Individualized stepped care of chronic illness. West J Med 2000;172(2):133–7.

89. Kroenke K, Spitzer RL, Williams JB. The PHQ-9: validity of a brief depression severity measure. J Gen Intern Med 2001;16(9):606–13.

90. Löwe B, Unützer J, Callahan CM, et al. Monitoring depression treatment outcomes with the Patient Health Questionnaire-9. Med Care 2004;42(12): 1194–201.

91. Kupfer DJ, Frank E, Perel JM, et al. Five-year outcome for maintenance therapies in recurrent depression. Arch Gen Psychiatry 1992;49(10):769–73.

92. Roy-Byrne P, Craske MG, Sullivan G, et al. Delivery of evidence-based treatment for multiple anxiety disorders in primary care: a randomized controlled trial. JAMA 2010;303(19):1921–8.

93. Williams JW, Gerrity M, Holsinger T, et al. Systematic review of multifaceted interventions to improve depression care. Gen Hosp Psychiatry 2007;29:91–116.

94. IMPACT evidence-based depression care. AIMS Center; 2011. Available at: http://impact-uw.org. Accessed October 29, 2011.

95. Levine S, Unutzer J, Yip JY, et al. Physicians' satisfaction with a collaborative disease management program for late-life depression in primary care. Gen Hosp Psychiatry 2005;27(6):383–91.

96. Richardson L, McCauley E, Katon W. Collaborative care for adolescent depression: a pilot study. Gen Hosp Psychiatry 2009;31(1):36–45.

97. Dwight-Johnson M, Ell K, Lee PJ. Can collaborative care address the needs of low-income Latinas with comorbid depression and cancer? Results from a randomized pilot study. Psychosomatics 2005;46(3):224–32.

98. Ell K, Xie B, Quon B, et al. Randomized controlled trial of collaborative care management of depression among low-income patients with cancer. J Clin Oncol 2008;26(27):4488–96.

99. Ell K, Katon W, Xie B, et al. Collaborative care management of major depression among low-income, predominantly Hispanic subjects with diabetes: a randomized controlled trial. Diabetes Care 2010;33(4):706–13.

100. Katon WJ, Russo JE, Von Korff M, et al. Long-term effects on medical costs of improving depression outcomes in patients with depression and diabetes. Diabetes Care 2008;31(6):1155–9.

101. Gilmer TP, Walker C, Johnson ED, et al. Improving treatment of depression among Latinos with diabetes using project dulce and IMPACT. Diabetes Care 2008;31(7):1324–6.

102. Unutzer J, Katon WJ, Fan MY, et al. Long-term cost effects of collaborative care for late-life depression. Am J Manag Care 2008;14(2):95–100.

103. Katon WJ, Roy-Byrne P, Russo J, et al. Cost-effectiveness and cost offset of a collaborative care intervention for primary care patients with panic disorder. Arch Gen Psychiatry 2002;59(12):1098–104.

104. Grypma L, Haverkamp R, Little S, et al. Taking an evidence-based model of depression care from research to practice: making lemonade out of depression. Gen Hosp Psychiatry 2006;28(2):101–7.

105. Reiss-Brennan B, Briot PC, Savitz LA, et al. Cost and quality impact of Intermountain's mental health integration program. J Healthc Manag 2010;55(2): 97–113 [discussion: 113–4].

106. Glied S, Herzog K, Frank R. Review: the net benefits of depression management in primary care. Med Care Res Rev 2010;67(3):251–74.

107. Mental health: a report of the Surgeon General—executive summary. U.S. Department of Health and Human Services; 1999. Available at: http://www.surgeongeneral.gov/library/mentalhealth. Accessed October 30 2011.

108. New Freedom Commission on Mental Health. Achieving the Promise: Transforming Mental Health Care in America, Final Report. Vol DHHS. PMID: SMA-03–3832.2003.

109. Engaging large employers regarding evidence-based behavioral health treatment. National Business Group on Health; 2010. Available at: http://www.businessgrouphealth.org/benefitstopics/et_mentalhealth.cfm. Accessed October 31, 2011.

110. Butler M, Kane RL, McAlpine D, et al. Integration of mental health/substance abuse and primary care. Evid Rep Technol Assess (Full Rep) 2008;(173):1–362.

111. Wagner EH, Austin BT, Von Korff M. Organizing care for patients with chronic illness. Milbank Q 1996;74(4):511–44.

112. Trivedi MH, Daly EJ. Measurement-based care for refractory depression: a clinical decision support model for clinical research and practice. Drug Alcohol Depend 2007;88(Suppl 2):S61–71.

113. Institute for Clinical Systems Improvement (ICSI). Available at: http://www.icsi. org/health_care_redesign_/diamond_35953/. Accessed July 10, 2011.
114. Korsen N, Pietruszewski P. Translating evidence to practice: two stories from the field. J Clin Psychol Med Settings 2009;16(1):47–57.
115. MHIP for behavioral health (mental health integration program). AIMS Center; 2011. Available at: http://integratedcare-nw.org/. Accessed October 30, 2011.
116. United States Department of Defenses' Deployment Health Clinical Center (DHCC). RESPECT-Mil. Available at: http://www.pdhealth.mil/respect-mil/index. asp. Accessed October 30, 2011.
117. Collaborative care for depression in the primary care setting. US Department of Veterans Affairs, Health Services Research and Development Service. Washington (DC); 2008.
118. Kathol RG, Butler M, McAlpine DD, et al. Barriers to physical and mental condition integrated service delivery. Psychosom Med 2010;72(6):511–8.
119. Unützer J, Choi Y, Cook IA, et al. A web-based data management system to improve care for depression in a multicenter clinical trial. Psychiatr Serv 2002; 53(6):671–3, 678.

Community-Based Partnerships for Improving Chronic Disease Management

James Plumb, MD, MPH[a,b,]*, Lara Carson Weinstein, MD, MPH[a],
Rickie Brawer, PhD, MPH[a,b], Kevin Scott, MD[a]

KEYWORDS

- Chronic disease • Community engagement • Partnerships • Chronic care model
- Diabetes • Refugee • Homeless

KEY POINTS

- A social ecology approach to chronic disease calls for the development of new collaborations between the traditional medical system (outpatient physicians, emergency care, and inpatient facilities) and economic development, housing, zoning, and access to healthy and affordable food.
- To improve chronic disease management, physicians and the health systems in which they work need to understand the principles of community engagement and proactively join in efforts under way in communities in which they serve.
- Future directions for research include rigorous testing of the Expanded Chronic Care Model (ECCM) from a cost-effectiveness perspective, mixed-method evaluation strategies that involve community members, such as participatory action research, and evaluation of processes designed to enhance coordination between community-based programs and health care providers through data sharing and collaborative planning.

Chronic diseases, such as heart disease, cancer, hypertension, stroke, and diabetes, now account for 80% of deaths in the United States and 75% of health care costs.[1] In 2005, 44% of all Americans had at least 1 chronic condition and 13% had 3 or more. By 2020, an estimated 157 million US residents will have 1 chronic condition or more.[1] With this growing burden of chronic disease, the medical and public health communities are re-examining their roles and envisioning innovative partnership opportunities for more effective interventions for chronic disease prevention and management at a population level.

The authors have nothing to disclose.
[a] Department of Family and Community Medicine, Jefferson Medical College of Thomas Jefferson University, 1015 Walnut, Philadelphia, PA 19107, USA; [b] Center for Urban Health, Thomas Jefferson University and Hospitals, 1015 Chestnut, Philadelphia, PA 19107, USA
* Department of Family and Community Medicine, Jefferson Medical College of Thomas Jefferson University, 1015 Chestnut, Suite 617, Philadelphia, PA 19107.
E-mail address: james.plumb@jefferson.edu

Prim Care Clin Office Pract 39 (2012) 433–447
doi:10.1016/j.pop.2012.03.011
0095-4543/12/$ – see front matter © 2012 Elsevier Inc. All rights reserved.

primarycare.theclinics.com

The potential to significantly improve chronic disease prevention and have an impact on morbidity and mortality from chronic conditions is enhanced by adopting strategies that integrate population health and social ecologic perspectives into the Chronic Care Model (CCM), realigning the patient-physician relationship, and effectively engaging communities.

THE EXPANDED CHRONIC CARE MODEL

From a health care system perspective, the CCM, as developed originally by Wagner,[2] identifies the essential elements that encourage high-quality care for individuals suffering from chronic disease. These elements are the health system, self-management support, delivery system design, decision support, clinical information systems, and individuals' communities. This model was later refined to incorporate more specific concepts in each of those 6 elements—patient safety in health systems, cultural competency and care management in delivery system design, care coordination in health system and clinical information systems, and an emphasis on leveraging community policies and community resources to address individual needs and care goals.

Because the CCM is geared to clinically oriented systems and difficult to use for broader prevention and health promotion practices, Barr and colleagues[3] proposed the ECCM in 2003 to include elements of the population health promotion field so that broadly based prevention efforts, recognition of the social determinants of health, and enhanced community participation could also be integrated into the work of health system teams as they seek to address chronic disease issues. The ECCM includes 3 additional components in terms of community resources and policies. These are building healthy public policy, creating supportive environments, and strengthening community action **Fig. 1**.[3]

The ECCM represents a shift from primary care and hospital based care focused on illness and disability to community-oriented services that focus on the prevention of illness and disability before they have a chance to occur. This shift is a vital aspect

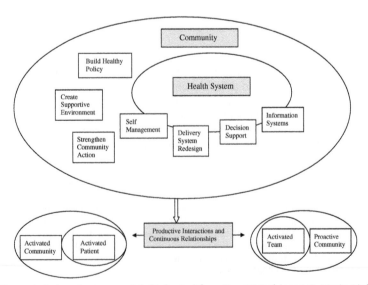

Fig. 1. Expanded chronic care model. (*Adapted from* Barr V, Robinson S, Marin-Link B. The expanded chronic care model: an integration of concepts and strategies from population health promotion and the chronic care model. Hosp Q 2003;7[1]:73–82; with permission.)

of responsible and accountable health care management in today's climate of health care reform with a strong emphasis on ensuring that community members are involved in planning for new services.[3]

REALIGNING THE PATIENT-PHYSICIAN RELATIONSHIP

Because chronic disease management is complex, it also requires a new view of the patient-provider relationship in addition to enhanced community-based partnerships. Collaborative care is a partnership paradigm that credits patients with an expertise that is similar in importance to the expertise of professionals.[4]

According to Holman and Loring, [5] health care can be delivered more effectively and efficiently if patients are full partners in the process. When acute disease was the primary cause of illness, patients were generally inexperienced and passive recipients of medical care, particularly because longitudinal follow-up was not required for these episodes. Now that chronic disease has become the principal medical problem for so many, patients must become partners in the care process, contributing their knowledge, preferences, and personal/social contexts at each decision or action level.[5]

RATIONALE FOR COMMUNITY PARTNERSHIPS IN CHRONIC DISEASE MANAGEMENT

Chronic conditions are rooted not only in physiologic processes but also in sociocultural and political contexts. Medical providers and programs, however, primarily consider chronic conditions at the individual or intrapersonal level. Chronic conditions are difficult to manage, much less cure, through a series of disconnected interventions, such as brief office visits, public health announcements, government funded programs, individual service programs, or the establishment of community advocacy groups. A more comprehensive approach to address root determinants of these chronic conditions is required, one involving community engagement in defining a problem and developing partnerships to identify and implement effective and sustainable solutions and management strategies.

According to Green and colleagues,[6] past public health efforts focused primarily on communicable disease. Chronic diseases exist, however, within the context of a wider array of lifestyle and social circumstances, each of which has an impact on the cause and course of disease. Thus, a comprehensive, multilevel, multipartner approach is required to develop the capacity to implement effective chronic illness prevention and health promotion programs that link traditional health care and socioenvironmental and political efforts.[6] The healthy community model for the 21st century should bridge disease prevention and management efforts that are often developed, implemented, and evaluated in silos. It should also connect health promotion and management efforts across chronic diseases that often share the same underlying root causes of disease, such as smoking, overweight/obesity, and limited physical activity.

SOCIAL ECOLOGY THEORY AND COMMUNITY PARTNERSHIPS

The Social Ecology Model[7] of health promotion provides an important framework for integrating community partnerships and chronic disease management. According to social ecology theory, the potential to change individual risk behavior is considered within the social and cultural context in which it occurs.[8] The Social Ecology Model describes several levels of influence that are critically interrelated and that must be recognized and addressed to effect positive health change, including intrapersonal factors, interpersonal factors, institutional and organizational factors, community factors, public policies, and broader structural or social factors.[7] Within the context of the Social Ecology Model, individuals, social support systems, community organizations, informal networks, and public policy leaders must be engaged and collaborate for successful health promotion and chronic disease management.

One example of the Social Ecology Model is the Building Community Supports for Diabetes Care (BCS) of the Robert Wood Johnson Foundation.[9] The BCS required that projects build community supports for diabetes care through clinic-community partnerships, by addressing 4 key areas: (1) working with existing services, encouraging use of these services, and enhancing access to them; (2) working together to identify gaps and create new programs, services, or policies that complement existing services; (3) providing leadership and a forum to raise awareness about diabetes and create consumer demand for resources and supports; and (4) providing a forum for community input and participation.[9] Examples of BCS interventions by ecologic level are found in **Table 1**.

Brownson and colleagues[9] conclude that BCS projects using partnership approaches show promise for building community support for diabetes care. Chronic illness care and patient self-management for diabetes and other chronic conditions benefit from continued support for implementation and evaluation of partnerships to build community network for self-management.

COMMUNITY ENGAGEMENT AND COMMUNITY CAPACITY BUILDING

According to the Centers for Disease Control and Prevention (CDC),[10] community engagement is defined as the process of working collaboratively with groups of people who are affiliated by geographic proximity, special interests, or similar situations with respect to issues affecting their well-being. It is helpful to consider the concepts of *community* and *capacity building* to help shape the community engagement process. First, the term, *community*, is a complex and fluid concept that needs to be defined. Some factors to consider when defining a community include socioeconomics, demographics, health status indices, ethnic and cultural characteristics, geographic boundaries, community norms, formal and informal power and authority figures, stakeholders, communication patterns, and existing assets and resources.[3]

Second, when considering a community collaborative approach to addressing specific health concerns, it is important to also consider the process of *capacity building*. Capacity building accounts for current resources available to a particular

Table 1
Examples of BCS interventions by ecologic level

Ecologic Level	BCS Interventions
Individual	Diabetes education classes, supermarket tours, case management, community walking maps, cooking demonstrations
Family, friends, and peers	Family diabetes curriculum, support groups, peer-led education classes
Systems/organizations	Office staff training to enhance capacity to support diabetes self-management, physician prescription pads for referrals to walking clubs, creation of health care performance goals
Community/policy	Advocacy training for project workers, securing indoor spaces for physical activity, diabetes materials in public libraries, presentations to community organizations to increase awareness of diabetes, improved selection of fresh produce at local markets

group as well as additional knowledge, skills, and resources that may need to be made available to community members in order for them to participate in meaningful community engagement. Capacity building is more complex and time consuming than approaching superficial community engagement in a manner that simply seeks community buy-in to a predetermined intervention. The effort spent on capacity building, however, is more likely to ensure a viable program in the long run (ie, sustainability). For example, true capacity building in a coalition with diverse membership whose focus is to address diabetes management and prevention might include diabetes training for community leaders and lay health workers, assistance with survey development, programs to improve coalition members' understanding of community-based education, facilitating the identification of community goals and potential strategies to achieve those goals, and strengthening relationship networks with grant writing skills and with government program planners and funders.

The CDC/Agency for Toxic Substances and Disease Registry Committee Task Force on the Principles of Community Engagement[10] has developed and refined principles for community engagement that incorporate key concepts to "assist public health professionals and community leaders interested in engaging the community in health decision making and action." These principles are summarized in **Table 2**. The principles of engagement can be used by people in a range of roles, from a program funder who needs to know how to support community engagement to a researcher or community leader who needs hands-on practical information on how to mobilize the members of a community to partner in research initiatives.

COMMUNITY-BASED PARTNERSHIPS: LOCAL AND NATIONAL CASE EXAMPLES
Thomas Jefferson University Department of Family and Community Medicine and Jefferson Center for Urban Health

The Thomas Jefferson University (TJU) Department of Family and Community Medicine (DFCM) is focusing on delivering a new model of care that provides state-of-the-art, comprehensive primary care in a variety of settings, from community to hospital, and engages communities in improving health indices. This new model of care, built on DFCM and TJU Hospitals (TJUH) resources and well-established links to community partnerships, integrates the best of family medicine, community, and public health principles and practice. The DFCM faculty, fellows, residents, and staff are committed to participating more actively in reducing inequalities in health, creating environments supportive of health, strengthening community action, building healthy public policy, and reorienting health services.

The Jefferson Center for Urban Health (CUH), directed by a DFCM faculty member, builds on the work of the DFCM and multiple TJUH community outreach activities. The mission of the center is to improve the health and well-being of Philadelphia citizens throughout the lifespan by marshalling the resources of TJUH and TJU and its DFCM and partnering with community organizations and neighborhoods. The center's goal is to improve the health status of individuals and targeted communities and neighborhoods through a multifaceted initiative, the ARCHES Project, which focuses on 6 domains/themes, including (1) access and advocacy; (2) research, evaluation, and outcomes measurement; (3) community partnerships and outreach; (4) health education, screening, and prevention programs; (5) education of health professions students and providers; and (6) service delivery systems innovation.

Through the ARCHES Project, the center's many partners include schools, homeless shelters, senior centers, faith-based communities, and other broad-based collaborative efforts that recognize neighborhood economic, social, and physical environments

Table 2
Principles of community engagement

Principle	Key Elements
Set goals	• Clarify the purposes/goals of the engagement effort • Specify populations and/or communities
Study community	• Economic conditions • Political structures • Norms and values • Demographic trends • History • Experience with engagement efforts • Perceptions of those initiating the engagement activities
Build trust	• Establish relationships • Work with the formal and informal leadership • Seek commitment from community organizations and leaders • Create processes for mobilizing the community
Encourage self-determination	• Community self-determination is the responsibility and right of all people • No external entity should assume that it can bestow on a community the power to act in its own self-interest
Establish partnerships	• Equitable partnerships are necessary for success
Respect diversity	• Use multiple engagement strategies • Explicitly recognize cultural influences
Identify community assets and develop capacity	• View community structures as resources for change and action • Provide experts and resources to assist with analysis, decision-making, and action • Provide support to develop leadership training, meeting facilitation, skill building
Release control to the community	• Include as many elements of a community as possible • Adapt to meet changing needs and growth
Make a long-term commitment	• Recognize different stages of development and provide ongoing technical assistance

Data from Principles of community engagement: 2nd edition. Clinical and Translational Science Awards Consortium Community Engagement Key Function Committee Task Force on the Principles of Community Engagement. 2011;11–7782. Available at: http://www.atsdr.cdc.gov/communityengagement/index.html. Accessed July 26, 2011.

as underlying determinants of health and disease. In addition, the center undertakes more extensive assessments in partnership with community-based organizations to create programs that reflect community need, voice, and culture. Projects are planned and evaluated individually based on established baselines set from existing data; information gleaned from key stakeholders through interviews, focus groups, and surveys that address critical attitudes, beliefs, and behaviors; and assessment of community assets/resources, such as human, economic, and social capital. Project planning and evaluation are driven by community members rather than the center, which provides technical expertise, linkages, and other support throughout the ongoing iterative processes.

Specifically, the Jefferson CUH facilitates academic-community partnerships by serving as a bridge between TJU/TJUH and urban neighborhoods to improve health outcomes through the following mechanisms: (1) facilitating collaborations around research, community projects, program planning/implementation, and evaluation; (2) strengthening the capacity of Philadelphia neighborhoods to address community identified needs; and (3) initiating and monitoring sustainable, collaborative interventions.

Additional DFCM/CUH community partnerships are summarized in **Table 3**, including the Center for Refugee Health, JeffHOPE,[11,12] Wellness Center, Pathways to Housing,[13–17] and the Stroke, Hypertension, and Prostate Education Intervention Team.[18] The Job Opportunities Investment Network Education on Diabetes in Urban Populations (JOINED-UP), CAPP,[19] and the Healthy Eating Active Living Convergence Partnership[20] are described in detail later to provide examples of successful, community-driven local and national efforts. These programs illustrate the opportunity to engage with communities and community organizations to enhance chronic disease management. Without this engagement, vulnerable populations would not have the advantage of chronic disease prevention, detection or management.

The Job Opportunity Investment Network Education on Diabetes in Urban Populations Project

JOINED-UP was built on a partnership between CUH and the Philadelphia Federation of Neighborhood Centers (FNC).[21] Founded in 1906, FNC is an umbrella organization for 15 community-based organizations, with deep roots in the community in the tradition of the Jane Adams Settlement House Movement.[21] The Federation's member agencies provide services to more than 100,000 children, adults, and families per year and have developed relationships with multiple generations of families.[21]

JOINED-UP was a diabetes and obesity healthy lifestyle education program embedded into a green jobs workforce development training program held at 2 FNC member agencies that targeted low-skilled, low-resourced residents in Philadelphia. As part of the comprehensive job training program, participants in the program were required to attend 6 Healthy Lifestyle workshops that were based on principles of the chronic disease self-management model and that used an example patient case study (whose attributes were created by program participants) as a means to encourage sharing of real-life experiences related to incorporating healthier behaviors onto daily life. Participants met individually with a professional health educator to review screening/survey results, discuss personal health concerns, and create a personal action plan. Motivational interviewing techniques guided this discussion. A certified diabetes educator met individually with individuals whose screening results indicated prediabetes and provided information about diabetes as well as suggestions for risk reduction. The certified diabetes educator counseled diagnosed diabetics about managing diabetes and preventing complications. A key component of the JOINED-UP program was facilitating patient activation and linkage to primary care. This provided an opportunity to engage and educate patients in a trusted setting to improve interaction between patients and their primary care providers.

The JOINED-UP program exemplifies a community-hospital outreach partnership that educated participants about diabetes prevention and control and linked them to community resources, including primary health care providers. The JOINED-UP project has resulted in several successful outcomes, including (1) integrating a diabetes prevention and management program into a workforce development program, which is a feasible and effective method of recruiting and engaging African American men in a disease self-management program; (2) directly linking the management of client health to attaining and retaining a job, which enhances the motivation of clients to better manage their chronic health conditions because they develop a clear

Table 3
Examples of TJU community partnerships facilitating chronic disease management

Program	Community Partners	Description	Outcomes	Funding Sources
JeffHOPE	Salvation Army Resources for Human Development Prevention Point Acts of the Apostles II Bethesda Project	• TJU medical student outreach program[11] • Provides free health care, health education and social advocacy services to homeless or otherwise medically underserved individuals	• 2000 Visits per year • Screened 300 men for cardiovascular disease,[12] colorectal cancer, prostate cancer, and hepatitis C	• Student fundraising • TJUH contribution • Association of American Medical Colleges • Caring Community grants • TJUH Women's Board • Civic Foundation
Wellness Center	Project H.O.M.E. Wellness Center Ridge Avenue Business Association Women Against Abuse Pro-Act Council for Relationships	• Primary medical care, behavioral health care, nutrition education, rehabilitative services, case management, and peer-led health promotion • Direct linkage to supportive housing, neighborhood-based affordable housing, economic development, access to employment opportunities; adult and youth education	• 800 Visits/year • Implementation of diabetes registry	• Independence Blue Cross Foundation • Medicaid Managed Care

Pathways to Housing	Pathways to Housing PA	• Housing First model, which ends chronic homelessness for individuals with serious mental illness[13,14] • Scattered site permanent supportive housing • Transdisciplinary care management team[15] • Novel integrated care program through a unique partnership with the DFCM[17]	• Chronic disease registry[16] • Ongoing tracking of standard health indicators • Integrated health record • Medication management and e-prescribing • On-site adult vaccines	• Housing: Philadelphia Office of Supportive Housing • Intensive care management: Philadelphia Department of Behavioral Health
Center for Refugee Health	Nationalities Service Center Lutheran Family and Children's Services Hebrew Immigrant Aid Society	• Partnership facilitates communication between the resettlement agencies and DFCM to assist refugees navigate through the health care system (laboratories, imaging, specialists, pharmacies, etc.)	• Since 2009, more than 700 refugees have received comprehensive screening and follow-up at DFCM	• Barra Foundation • Pennsylvania Refugee Coordination Center
Stroke, Hypertension, and Prostate Evaluation and Intervention Team (SHAPE-IT)	DFCM CUH Philadelphia Department of Health Health Promotion Council Community Partners	• Reduce the incidence of stroke and morbidity and mortality from prostate cancer in high-risk African American men • Development of Project Advisory Council	• Screening/education for 7019 men in high risk zip codes • Targeted population linked to primary care services	• Pennsylvania Department of Health

understanding that they must stay healthy to secure and keep a job; (3) providing healthy lifestyle education in a familiar community center rather than a health care facility, which helps build trust between health educators and other members of the health care team and their client partners—"going to where men are" is crucial to effective engagement; (4) providing wrap-around services (ie, job training, transportation, child care, emergency assistance, and housing assistance) in a central location where disease self-management programming and support are also delivered, which helps keep clients engaged in the self-management program as well as the job training program and allows clients to incorporate disease management into their day-to-day routines; this strategy offers synergistic rather than merely additive benefit; (5) recognizing the high prevalence of prediabetes (44%), which provides an opportunity to have an impact on further progression of disease in participants; and (6) providing healthy lifestyle education as part of a workforce development program, which can be an important factor in improving the health of children and families.

Community Asthma Prevention Program of Philadelphia

The Community Asthma Prevention Program of Philadelphia (CAPP)[19] provided community-based education for asthmatic children; however, this community-driven intervention was also designed to create community lay asthma experts who could sustain prevention and disease management efforts.

The CAPP, based on the *You Can Control Asthma*–validated curriculum developed by Georgetown University, was initiated in Philadelphia in 1997 by the Children's Hospital of Philadelphia (CHOP) through a cooperative agreement with the US Department of Health and Human Services.[22] This program involved a collaborative of more than 20 community-based organizations, including primary care providers, hospitals, health care insurers, faith-based institutions, recreation centers, and schools, that combined science with community assets, interests, and preferences to address poorly controlled asthma among children. This evidence-based, multifaceted, comprehensive program included opportunities for parents/caregivers and children to learn about asthma self-management and control and education for primary care providers and provided home visits conducted by trained lay-health-educators to assess environmental triggers. Community involvement ensured that interventions were acceptable and accessible to the community as well as integrated with other community efforts related to asthma management.

Educational programs for asthmatic children and their caregivers were held in community sites, such as schools, daycare centers, and churches, and were taught by trained peer educators, including parents of asthmatic children as well as asthmatic teenagers and college students. Students received free asthma devices, such as peak flow meters, and mattress and pillow covers to reduce environmental triggers. More than 3500 members of the community contributed to and participated in the program over a 4-year period.[23] In a study of 267 participants, knowledge, quality of life, and asthma control significantly improved compared with preprogram measures.[23] Moreover and notably, these gains were retained for at least 1 year.[23] In addition, workshops for school personnel were conducted for classroom teachers, health and physical education teachers, coaches, and school nurses to convey information about asthma symptoms and treatment and the impact of asthma on school performance and attendance.

Finally, CAPP and CHOP, through the Controlling Asthma in American Cities Project, offered 3 levels of primary care provider education based on National Heart, Lung, and Blood Institute guidelines and the needs of practitioners and their staffs. Using a modified Physician Asthma Care Education curriculum, level one focused on asthma knowledge and patient-provider communication; level two facilitated practice system changes by creating physician and nurse asthma champions in practices, integrating support from CAPP's clinical coordinator through monthly case discussions and tele-conferences, and using an asthma toolbox and patient education materials designed by literacy experts; and in level three educational programs, quality improvement methods were integrated into practices through site-specific interventions.

To build a more robust system of coordinated services, CAPP's efforts have been linked to other asthma education programs through the efforts of Philadelphia Allies Against Asthma (PAAA).[24] The Child Asthma Link Line developed by PAAA connects asthmatic children seen in Philadelphia's pediatric emergency departments or referred by schools to CAPP's community and school-based programs. The CAPP and PAAA programs demonstrate how multisector community involvement helps create realistic approaches to disease management, reduce barriers to care, and reduce duplicative efforts by bridging and integrating multiple existing efforts aimed at improving health outcomes and reducing health disparities, thereby leveraging available community resources and assets.

Reducing or eliminating health disparities, such as those seen with the burden of asthma morbidity, among different ethnic and racial groups remains a challenge. Primary care interventions that are linked with community-based interventions that address family, social, and behavioral factors are essential in meeting this challenge. Comprehensive systematic approaches that connect diverse community partners, raise awareness and knowledge about health concerns, and support policies address-ing fragmented systems that affect health, including health insurance, school systems, and housing, are needed to support and improve on the results of traditional primary care efforts. Current efforts to reduce obesity and its underlying root causes provide the context for the final case study.

Healthy Eating Active Living Convergence Partnership

Obesity is a complex health issue, and as such, requires complex solutions that involve diverse individuals and institutions across multiple levels of society and that leverage public-private partnerships. More than one-third of adults and 17% of chil-dren in the United States are obese.[25] Obesity is a risk factor for many health condi-tions, including heart disease, stroke, hypertension, type 2 diabetes mellitus, some cancers, liver and gall bladder disease, sleep apnea, respiratory problems, osteoar-thritis, fertility problems, and mental health conditions. Like asthma, obesity cannot be managed by interventions focused on the individual level alone. Scientists, the medical community, government, schools, business, and other community partners must coordinate responses designed to reverse this growing epidemic. Efforts to reduce and control obesity are currently being implemented at the local, state, and national levels and involve partners who may have little or no tradition of working together on health issues. These nontraditional partners include societal sectors, such as food supply and distribution systems; school food systems and policies; food outlets, such as supermarkets and corner stores; health care; urban planning and zoning departments; transportation; recreation and parks departments; and community-based organizations, such as the YMCA, bicycle coalitions, neighborhood centers, and faith-based institutions, among many others.

In 2006, a collaboration of funders (the California Endowment, Kaiser Permanente, the Kresge Foundation, Nemours, the Robert Wood Johnson Foundation, and the W.K. Kellogg Foundation) created the Healthy Eating Active Living Convergence Part-nership.[20] These national organizations were funding initiatives focused on healthy eating and active living as strategies to address overweight and obesity and were interested in developing a more coordinated approach for improving healthy food and physical activity norms and environments. The CDC provided technical assistance, and PolicyLink, a national research and action institute devoted to economic and social equity, served as the program director for the Healthy Eating Active Living Convergence Partnership. The Prevention Institute, a nonprofit organization that promotes and advocates for policies, organizational practices, and collaborative efforts that improve health and the quality of life, provides policy research, analysis, and strategic support for the Healthy Eating Active Living Convergence Partnership. The Convergence Partnership is committed to promoting and leveraging work across multiple fields and sectors to advance knowledge, resource sharing, and policy and environmental change that will help build a national movement toward healthy people in healthy places. The Healthy Eating Active Living Convergence Partnership supports each partner's efforts and seeks to build new internal and external relationships to build synergy across multiple disciplines and to strengthen local, regional, and national policy and system change efforts that support fresh, local healthy food and safe places to play and be active.[20] The Convergence Partnership has developed a 10-point vision to promote healthy eating and active living. This vision is summarized in **Box 1**.[20]

Health care organizations and providers play an important role in reducing obesity. Primary care providers need to adopt and implement standard practices for routine body mass index screening and counseling that supports healthier food choices and physical activity at every visit. Hospitals and other health care employers need to set an example for other employers by promoting physical activity, such as taking the stairs and improving food choices in cafeterias and vending machines. Primary

---

Box 1
Convergence partnership vision

- Safe neighborhoods, communities, and buildings support physical activity as part of everyday life.
- Fresh, local, and healthy food is available and affordable in all communities and neighborhoods.
- Healthy foods and beverages are promoted in grocery and other food stores, restaurants, and entertainment venues.
- Schools offer and promote healthy foods and beverages to students.
- Schools promote healthy physical activities and incorporate them throughout the day, including before and after school.
- Workplaces and employers offer and promote access to healthy foods and beverages and opportunities for physical activity.
- Health care organizations and providers promote healthy eating and active living in their own institutional policies and in their clinical practices.
- Government and the private sector support and promote healthy eating and active living environments.
- Organizations, institutions, and individuals that influence the information and entertainment environments share responsibility for and act responsibly to promote healthy eating and active living.
- Childcare organizations, including preschool, afterschool, and early childhood settings, offer and promote only healthy foods and beverages to children and provide sufficient opportunities for and promote physical activity.

care providers and hospitals should also support breastfeeding initiation, duration, and exclusivity, one of the 5 target areas identified by the CDC state-based Nutrition and Physical Activity Program to Prevent Obesity and Other Chronic Diseases.[25] Finally, physicians and other health care providers can refer patients to community organizations that promote healthy eating and physical activity and can advocate for system and policy changes that make healthy choices the easier choices for their patients.

SUMMARY

With the growing burden of chronic disease, the medical and public health communities are re-examining their roles and exploring opportunities for more effective prevention and clinical interventions. There is growing recognition of the need to address the underlying root causes/contributing factors that cross multiple chronic diseases and to integrate the silos in which chronic diseases are addressed. A social ecology approach to chronic disease calls for the development of new collaborations between the traditional medical system (outpatient physicians, emergency care, and inpatient facilities) and economic development, housing, zoning, and access to healthy and affordable food. As professionals and citizens,[26] providers can become directly involved in providing technical expertise and/or advocating in a variety of ways for changes in social polices that effect health.[27] The ECCM provides a foundation to explore these expanded roles and to operationalize the social ecology approach. The established principles of community engagement detail a methodology to work with communities to organize a more comprehensive approach to chronic disease prevention and management.

To improve chronic disease management, physicians and the health systems in which they work need to understand the principles of community engagement and proactively join in efforts under way in communities in which they serve. Multiple examples of community engagement have been provided highlighting the impact that can be realized through collaboration with agencies that interface with populations at levels that are not traditionally health related. This impact has been most evident in improving chronic disease management and outcomes in diabetes, asthma, obesity, and hypertension.

Future directions for research include rigorous testing of the ECCM from a cost-effectiveness perspective; mixed-method evaluation strategies that involve community members, such as participatory action research; and evaluation of processes designed to enhance coordination between community-based programs and health care providers through data sharing and collaborative planning.

REFERENCES

1. Tackling the burden of chronic diseases in the USA. Lancet 2009;373(9659):185.
2. Wagner EH, Austin BT, Davis C, et al. Improving chronic illness care: translating evidence into action: interventions that encourage people to acquire self-management skills are essential in chronic illness care. Health Aff 2001;20(6):64–78.
3. Barr VJ, Robinson S, Marin-Link B, et al. The expanded chronic care model: an integration of concepts and strategies from population health promotion and the Chronic Care Model. Hosp Q 2003;7(1):73–82.
4. Bodenheimer T, Lorig K, Holman H, et al. Patient self-management of chronic disease in primary care.see comment. JAMA 2002;288(19):2469–75.
5. Holman H, Lorig K. Patients as partners in managing chronic disease. Br Med J 2000;320(7234):526–7.

6. Green L, Daniel M, Novick L. Partnerships and coalitions for community-based research. Public Health Rep 2001;116(Suppl 1):20–31.

7. McLeroy KR, Bibeau D, Steckler A, et al. An ecological perspective on health promotion programs. Health Educ Q 1988;15(4):351–77.

8. Goodman RM, Wandersman A, Chinman M, et al. An ecological assessment of community-based interventions for prevention and health promotion: approaches to measuring community coalitions. Am J Community Psychol 1996;24(1): 33–61.

9. Brownson CA, O'Toole ML, Shetty G, et al. Clinic-community partnerships: a foundation for providing community supports for diabetes care and self-management. Diabetes Spectr 2007;20(4):209–14.

10. Principles of Community Engagement: 2nd edition. Clinical and Translational Science Awards Consortium Community Engagement Key Function Committee Task Forse on the Principles of Community Engagement. 2011;11–7782. Available at: http://www.atsdr.cdc.gov/communityengagement/index.html. Accessed July 26, 2011.

11. Hemba K, Plumb JD. JeffHOPE: the development and operation of a student-run clinic. J Community Med Prim Health Care 2011;2(3):167.

12. Kim DH, Daskalakis C, Plumb JD, et al. Modifiable cardiovascular risk factors among individuals in low socioeconomic communities and homeless shelters. Fam Community Health 2008;31(4):269–80.

13. Tsemberis S, Stefancic A. Pathways' Housing First Program. NREPP: SAMHSA's national registry of evidence-based programs and practices. Rockville (MD): United States Department of Health and Human Services, Substance Abuse and Mental Health Service Administration; 2008. Available at: http://homeless.samhsa.gov/channel/housing-first-447.aspx. Accessed July 7, 2011, December 16, 2011.

14. Tsemberis S, Gulcur L, Nakae M. Housing first, consumer choice, and harm reduction for homeless individuals with a dual diagnosis. Am J Public Health 2004;94(4):651–6.

15. Weinstein LC, Henwood BF, Cody J, et al. Transforming assertive community treatment into an integrated care system: the role of nursing and primary care partnerships. J Am Psychiatr Nurses Assoc 2011;17(1):64–71.

16. Weinstein LC, Henwood BF, Matejkowski J, et al. Moving from street to home: health status of entrants to a housing first program. J Prim Care Commun Health 2011;2(1):11–5.

17. Henwood BF, Weinstein LC, Tsemberis S. Creating a medical home for homeless persons with serious mental illness. Psychiatr Serv 2011;62(5):561–2.

18. Weinstein LC, Plumb JD, Brawer R. Community engagement of men. Prim Care Clin Off Pract 2006;33(1):247–59.

19. Community Asthma Prevention Program (CAPP). Available at: http://www.chop.edu/service/community-asthma-prevention-program-capp/home.html. Accessed December 16, 2011.

20. Lee V, Mikkelsen L, Srikantharajah J, et al. Promising strategies for creating healthy eating and active living environments. A document from the Prevention Institute; 2008.

21. Philadelphia Federation of Neighborhood Centers. Available at: www.federationnc.org/About-Us.page. Accessed December 16, 2011.

22. Bryant-Stephens T. Asthma disparities in urban environments. J Allergy Clin Immunol 2009;123(6):1199–206.

23. Bryant-Stephens T, Li Y. Community asthma education program for parents of urban asthmatic children. J Natl Med Assoc 2004;96(7):954–60.

24. Rosenthal MP, Butterfoss FD, Doctor LJ, et al. The coalition process at work: building care coordination models to control chronic disease. Health Promot Pract 2006;7(Suppl 2):117S–26S.

25. Obesity—halting the epidemic by making health easier. Centers for Disease Control and Prevention. Aat a Glance 2011. Available at: http://www.cdc.gov/chronicdisease/resources/publications/AAG/obesity.htm. Accessed December 22, 2011.

26. Gruen RL, Pearson SD, Brennan TA. Physician citizens—public roles and professional responsibilities. JAMA 2006;291(1):94–8.

27. Woolf S. Social policy and health policy. JAMA 2000;11:1166–9.

Index

Note: Page numbers of article titles are in **boldface** type.

A

doi:10.1016/S0095-4543(12)00037-1
0095-4543/12/$ – see front matter © 2012 Elsevier Inc. All rights reserved.
primarycare.theclinics.com

Printed and bound by CPI Group (UK) Ltd, Croydon, CR0 4YY

03/10/2024

01040460-0006